Clinical Phonology

Assessment and Treatment
of Articulation Disorders in
Children and Adults

Clinical Phonology

Assessment and Treatment of Articulation Disorders in Children and Adults

Edward S. Klein, Ph.D.
Associate Professor
Department of Communication Disorders
University of Utah

S

SINGULAR PUBLISHING GROUP, INC.
SAN DIEGO · LONDON

Singular Publishing Group, Inc.
4284 41st Street
San Diego, California 92105–1197

19 Compton Terrace
London, N1 2UN, UK

Typeset in 10/12 Palatino by So Cal Graphics
Printed in the United States of America by McNaughton & Gunn

Library of Congress Cataloging-in-Publication Data

Klein, Edward S.
    Clinical phonology: assessment and treatment of articulation disorders
in children and adults / Edward S. Klein
      p.   cm.
    Includes bibliographical references and index.
    ISBN 1-56593-602-7
    1. Articulation disorders.   I. Title.
    [DNLM: 1. Articulation Disorders.   2. Speech-Language Pathology.
WL 340.2 K64c 1995]
RC424.7.K58   1995
616.85'5—dc20   95-31735
for Library of Congress   CIP

Contents

Preface

Prior to publication of this book, I asked several people that I respect highly in the field of phonology to read and comment upon the material presented herein. Most comments were quite positive. One was not. This one person, one of the people I respect most in the areas of phonology and child language, related to me some deeply felt concerns about the tone of the book. It wasn't nearly scholarly enough; there were too many offhand, flippant or humorous comments that could be offensive to the "serious, scholarly" readers in the field.

I was initially devastated. First of all, I didn't disagree with this reviewer. The entire purpose of this text was to take some of the mystery, some of the complexity out of the discussion of clinical phonology, a complex topic indeed. I felt readability and comprehension would be enhanced if I wrote as if I was talking to a group of clinicians learning much of the material for the first time. But I certainly had no desire to offend anyone, especially those readers who already had a substantial background in the area of clinical phonology. Second, I was committed to avoiding some of the more contentious, theoretical and currently unresolved issues in clinical phonology in favor of a more practical presentation based on what we know, not what we hypothesize to be true. As such, several interesting and perhaps important subjects were not addressed in this text. Nowhere was there a discussion of various theories of phonological development nor was there any use of the terms naturalness, underlying representations or phonological knowledge. This lack of discussion was not meant to imply a lack of interest in these topics on my part. (Some of you who have heard my clinical workshops may remember my answering a question of "why" with a brief synopsis of my "Hansel and Gretel theory of phonological development"). It's just that I believed that the concepts of clinical phonology presented herein could stand by themselves without any discussion of those more theoretical issues. Yet the last thing I wanted was for scholars in the field, my peers, to dismiss this text because I refrained from a discussion of these issues. I was faced with a dilemma.

In the end, I decided that I had to stay true to the students and clinicians in the field for whom I wrote this book to begin with: those of you who have heard about clinical phonology have learned about it to some extent and have tried to use its concepts in your clinical work, but have remained frustrated by the lack of practical, clinically relevant guidance available to help you "put it all together" from a phonological perspective. I hope I have accomplished at least this in this text. If any of you are offended by anything I have written, I apologize. My only goal has been to enhance readability and understanding, and perhaps leave a small smile on the reader's face at the same time. If any of you are disappointed by the lack of weighty discourse, again I apologize. This text has had a different purpose. To the rest of you, I hope this textbook helps to open at least some windows and shed some light on a complex topic.

We are, I believe, only at the beginning of an exciting new time in the field of treatment for articulation disorders. The book by David Ingram (1976) was the first glimpse of this

new time and the work of Barabara Hodson (e.g. Hodson and Paden, 1983) brought clinicians in the field into this new era for perhaps the first time. The purpose of this book is to
continue the teaching process begun by my esteemed colleagues. It is certainly not the last
word on clinical phonology. The final work is many years off and will probably come from
someone less bound to traditional thinking than this author, perhaps a student reading
about clinical phonology today for the first time. I do hope, however, that you will see this
book as a valuable step along the long road that still remains to be traveled. Happy reading!

Acknowledgments

The most overwhelming realization I have as this book goes to press is that we are all nothing without our teachers, our students, our clients and our friends (also our editors, if we write). The bottom line is, I could not have even come close to writing this book if it were not for some very special people.

For example, take my past graduate students at Whittier College. (*Please* take them). Without these students, (Linda, Kathy, Terri, Jeannie, Vicki, Barbara, Stephanie and all the others) I would never have developed as a teacher sufficiently to be able to turn my concepts of phonology into a cohesive program. They asked questions, never accepted anything on faith alone and forced me to come up with alternatives when problems arose. This book would not have happened without them.

And then there are my teachers and mentors. Joan Regnell and Dr. Jim Hillis deserve special mention during my early growth in the field. Joan was the primary reason I came into the field and her enthusiasm helped stimulate my first academic excitement. Jim pushed me to be as good as I could be at the masters level and has remained an important source of advice and academic stimulation for me since that time. Thank you both. Dr. Fred Weiner introduced me to clinical phonology and provided the initial spark of excitement and motivation that has sustained me in this area for close to 20 years. Dr. Jim Shanks remains not only a close friend but is my model for the best pure clinician I have ever seen or known. He has helped me immeasurably in my growth as a scholar who is a clinician first. Finally, Dr. Paul Sindelar is a mentor and friend who has served as my primary academic model since my Penn State days. Thanks to his teaching, a little bit ot his insight, wisdom, creativity and sheer brilliance accompanies me in all my own academic and clinical endeavors.

There are many other people without whom this text would not have been written. Dr. Mike Moran has been a respected colleague and friend since our days in Pennsylvania. His advice over the years and his support and words of wisdom regarding this manuscript have been invaluable and his chapter contribution to this text has strengthened it greatly. Thanks, Mike. Maria Sarro (wherever you are) was the first editor to believe in this project and her support gave me the impetus to begin the long manuscript preparation process. Marie Linvill has been the editor during the completion and final preparation of the text and Sandy Doyle has spent much time and energy helping me to survive the editing process. Without her support, insight and help, you would never be reading these words today.

Finally, I'd like to thank several thousand clinicians from across the country and Canada who have attended my workshops on clinical phonology and have provided important feedback which has helped to crystallize my thinking and improve my presentation. Super special among this group is Beth Collins Rivera and her colleagues in the Orange County School District in Orlando, Florida. Thanks to all of you from the bottom of my heart.

Dedication

To my wife Joy, who kept me going during some fairly dark times and helped me make the transition from the halls of academe to the kitchens of freshly baked croissants and back again with relative ease. Thank you, my love.

✦ PART I ✦

From Articulation to Clinical Phonology: Development of a Discipline

CHAPTER 1

Introduction to Clinical Phonology

Message From the Author

haɪ ɛdadi, maɪ nen it ɛd aɪn, æn aɪm hioʊ de hu hɔk hu jʉ daʊt hapi dæt aɪ hop jʉoʊ ɪtɛd ɪn—hɪdetən. I dɪt ʌdʌ mek jʉoʊ hʌm æ hɪdo hɪtʃ ɪn haɪt, jʉ naɪt æt wɛoʊ hek jʉoʊ dɛdoʊ hɛto æn wioʊ daɪt aʊt hioʊ.

(NOTE: Okay, calm down . . . I promise that we will soon revert to English rather than phonetics. However, the remainder of this introductory message is important to some of the issues to be discussed in this and the next chapter. So here goes . . . and feel free to "cheat" by looking at the translation in the footnote below.)

Naʊ, do dʌt jʉoʊ dənidɨ. No dʌn ɪt ho dʌn, oʊ naɪt, oʊ idən heoʊ hɪdoʊ hu jʉoʊ dɪtoʊ. ɪt jʉ dædoʊ bi æt jʉoʊ haʊt, ɪn jʉoʊ dænə, hip ɪn jʉoʊ dɛd; ɪt jʉ dædoʊ bi ɪn jʉoʊ dætʌ, hek æ baɪ dæt oʉ dɪdo (o he, mebɨ aɪ æ dʌt aʊt ɪdoʊ); ɪt jʉ dædoʊ bi hɪt aɪ hoʊtʃ, oʊ hʌt hɔ dædɪt oʊ dɪdoʊ ɪ dʌt—den, baɪ ɔoʊ min, dʌn ʌp jʉoʊ hʌdədʒ, hʌboʊ jʉoʊ hepoʊ æ nætʃ gɛdoʊ, æ he daɪd ɪn jʉoʊ haoʊ, hen, dædən, bækʉm oʊ dʌdət ɛ hek jʉ hʉ wʌk. It, an ʌdoʊ hæn, jʉ aoʊ ɪtɛd in hɪdetən, æn jʉ wioʊ na bi din hætə hɔt, jʉoʊ hɪtɪt hi, dot hɪkən didaʊt hɛdoʊ æn hɪd adən hædɪt an hob, den hʊt jʉoʊ hʌ daʊn, æn web hæg. no ni dɪt ʌ nɛnoʊ hatoʊ an heton. dɪ bʉ hot ɪt obo.[1]

---

[1]Hi everybody. My name is Ed Klein and I'm here today to talk to you about a topic that I hope you're interested in—articulation. If this doesn't make your *thumb* and *fingers* twitch in excitement, you might as well take your *yellow pencils* and *wheel* right out of here. Now, don't duck your responsibility. No one is holding a *gun* or *knife* or even a pair of *scissors* to your *zippers*. If you'd rather be at your *house* in your *pajamas*, *sleeping* in your *bed*; if you'd rather be in your *bathtub* taking a *bath* by a *lamp* or *window* (OK, maybe I am *jumping* around a little); if you'd rather be *fishing* by the *church*, or hunting for a *rabbit* or *squirrel* in the *brush*—then, by all means, *drum* up your courage, *shovel* your *papers* and *matches* together and return to your *car*, *plane*, *wagon*, *vacuum* or whatever else takes you to this work.

If, on the other hand, you are interested in articulation and you will not be dreaming of *Santa Claus*, your *Christmas tree*, roast *chicken* without *feathers* and a sizzling *orange carrot* on the *stove*, then put your *cup* down and wave the *flag*. No need to *ring* up the mental hospital on the *telephone*. This *blue* prose is over.

What you've just read (or haven't read, as the case may be) is an attempt to simulate a 4-year-old child with lousy articulation (forgive the technical term). Of course, no 4-year-old would talk like that; the language structure in most cases is consistent with that of an adult. But the phonological behaviors *are* typical of a child with phonological disorders. Now, some of you may have noticed something about the underlined words in the sample. These words represent most of the items from the *Goldman-Fristoe Test of Articulation* (Goldman & Fristoe, 1986) and they'll be referred to frequently in the first few chapters of this book—to help in our comparison of traditional and newer phonological approaches to working with children with speech disorders.

In fact, a good case can be made that more has changed in our understanding of speech disorders since 1976 (when Ingram published his landmark work *Phonological Disability in Children*) than in the 40 years before that time. In short, speech-language clinicians are being cautioned against focusing on each specific sound error in the client as a separate distinct entity. Instead, they are being urged to try to find underlying patterns of productions that could account for several errors at one time. This recent methodology has been alternately called *phonological process analysis*, *phonological rule analysis*, or simply, *phonological analysis*—the term that will be used throughout this text.

Concurrent with the development of procedures for phonological analysis, there has been a change in the focus of therapy for these children (and adults) with speech disorders. Briefly, there has been a growing tendency to de-emphasize traditional approaches stressing motoric manipulation of the articulators (e.g., Van Riper, 1972; McDonald, 1964) in favor of more conceptually based programs (Ferrier & Davis, 1973; Klein, 1985, Weiner, 1981; Young, 1983).

For several years now, proponents of phonological analysis and intervention have reported remarkable results for their clients who have undergone therapy based on this newer approach. Specifically, numerous children have been described who previously might have been in therapy for many years given the severity of their speech disorders, but have been dismissed in 12–18 months after undergoing phonologically based assessment and therapy (Hodson & Paden, 1983; Hodson, 1992; Klein, in press; Monahan, 1986; Weiner, 1981; Young, 1983).

Unfortunately, as positive as all this sounds, there's been a real downside to these changes. In short, many clinicians have been left behind in this revolution. Things have changed enough such that a large number of clinicians in the field don't even know the current terminology, much less how to use the currently accepted procedures with their clients. As an example, I have given numerous 2-day workshops on clinical phonology to public school, hospital, and private practice clinicians across the United States and Canada. Overall, fewer than 10% of the more than 1,500 clinicians attending these workshops have reported using phonologically based approaches with their clients prior to the workshop. Fewer than 30% have known enough about clinical phonology to identify even the most basic concepts. Hodson (1992) reported similar data, and Fey (1985) noted that in his interactions with clinicians in the field, clinical phonology was a "source of . . . bewilderment" (p. 225) for many clinicians. What this indicates is a large problem in our field: Although many leading scholars now agree that a phonological framework is preferred in working with individuals with speech disorders, the methodology is not yet filtering down to the very people serving these individuals.

This book has been written to try to help overcome this problem. It's been written for speech-language clinicians in the field who have heard about the many benefits of clinical phonology but haven't yet found the right resource or person to help them learn how to use it in therapy. It's been written for those of you who have made attempts to learn about phonology only to get bogged down because of the complexity of the terminology or the inadequacy of the explanations. It's also for those of you who have felt somewhat threatened by the magnitude of the changes in the field, wondering if you would ever be able to learn how to use this new approach. Finally, this book has been written for college and university students who, after all, are the clinicians of tomorrow.

In order to make the learning process easier, a somewhat different approach has been taken than is normally the case in a textbook of this sort. Supplementing the textual material, a series of *Clinical Mastery Exercises* has been created in order to teach, in an orderly fashion, the performance aspects of phonological analysis and intervention. Although these exercises themselves will not make you immediate experts in clinical phonology, they will provide you with sufficient background, practice, and examples to learn the rest on your own.

It has been said that one of the curses of new learning is that, as part of the process, it requires us all to become students once again. I hope this text will make that process easier while at the same time helping to speed up the dissemination of this important new approach to those of you who are or will be working with children and adults with speech disorders.

CHAPTER 2

Articulation Analysis: Traditional, Distinctive Features, Phonological Analysis

An Attempted Synthesis

Problems Revisited

As stated in Chapter 1, even after close to 15 years of books, articles, tests, and workshops, phonological analysis and intervention is not yet "filtering down" to clinicians in the field. The question is, why? Several possible reasons are forwarded:

1. Déjà vu all over again? There's a feeling on the part of many people in the field, when they first start learning and understanding the methodology, of "So what? It's the same thing I've been doing for years." Many of these clinicians are excellent and highly respected professionals. Even some well-known investigators in the field of phonology have questioned the "differentness" of the approach (e.g., McReynolds & Elbert, 1981).

In reality, all of the various forms of phonological analysis and intervention are different from what has traditionally been done. The analysis is different; different parameters of the target word are being considered than previously. And, if done appropriately, therapy might be very different. It is hoped that this will become more obvious by the end of this chapter.

2. A brave new world? If some people have been too quick to label phonological analysis as not very different from what has been done before, others have presented the methodologies as totally new, with little connection to past modes of articulation analysis. As an example, consider this blurb from a recent workshop entitled "Phonological Process Analysis: The New Method of Treating Articulation Disorders":

> Phonological Process Analysis (PPA) is one of the most important new developments in the field of communication disorders. This exciting approach . . .

Of course, it's obvious that descriptions like this are advertising hyperbole— meant to increase workshop attendance. But perhaps it set up expectations in the minds of those attending that finally they were going to get "the pink pill."

As the chapter progresses, it will hopefully become clear that current modes of articulation analysis, while very different from what occurred previously, can be viewed as a logical outgrowth of previous modes of articulation analysis. In other words, phonological analysis is an advance in our concepts of articulation analysis; it is not the discovery of a new world.

3. Let the so-called experts get their act together first; then I'll learn about it. Sadly, there has been a lack of a unifying vision concerning how and where phonological analysis fits into the realm of speech-language pathology. As an example of this, many articles have been published over the last 15 years describing phonological "processes" used by various disorder groups—clients with aphasia, apraxia, cleft palate, or hearing loss, for example. What has been most interesting about these articles has been the underlying tone or message: "Can you believe it? We've actually found another group in which phonological 'processes' seem to be working." Well, what is so exciting about that? If phonological analysis is an advance in the methodology of articulation assessment (which it is), wouldn't one expect that this better methodology could be used for all people with deviant articulation, regardless of etiology? Of course.

The problem is, investigators have tended to blur the distinction between *theories of phonological development and theories of deviant phonology* on one hand, and our *methodology used to analyze deviant phonology*, on the other hand. As such, there has been a tendency for investigators to ignore areas of agreement and instead concentrate on areas of theoretical disagreement, overlooking the fact that our entire underlying model of articulation analysis has changed in the last 20 years. Investigators such as Hodson (1986), Ingram (1976), Shriberg and Kwiatkowski (1980), Gierut (1986), Schwartz (1992), or McReynolds and Elbert (1981) may all disagree on what has *caused* the articulation problem. Shriberg and Kwiatkowski may want to call the problem a "natural process" whereas McReynolds chooses to refer to it as a "pattern." They may all disagree on what they believe is going on in the child's head. But without a doubt, they would all agree that our typical way of analyzing articulation has changed.

The dilemma seems to come down to the fact that our model for analyzing articulation has changed, but no one has described the new model—at least as it relates to the traditional one. Unfortunately, this failure makes it easy for people to say phonological analysis and intervention is no different from what was done before—because in reality, part of it is no different. It has also been easy for people in the field to ignore the changes—because as one investigator stresses the importance of determining natural processes (Shriberg & Kwiatkowski, 1980), another is most concerned with phonological knowledge (Elbert & Gierut, 1986), still another recommends an analysis of homonymy (Ingram, 1981), and on and on. It becomes understandable that the perplexed clinician would be tempted to throw his or her hands up in despair and cry, "No more. Please get back to me when you agree on something."

Well, despite what it seems, we do agree. As the chapter progresses, a model of articulation analysis will be presented which will hopefully tie together past and present ways of analyzing articulation.

4. No, no, a thousand times no. Most clinicians look on their past training with various mixtures of awe, appreciation, and repugnance. At the least, even the best prepared of us have no desire to go back to the point of our first clinical session (and the accompanying anxiety and insecurity) any more than we have a wish to learn to drive a car for the first time again. Yet unfortunately, this is just what phonological analysis and intervention require, for at least a while. It's not really that difficult to learn—in fact, as we'll soon see, it less involves new learning than it does relearning what every clinician has learned at some point in his or her past training (but has forgotten through disuse). Unfortunately, however, it cannot be learned in a 2-hour or even 1-day workshop. And it does involve a period of insecurity during the initial learning stages. And it does require that the new learner practice many of the relearned and newly learned skills for several months before he or she can master the procedure.

One begins to see why phonological analysis and intervention has had such a tough time being disseminated. But there is one important thing to keep in mind: It can be learned. Every clinician willing to spend some time in learning and practice will learn how to use phonological analysis and intervention with speech-disordered clients. And, as we'll soon see, those clients will benefit immensely.

Objectives for Remainder of Chapter

In light of the problems just discussed, there are four objectives for the remainder of this chapter:

1. To demonstrate that phonological analysis is a different mode of articulation assessment from what has typically been done previously in the field of speech therapy.
2. To show that although phonological analysis is different, it is related to the types of articulation analysis done previously in the field.
3. To present a model that will tie together past and current methods of articulation analysis.
4. To show that phonological analysis is a more appropriate method for assessment of disordered articulation than any other method currently available.

A Traditional Analysis

Let's return briefly to the sample of reduced phonology that appeared at the beginning of Chapter 1. Since all of the words from the *Goldman-Fristoe Test of Articulation (GFTA)* have been used, it becomes rather easy to perform a traditional articulation analysis on the data. Figure 2–1 illustrates a properly filled-out *GFTA* response form and Table 2–1 shows a typical summary of the speech data. A number of factors immediately become apparent:

1. *Many sounds in error*—The "child" has 39 separate sound errors for the test items. This number, of course, excludes any possible vowel errors, which are not assessed on the *GFTA*.
2. *Inconsistency*—Only two sounds in the "child's" repertoire are consistently produced across all three word positions. The *d* sound is correctly articulated in all positions and the "child" demonstrates a consistent *b/v* substitution. Interestingly, however, *b* is never produced correctly in regular *b*-words *(bath, tub, rabbit)* although it is produced correctly in a *b*-cluster word *(blue)*.

   As another of what could be many more examples, *m* is never produced correctly in any of the GFTA words, yet look back at word 3 of the speech sample *(my)*—the *m* is articulated correctly here and in a number of other words throughout the conversational sample. What is the clinician to think? Inconsistency, without a doubt—at least according to a traditional analysis.
3. *Basic element of concern is the sound*—The major unit for analysis, according to a traditional framework, is the speech sound as a distinct entity, separate from all other speech sounds. Thus, all errors are described in terms of specific sounds (for example, "a *th* for *s* substitution").

As an example of how the basic unit of concern was the entire sound in a traditional analysis, consider for a moment one "diagram of errors" from Van Riper and Irwin's 1958 text, *Voice and Articulation* (see Figure 2–2). This type of error diagram

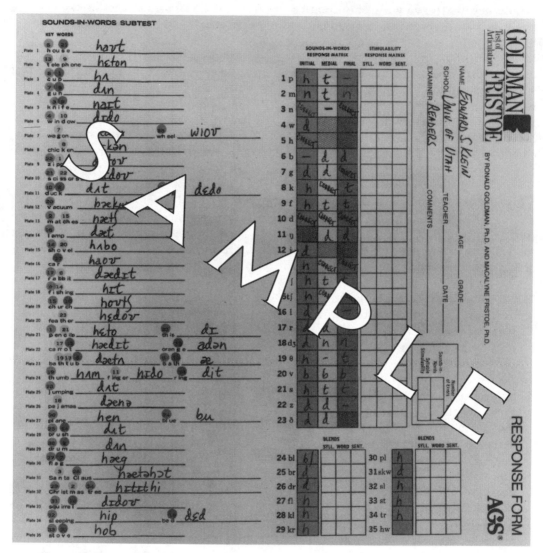

Figure 2–1. Completed Goldman-Fristoe response form for opening paragraphs. (Goldman-Fristoe Test of Articulation by Ronald Goldman & Macalyn Fristoe © 1986 by American Guidance Service, Inc., 4201 Woodland Road, Circle Pines, Minnesota 55014-1796. Reproduced with permission of the Publisher. All rights reserved.)

TABLE 2–1. Traditional description of speech errors from opening sample.

Traditional	
Inconsistent substitution of:	
d for *w, g, y, l, r, dj,* th(v), *z*	(initial)
d for *b, g, ng, l, r, v, z,* th(v)	(medial)
d for *b, ng*	(final)
h for *p, k, f, t, ch, s, sh,* th(u)	(initial)
**b* for *v*	(all pos.)
n for *m*	(init., fin.)
n for *dj*	(med., fin.)
t for *p, m, f, sh, s*	(medial)
t for *k, f, sh,* th(u), *a*	(final)
Inconsistent omission of:	
b	(initial)
n, th(u)	(medial)
p, l, r, z	(final)

*consistent error

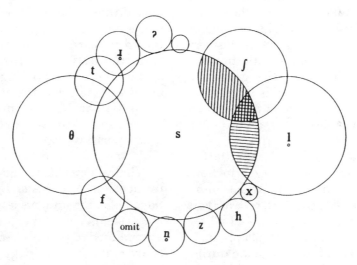

Key:

ʃ = *sh*	tʃ = *ch*
θ = unvoiced *th*	x = the velar fricative
l̥ = unvoiced *l*	ʔ = glottal stop
n̥ = unvoiced *n*	ɹ̥ = breathy unvoiced [r]

Figure 2–2. An error diagram showing common errors of the [s] phoneme. (From Van Riper, C., & Irwin, J. *Voice and Articulation,* p. 81 © 1958 Allyn & Bacon, Needham Heights, MA. All rights reserved. Reprinted with permission of Allyn & Bacon.)

appeared for all of the "standard sounds" and according to Van Riper and Irwin, "The intersection circles create areas which represent distortions and transitional sounds . . . and . . . the size of the circle represents the relative frequency of the type of error" (p. 79).

What is most interesting about these diagrams is that all errors were treated equivalently. Although some occurred more frequently than others, they all could be described in the same way—by a circle. All substitutions were alike. For example, *t* for *s* was viewed in the same way as *th* for *s*. In fact, both were called lisps—*th* for *s* was an interdental frontal lisp (a term that still has currency today), and *t* for *s* was called an occluded lisp (a term no longer in common use). Even omissions were pictured in the same manner, as a substitution of "nothing" for the intended sound.

As will become apparent, these diagrams were misleading. All substitutions are not alike—a *t* for *s* substitution is very different from a *th* for *s* substitution, for example—a distinction that has great clinical relevance. An omission is more properly regarded as a change in the structure of the target syllable—not as a substitution of nothing for the sound in error.

But from a traditional articulation framework, these and other distinctions were ignored during the assessment process. In fact, the entire analysis involved simply a compilation of all the errors into a list similar to what appears in Table 2–1. No attempt was made during the assessment period to analyze any structural or other difference between the target and what the client said. So if the client said /θIn/ for *sin*,[1] this was considered a *th* for *s* substitution only. Did labeling the error a substitution help us to determine what the client was doing

wrong? Did it help us realize that the client had a problem with placement (as opposed to, for example, manner or voicing)? Absolutely not. Of course, some of our therapy techniques showed an understanding of this being a placement problem (for example, asking the client to make the *s* sound with the teeth closed). However, other time-honored therapy techniques had the clinician instruct the client to "hiss the bad guy" or "make a sound like a snake"—which of course incorrectly stressed the manner feature of friction.

In short, during a traditional assessment, there was no systematic attempt to describe articulation errors in terms of the differences between the target and the client's production. Interestingly, even 20–40 years ago, most clinicians had the knowledge to conduct the beginnings of a systematic analysis, if we had wanted to, or had thought of it. How? By using the place-manner-voicing charts we were all forced to learn early on in our training. Unfortunately, the odds were stacked against this ever happening, because traditionally trained clinicians were taught two separate, parallel systems for studying articulation—one "theoretical," taught in basic science-type courses, and one "practical," taught in disorder courses and during clinical practicum. And "never did the twain meet." As one example of how traditionally taught students learned two separate systems, consider Figure 2–3, which is a reproduction of a place-manner-voicing chart appearing on page 80 of the Van Riper and Irwin (1958) book mentioned earlier. What is most astounding is the fact that nowhere in the text is there any reference to that chart! It's just there.

Eventually, because there was "no practical use" for place-manner-voicing information, most practicing clinicians ended

---

[1]A convention that will be used throughout this book will be the use of phonetics for a client's response while maintaining orthographics for the target word. This is being done so that reading is facilitated for those less familiar with phonetics, while ensuring the necessary precision during error description.

CONSONANTS

	Bi-labial	Labio-dental	Dental and Alveolar	Retroflex	Palato-alveolar	Alveolo-palatal	Palatal	Velar	Uvular	Pharyngal	Glottal
Plosive	p b		t d	ʈ ɖ			c ɟ	k g	q ɢ		ʔ
Nasal	m	ɱ	n	ɳ			ɲ	ŋ	N		
Lateral Fricative			ɬ ɮ								
Lateral Non-fricative			l	ɭ			ʎ				
Rolled			r						ʀ		
Flapped			ɾ	ɽ					ʀ		
Fricative	ɸ β	f v	θ ð s z	ʂ ʐ	ʃ ʒ	ɕ ʑ	ç j	x ɣ	χ ʁ	ħ ʕ	h ɦ
Frictionless Continuants and Semi-vowels	w ɥ	ʋ	ɹ				j (ɥ)	(w)	ʁ		

VOWELS

		Front	Central	Back	
Close	(y ʉ u)	i y	ɨ ʉ	ɯ u	
Half-close	(ø o)	e ø		ɤ o	
Half-open	(œ)	ɛ œ	ə	ʌ ɔ	
Open	(ɒ)	a		ɑ ɒ	

(Secondary articulations are shown by symbols in brackets.)

OTHER SOUNDS.—Palatalized consonants: ʈ, ɟ, etc. Velarized or pharyngalized consonants: ɫ, ɖ, ẓ, etc. Ejective consonants (plosives with simultaneous glottal stop): p', t', etc. Implosive voiced consonants: ɓ, ɗ, etc. ř fricative trill. σ, ʑ (labialized θ, ð, or s, z). ƫ, ʓ (labialized ʃ, ʒ). ɋ, ʓ (clicks, Zulu c, ɋ, x). l (a sound between r and l). ʍ (voiceless w). ɪ, ʏ, ʊ (lowered varieties of i, y, u). ɜ (a variety of ə). ɵ (a vowel between ø and o).

Affricates are normally represented by groups of two consonants (ts, tʃ, dʒ, etc.), but, when necessary, ligatures are used (ʦ, ʧ, ʤ, etc.), or the marks ‿ or ͡ (ʦ or ʧ, etc.). c, ɟ may occasionally be used in place of tʃ, dʒ. Aspirated plosives: ph, th, etc.

LENGTH, STRESS, PITCH.—ː (full length). · (half length). ' (stress, placed at beginning of the stressed syllable). ˌ (secondary stress). ˉ (high level pitch); ˍ (low level); ´ (high rising); ˎ (low rising); ˆ (high falling); ˏ (low falling); ˄ (rise-fall); ˅ (fall-rise). See Écriture phonétique internationale, p. 9.

MODIFIERS.— ˜ nasality. ˳ breath (l̥ = breathed l). ˬ voice (ş = z). ' slight aspiration following p, t, etc. ˌ specially close vowel (e̝ = a very close e). ˌ specially open vowel (e̞ = a rather open e). ˮ labialization (n̫ = labialized n). ̪ dental articulation (t̪ = dental t). ˈ palatalization (ż = ʒ). ˔ tongue slightly raised. ˕ tongue slightly lowered. ˒ lips more rounded. ˓ lips more spread. Central vowels i (= ï), u (= ü), e (= ë), ə (= ö), ɛ, ɔ. (e.g. n̩) syllabic consonant. ˘ consonantal vowel. ʃ variety of ʃ resembling s, etc.

Figure 2-3. Place-manner-voicing chart. (From Van Riper, C., & Irwin, J. Voice and Articulation, p. 80 © 1958 Allyn & Bacon, Needham Heights, MA. All rights reserved. Reprinted with permission of Allyn & Bacon.)

up forgetting these features of the sound and creating lists of sound errors instead— hence tests like the *Goldman-Fristoe Test of Articulation* (Goldman & Fristoe, 1986), the *Arizona Articulation Proficiency Scale* (Fudala, 1970), and most others of the time, which involved error compilation only, with no real analysis at all. (This problem, of course, continues today in training programs that remain tradition- ally based.) If there was any realization or usage of the place, manner, voicing or other differences between the target sound and the client's error, it occurred after the analysis, during therapy.

According to a traditional analysis, then, there were four ways of describing articu- lation errors:

1. *Substitution*—substitution of one stan- dard phonetic sound for another (e.g., /tµp/ for *soup*).
2. *Distortion*—substitution of a nonstan- dard phonetic sound for another in the word (e.g., /sµp/ with a lateral *s* for *soup*).
3. *Omission*—omission of a sound from the word (e.g., /µp/ for *soup*).
4. *Addition*—addition of an extra sound into the word (e.g., /stup/ for *soup*).

As stated, the purpose of an articulation assessment was to determine *all* errors made by the client, and describe them in list form (as in Table 2–1). Then, the thera- pist would begin with the sound that "developed earliest" in normal children (in this case, probably *m*), and teach the client how to produce the sound correctly, usually one sound at a time.

A Different Way of Looking at Things

During the late 1960s and early 1970s, the study of articulation disorders began to change. More and more speech-language pathologists began to realize that the place-

ment, manner, and voicing characteristics that contrasted the sounds of speech were more important than the sounds themselves. The concept of distinctive features was born. (Well, not really. Actually, in as early as 1958, Albright and Albright had implied the need for speech-language pathologists to consider the "systematic structure underlying the variability of forms" (p. 259) in the child's output. And, of course, Jakobson, Fant, and Halle (1952) had described a distinctive fea- ture system in 1952. But it was the 1970s before speech-language pathologists in any number began trying to incorporate the use of distinctive features into clinical practice with their clients with speech disorders.)

For the advocates of distinctive feature analysis, each speech sound was no longer a unitary segment, but instead was related to every other speech sound by means of whatever features were being described. The belief was that one might be able to find underlying patterns that would account for several sound errors at once. For example, if a child misarticulated *v*, *f*, *s*, *sh*, and *th*, perhaps his or her underlying problem was with the manner feature of frication, rather than with each of the sounds separately.

The first formal test to encourage analy- sis of these features underlying sound pro- duction was the *Fisher-Logemann Test of Articulation Competence* (Fisher & Loge- mann, 1971). Fisher and Logemann used the traditional distinctive feature system of place, manner, and voicing as the basis of their test. According to the authors, this type of analysis had two advantages:

1. It allowed one to determine the *nature* of the error made by the client.
2. It allowed one to find *patterns of feature errors* common to many sounds; this, they said, would facilitate therapy.

Interestingly enough, the Fisher- Logemann system of analysis never really caught on very widely in the field (interesting because the Fisher-Logemann system is much closer in design to current methods of phonological analysis than is the major distinctive feature system that followed it). In fact, most students in the 1970s, *if* they learned about distinctive features, never associated the Fisher-Logemann system with that term. Instead, the term was reserved for a theoretical system of supposedly idealized, universal distinctive features created by Chomsky and Halle (1968), which ultimately led to the creation of an assessment device—*the Distinctive Feature Analysis of Misarticulation* (McReynolds & Engmann, 1975).

It is clear now that the foray into "Chomsky and Halle-esque" distinctive feature analysis was a digression for the field of speech-language pathology. But it was an important digression because it helped educate speech pathologists to the possibility that the particular sounds a child misarticulated might be less important than the nature of the misarticulations. Clinicians became aware that by studying the nature of production for several error sounds in the child's speech, one might be able to find logical *patterns* to the errors that the child was making.

To illustrate some of the benefits that might have accrued given the changes during the 1970s, let's return once again to the sample of reduced phonology appearing at the beginning of Chapter 1. Figure 2–4 displays a *Fisher-Logemann* test form that might have been filled out for that speech sample. Table 2–2 compares a summary of the traditional analysis performed earlier with summaries of both Fisher-Logemann and McReynolds-Engmann distinctive feature analyses. Some differences immediately become apparent:

1. *Fewer errors in a distinctive feature analysis*—While the traditional description yielded 39 errors, a place-manner-voicing feature analysis results in 12 errors. Likewise, a McReynolds-Eng-

mann (Chomsky-Halle) feature analysis yields anywhere from 9–16 errors (depending on the percentage criterion used to define an error). The obvious conclusion? With fewer errors to work on, therapy would progress more quickly.

2. *Using a distinctive feature approach, the child's speech system is viewed as more consistent, less random*—This is a little less obvious but an important difference nonetheless. For example, the traditional description yielded 39 errors, with only 1 consistent (2.5%). On the other hand, the place-manner-voicing analysis resulted in 12 errors with 4 consistent (33%). Likewise, the McReynolds-Engmann analysis yielded 9–15 errors (depending on the criterion) with 4 or so consistent. In short, along with the use of distinctive feature methods of analysis, the child's speech system is beginning to be viewed as more reasonable, more orderly, and less random than might have been the case previously.

3. *The focus of the two types of analysis is different*—Look closely at the descriptions of the errors. In a traditional analysis, the focus is on the sounds in error. In a distinctive feature analysis, the focus is on the physiological and/or acoustic parameters of speech production that might be *responsible* for the child's errors. In a traditional analysis, there is no attempt to describe what articulatory features the child is or is not producing. The only question is a yes-no question. "Is the child producing the sound correctly or not?" Determination of what the child might be doing incorrectly is left until the beginning of therapy for a particular sound. In feature analysis, on the other hand, production or nonproduction of a given sound in a given word is unimportant. Instead, the attempt is made to find production factors that might be impeding correct articulation *across sounds*. Thus, the analysis of what the child is doing wrong that is impeding correct articu-

THE FISHER-LOGEMANN TEST OF ARTICULATION COMPETENCE

Screening ☐ Complete ☐

Record Form for the Picture Test

Name **EDWARD KLEIN** Date **11/18/83** Examiner **CONVENTION ATTENDEES**

Age_____ Grade (or Occupation)_____ School (or Employer)_____

Birthdate_____ Home Address_____

Native Dialect_____ Foreign Language in home_____

CONSONANT PHONEMES

Card	IPA Phoneme	Common Spelling	Dev. Age	Place of Articulation	Voicing	Stop Pre.	Stop Inter.	Stop Post.	Fricative Pre.	Fricative Inter.	Fricative Post.	Affricate Pre.	Affricate Inter.	Affricate Post.	Glide Pre.	Glide Inter.	Glide Post.	Lateral Pre.	Lateral Inter.	Lateral Post.	Nasal Pre.	Nasal Inter.	Nasal Post.
1	p	p	3		ⱴ	h /p	t /p	- /p	/mᴵ														
2	b	b	5																				
3	ʍ	wh	3	Bilabial																			
4	w	w			V	- /b	∂ /b	∂ /b							d /w	∗ /w					n /m	t /m	n /m
5	m	m	3																				
6	f	f	4	Labio-dental	ⱴ				h /f	t /f	t /f												
7	v	v	7		V				b /v	b /v	b /v												
8	θ	th	7	Tip-dental	ⱴ				ʜb /θ	-/θ	t /θ												
9	ð	th	8		V				∂ /ð	∂ /ð	/ð												
10	t	t	6	Tip-alveolar	ⱴ	h /t	/t²	/t															
11	d	d	5																				
12	l	l	6																				
13	n	n	3		V	/d	/d	/d										∂ /l	t /l	/l	/n	/n	/n
14	s	s	7	Blade-alveolar	ⱴ				h /s	t /s	t /s												
15	z	z	7		V	∂ /z	∂ /z	/z															
16	ʃ	sh	6	Blade-prepalatal	ⱴ				b /ʃ	t /ʃ	t /ʃ	h /tʃ	/tʃ	/tʃ									
17	ʒ	zh	7																				
18	tʃ	ch	6		V				/ʒ	/ʒ²		d /dʒ	n /dʒ	/dʒ									
19	dʒ	j	7																				
20	j	y	5	Front-palatal	ⱴ										∂ /j	/j							
					V																		
21	r	r	6	Central-palatal	ⱴ										∂ /r	∂ /r	/r⁴						
					V																		
22	k	k	4	Back-velar	ⱴ	h /k	/k	t /k															
23	g	g	4																				
24	ŋ	ng	5		V	∂ /g	∂ /g	/g													ʜ /ŋ	∂ /ŋ	
25	h	h	3	Glottal	ⱴ				/h	/h													

SUMMARY OF MISARTICULATION PATTERNS:

MANNER OF FORMATION ERRORS: *Probs. w/ fricatives except in initial, voiceless ; problems w/ glides, probs. - voiceless stops*

PLACE OF ARTICULATION ERRORS: *Probs: w/ dental, many bilabial, many back-velar - but not all*

VOICING ERRORS:

Notes: (These and additional notes are discussed in the Manual under "Dialectal Variations")
1. Either /m/ or /w/ 3. Either /ʒ/ or /dʒ/.
2. Either /t/ or /d/ 4. Either /r/ or /ɚ/ or lengthening of the preceding vowel.

Figure 2–4. Completed Fisher-Logemann test form. (From Fisher, H. B., & Logemann, J. A. 1971, *The Fisher-Logemann test of articulation competence*, copyright © 1995 by Pro-Ed, Austin, Texas. Reprinted with permission.)

TABLE 2–2. Comparison among traditional, place-manner-voicing distinctive feature, and McReynolds and Engmann distinctive feature systems of articulation analysis.

Traditional	Place, Manner, Voice

Traditional

Inconsistent substitution of:

d for *w, g, y, l, r, dj, th*(v), *z*	(initial)
d for *b, g, ng, l, r, v, z, th*(v)	(medial)
d for *b, ng*	(final)
h for *p, k, f, t, ch, s, sh, th*(u)	(initial)
*b for *v*	(all pos.)
n for *m*	(init., fin.)
n for *dj*	(med., fin.)
t for *p, m, f, sh, s*	(medial)
t for *k, f, sh, th*(u), *s*	(final)

Inconsistent omission of:

b	(initial)
n, th(u)	(medial)
p, l, r, z	(final)

Place, Manner, Voice

Manner

 – Stopping fricatives except initial voiceless and *h*.
* – Stopping glides and laterals in initial, medial.
 – Stopping nasals in medial inconsistently.
* – Fricating voiceless stops.
 – Nasalizing voiced affricates, medial and final.
 – Stopping voiced affricates, initial.
* – Unstopping voiceless affricate, initial.

Place
* – Glottalizing voiceless stops and fricatives, initial.
* – Bilabializing voiced labiodentals.
 – Alveolarizing velar stops, nasals, palatals.

Omissions

 – Bilabial stop.
 – Voiced alveolar nasals, fricatives, and laterals.

Chomsky-Halle D.F.
(a la McReynolds/Engmann)

	% incorrect
+ vocalic (no vowels tested)	100
– vocalic	0
+ consonantal	14
– consonantal	50
*+ high	80
– high	0
*+ back	77
– back	0
+ low	0
– low	13
+ anterior	13
– anterior	64
+ coronal	13
– coronal	67
+ voice	3
– voice	0
*+ continuant	82
– continuant	15
+ nasal	43
– nasal	5
*+ strident	90
– strident	0

*=consistent error

lation is moved up to the assessment stage, so that patterns of production errors can be found.

Regrouping for a Moment

The development of feature analysis was valuable because it allowed us to study three parameters of speech production in which errors could occur, impeding correct articulation. These three parameters of possible constraint on articulation were:

1. *Placement*—constraints caused by inappropriate location of articulatory valving within the vocal tract.
2. *Manner*—constraints caused by inappropriate degree or type of articulatory constriction.
3. *Voicing*—constraints caused by inappropriate timing or use of vocal cord vibration.

Although this type of feature analysis was valuable, it still didn't provide us with the total picture. Why? Because the distinctive feature systems only allowed for analysis of the phonetic[2] or production parameters of possible constraint on articulation. This emphasis on the study of only phonetic factors impeding articulation was underlined in an interesting article by Ladefoged (1980) where he stated "the production of speech is constrained by the articulatory parameters that people can vary" (p. 25). He then went on to describe what he called a "necessary and sufficient set" (p. 27) of articulatory parameters affecting speech production. A listing of this set appears in Figure 2–5.

Toward a Comprehensive Articulation Analysis

What Ladefoged and earlier distinctive feature advocates did not account for were the *phonemic factors* that could impede correct articulation. As such, feature systems could not deal with omissions, which were either ignored in the analysis, or analyzed as if a sound had been produced that lacked all the necessary place, manner, and voicing features! Errors of assimilation (errors due to the context of a sound) were analyzed in the same way as other substitution errors, although this would have to muddy the analysis.

In short, what was not realized was that there are at least seven parameters of possible constraint on articulation. These parameters are illustrated in the Model of Parameters of Articulatory Constraint which appears in Figure 2–6. As can be seen, in addition to the placement, manner, and voicing categories introduced earlier, there are the following four parameters of possible articulatory constraint:

1. *Contextual*—constraints caused by the influence of other sounds on the target sound (assimilation).
2. *Structural*—constraints caused by the phonemic structure of the intended word. This category has three levels:
   a. Position of the sound within a word (initial, medial, final)
   b. Syllable structure of the intended syllable housing the sound
   c. Number of syllables in the utterance.
3. *Semantic*—constraints on correct articulation due to lexical limitations.

---

[2]A full discussion of the differences between the terms *phonetic* and *phonemic* is outside the purview of this book. Besides, there's little agreement as to the exact use or value of those terms anyway. For our purposes, phonetic parameters are those that concern the motoric act of speaking, whereas phonemic parameters are those that pertain to cognitive or linguistic activities involved in speaking. Contrary to many sources, however, no etiological significance is implied here in using those terms. For example, although a placement problem concerns the "motor act if speaking," it is not the intention to imply that this problem is "motorically caused." Sufficiently confused? Serves you right for reading footnotes!

A necessary and sufficient set of articulatory parameters

1. Front raising
2. Back raising
3. Tip raising
4. Tip advancing
5. Pharynx width
6. Tongue bunching
7. Lateral tongue contraction
8. Lip height

9. Lip width
10. Lip protrusion
11. Velic opening
12. Larynx lowering
13. Glottal aperture
14. Phonation tension
15. Glottal length
16. Lung volume decrement

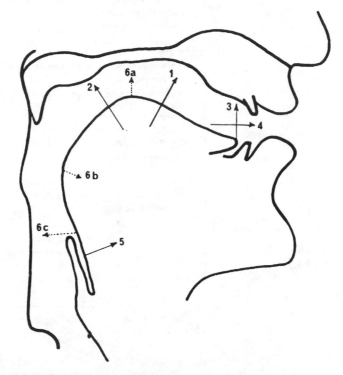

Figure 2–5. Description of "full" set of articulatory parameters. (From Ladefoged, P. [1980]. Articulatory parameters. *Language and Speech, 23,* 25–30. Reprinted with permission.)

4. *Linguistic*—phonological constraints imposed by morphological or syntactic deficiencies.

It becomes clear that the only way to conduct a total analysis of an individual's phonological system is to consider all of these parameters in a systematic fashion.

Presumably, someone should be able to come up with a formal test that would thoroughly evaluate each of these parameters. However, don't expect it soon . . . because it would weigh 200 pounds, it would cost $10,000 to buy, and it'd take several years to administer. To understand why, it's important to look a little more closely at each of the parameters.

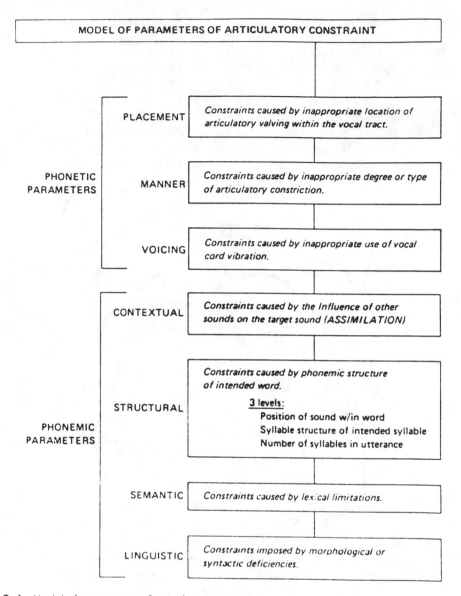

Figure 2–6. Model of parameters of articulatory constraint.

The voicing parameter is probably the easiest to discuss, because there are only two alternatives—voiced and voiceless.[3] (See Figure 2–7.) The manner parameter is a bit more complex. There are at least seven possibilities or alternatives in nor-mal adult American English phonology—fricative, stop, affricate, lateral, retroflex (rhotic), nasal, glide. (See Figure 2–8.)

If one tried to construct a formal assess-ment device that would systematically consider each of the alternatives in one

[3]Actually, this is not totally true. In American English Phonology, we have a sound that is "somewhere between" voiced and voiceless—the medial sound in *butter* or *rubber*, for instance. Although it is important to realize this for therapy, however, we will stick to just considering the voiced/voiceless distinction here.

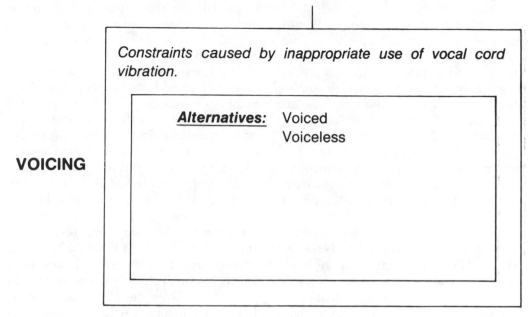

Figure 2–7. Alternatives available in voicing parameter.

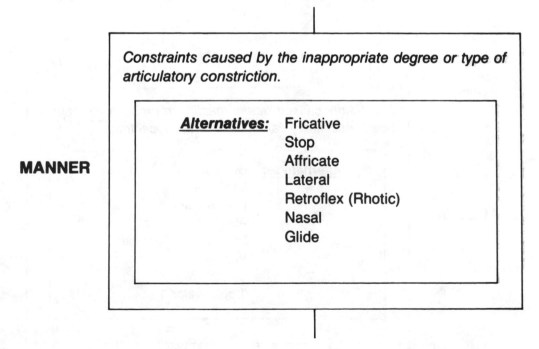

Figure 2–8. Alternatives available in manner parameter.

21

parameter in combination with each alternative in the other parameter, one would need a test having 2 × 7 or 14 items. "No problem," you say. Besides, you think you've found a flaw. "Aha," you argue, "there's no need to consider every combination. After all, there's no voiceless lateral in English." True . . . if we're testing only people with adult American English phonology. Unfortunately, we're not. The children who we see often have phonological systems that are very different from the adult phonological model. And, of course, in deviant phonology, there is one very common voiceless lateral that occurs—the lateral *s*, also known as the lateral lisp. If we don't have a framework that allows us to consider and explain this error, then the lateral *s* becomes that glorious wastebag term that we as speech-language pathologists have traditionally used when we couldn't explain what was happening—*distortion*. Now, we may not need to test specifically for every combination

of production alternatives (more on this soon), but we *must* have a framework or a model of analysis that allows us to consider them.

So far, we've only considered two parameters. Figure 2–9 illustrates the placement parameter, in which there are at least seven (and perhaps eight) alternatives in adult American English phonology—bilabial, labiodental, interdental, alveolar, platal, velar, and glottal. (Additionally, Kent (1993) labeled *w* as labial-velar, because the tongue is constrained in the back of the mouth while the lips move for the *w* sound. Although most texts ignore this distinction, Kent is unquestionably correct and clinicians would do well to learn this distinction between *w* and the bilabials.) To consider all of these alternatives in combination with the alternatives available in the voicing and manner categories, we now need a test that has 2 × 7 × 7 or 98 items—to assess for each possible combination *just once*. This is still within

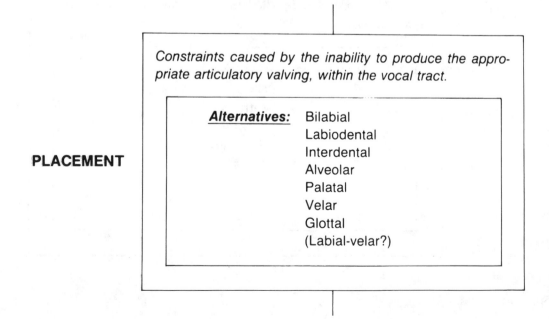

PLACEMENT

Constraints caused by the inability to produce the appropriate articulatory valving, within the vocal tract.

Alternatives: Bilabial
Labiodental
Interdental
Alveolar
Palatal
Velar
Glottal
(Labial-velar?)

Figure 2–9. Alternatives available in placement parameters.

reason test-wise, but we haven't dealt with the phonemic parameters of constraint yet.

Attempting to tackle the contextual parameter is not easy, because assimilation is known to occur across several sounds in an utterance (Zemlin, 1988). To make it simpler, let's just consider context as being the effect of adjacent sounds. With approximately 40 different possible contexts before the target and the same 40 possible after (see Figure 2–10), the same problem of unwieldiness that anyone who has administered McDonald's Deep Test of Articulation (1964b) can remember vividly, begins to grow. When one adds the structural parameter (see Figure 2–11), including perhaps 4 alternatives for word length, 10 for syllable structure, and 3 for word position, we've suddenly created a test of $2 \times 7 \times 7 \times 40 \times 40 \times 4 \times 10 \times 3$ or 18,816,000 items—if we want to test for

every possible error just once! And we haven't yet even begun to consider the possibility of phonological variations caused by semantic or linguistic factors (and they both occur on occasion—e.g., Schwartz, Messick, & Pollock, 1983).

It is obviously impossible to construct a formal test that can consider every possible error. But that's just as well, because you'd never have time to give it. Also, it's unnecessary to test for every possible error. Why? Because the phonological systems of most children are consistent enough such that usually a limited number of rules will describe a given child's system (usually no more than 12–15; often less). But even though it is unnecessary to test for every possibility, in reality any of those 18,000,000 errors can conceivably occur in a given child. And as we've all learned, much to our chagrin, some chil-

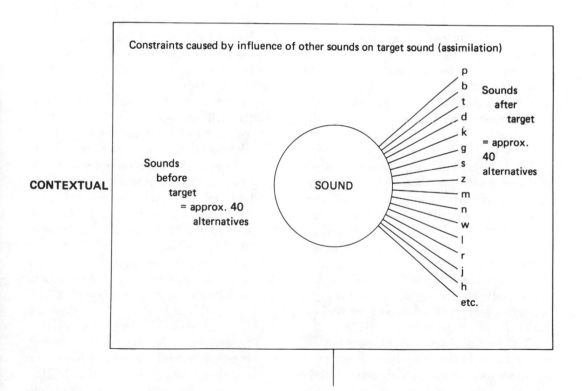

Figure 2–10. Alternatives available in context parameter.

	Constraints caused by phonemic structure of intended words		
	Levels:	WORD LENGTH	SYLLABLE STRUCTURE	WORD POSITION
STRUCTURAL	Alternatives:	One-Syllable	C	Prevocalic
		Two-Syllable	CV	Intervocalic
		Three-Syllable	VC	Post-vocalic
		Four-Syllable	CVC	
			CVCV	
			CCVC	
			CVCC	
			CCCVC	
			CCVCC	
			CCCVCC	

Figure 2–11. Alternatives available in structural parameter.

dren do, indeed, make some very strange errors.

So what do you do? It's a big problem. Traditional tests (e.g., the *Templin-Darley Tests of Articulation*, Templin & Darley, 1969, or the *Arizona Articulation Proficiency Scale*, Fudala, 1970) are not organized to provide information on any of the parameters of constraints; they're just organized to give information on sounds. Tests based on distinctive features (e.g., the *Fisher-Logemann Test of Articulation Competence*, Fisher & Logemann, 1971) are organized to provide information on place, manner, and voicing parameters, but do not consider the phonemic parameters of constraint. Unfortunately, in most unintelligible children, context and structural factors predominate.

One partial solution to this problem has come with the recent development of "phonological process" assessment devices, many of which are now available on the market. (A full discussion of these tests is undertaken in Chapter 10.) All of these devices allow for analysis of more parameters of constraint than traditional or distinctive feature tests. In fact, what the

authors have done is to organize their devices to assess the most commonly occurring errors in each of the parameters. The tests differ from one another in the errors or phonological rules that are evaluated—but the purposes are the same: to try to get a better idea of the child's phonological system, considering more parameters of constraint than traditional or distinctive feature methodologies.

Now, each of these newer systems of articulation analysis is better than and different from earlier methods of evaluation because a more accurate picture of the child's problems can be obtained. But all of these devices have one problem: Remember, a child might theoretically have over 18,000,000 possibilities for errors. What if the child has a pattern of errors or a rule that is not considered on the assessment device? This can happen in two ways:

1. *Idiosyncratic Rules*—These are, simply, unusual phonological rules that are seen infrequently, and are not considered on formal assessment devices. Recent literature is replete with descriptions of children who demonstrated rules that are

not in the "top 10" (e.g., see Camarata & Gandour, 1984, or Leonard, 1985). In fact, the possibilities for variation seem endless. Some examples:

a. *H'ing of stops*—Weiner (1981b) called this type of rule, where an entire class of sounds goes to one "favored" sound, a "systematic sound preference" (p. 281). In this case, all stops turn into the *h* sound, so that

> cow → /haʊ/
>
> gun → /hʌn/
>
> day → /he/
>
> pass → /hæs/
>
> boy → /hɔɪ/.

b. *Nasal snorting*—Substitution of a nasal snort for various sounds in the child's repertoire (usually fricatives).

c. *"Buddy Hackett Rule"*—This tongue-in-cheek label refers to a very real phonological problem first seen several years ago and since reported a number of times by speech pathologists across the country. Anybody who has seen comedian Buddy Hackett should be able to visualize what Kim, a 4-year-old girl, was doing. On all *s*, *z*, and *sh* sounds, Kim's lip and lower jaw deviated as far as possible to the left. Surprisingly, her intelligibility was unaffected, with only a slight distortion of these sounds heard. However, her parents were concerned about how she looked and listeners expected her to launch into a punch line at any minute, so we saw her for therapy. The "Buddy Hackett Rule" was born.

2. *Limited Rules*—These are rules that are just as predictable and consistent as other rules, but occur only in limited contexts or within limited parameters. For example, while we have seen *h'ing*

of all stops only once in 15 years, *h'ing of initial voiceless stops* has occurred several times. This latter rule is limited because it only applies to a certain type of stop (voiceless) and only in one position (initial). But it is just as consistent as any other rule the child might exhibit. Some other possibilities for limited rules:

a. Cluster reduction of fricative-liquid clusters.

b. Labial assimilation in words with the vowels /u/ and /o/.

c. Stopping of medial voiced fricatives. In fact, limited rules come in all sizes and shapes and are extremely important because they are the major contributors to what *looks like* inconsistency in children's speech.

A more complete discussion of idiosyncratic and limited rules will appear in a later chapter. What's important at this point is the understanding that although idiosyncratic and limited rules might be very important causes of a child's unintelligibility, current formal phonological assessment devices will miss them (unless additional analysis is undertaken).

What's the answer? *Any valid analysis of articulation must be done by the tester, not the test.* No formal test can evaluate 18,000,000 possibilities. But we have the best little analytical device available right above our shoulders. And once we have internalized the possible parameters of articulatory constraint along with all alternatives available in each parameter, we can quickly perform all of the operations that will allow us to discard more than 17,999,900 possibilities that do not relate to the child we are analyzing. The name of this analytical procedure? *Generative analysis*, and it has been around for many more years than have the formal tests of phonology listed earlier in the chapter. In fact, it might even be suggested that development of those tests has represented yet another detour in our long road toward a complete understanding of speech disorders.

Time for a Small Break

Several things may be going through your head at this point:

> "Generative analysis . . . I don't like the sound of that."

> "It sounds complicated and worse, it sounds like it'll take a long time."

> "With my caseload, I don't have weeks to spend on one evaluation."

Well, please rest assured that you will *not* be asked to spend an overwhelming amount of time in analyzing articulation. In fact, the bulk of your time will be spent in first *learning* how to perform a generative analysis. Chapters 5 through 10 are designed to teach you just that. But as you become more proficient, you'll begin to notice that much of the process is just bookkeeping; that what is being learned is not so much a tool as it is a different way of thinking. Once you learn this different way of thinking, the analysis is not only do-able, it's also interesting and in some ways, fun!

And the time problem? One of the most frequent complaints of clinicians who have tried to use phonological analysis is that "It takes too long." Perhaps true—if you use one of the formal tests on the market. But once you learn how to do a generative analysis, time will not be a problem. In fact, the *speed with which you can do a good phonological analysis is directly correlated with your level of familiarity with the parameters of articulatory constraint*. In other words, the more familiar you are with the alternatives available under the parameters of place, manner, voicing, context, and the others, the more quickly you can do the analysis. Unfortunately, as mentioned earlier in this chapter, many clinicians have left terms like

voiceless labiodental fricative back in introductory phonetics. Just as unfortunately, many clinicians no longer do any phonetic transcription. The problem is, whether we like it or not, knowledge of the parameters of articulatory constraint and ability to do phonetic transcription constitute the "tools of our trade" if we are working with children or adults who have articulation disorders. To work with individuals with phonological disorders without these tools is not that different from a surgeon trying to do surgery without the knowledge of what a scalpel is or how to use it.

If, indeed, our field is going to reap the possible benefits of phonological analysis and intervention, clinicians are going to have to redevelop these lost tools. Essentially, you have to know the inside of your mouth like the back of your hand. And what are these benefits?

Benefits of Phonological Analysis

1. Phonological analysis provides a better and more accurate idea of a child's (or adult's) problems in articulation. Because all relevant parameters are being considered, phonological analysis results in fewer errors and more consistent errors. (We'll see a dramatic example of this soon.)

2. Phonological analysis allows for development of more appropriate therapy techniques, better geared toward the child's real problem. Traditionally, if a child deleted a final *t* sound, the clinician might have tried to instruct the child to put his or her tongue to the roof of the mouth; in other words, he or she might have worked on *t* placement or production. Using a phonological framework, however, it is clear that the child has a problem with the concept of syllable structure. So there is no reason and no need to teach *t* placement. In short, if there isn't a problem with the placement constraint, why teach as if there is? Use of a phonological framework helps to avoid therapeutic miscalculations of this type.

3. A phonological framework leads to greatly decreased time in therapy. Of course this is the bottom line. Before any competent speech pathologist is going to use a new therapeutic procedure, he or she will rightfully demand some measure of that procedure's greater effectiveness. On all counts, a phonological framework meets this test. For several years now, proponents of phonological analysis and intervention have reported remarkable results for their clients who have undergone therapy based on this newer approach. Specifically, numerous children have been described who previously might have been in therapy for many years given the severity of their speech disorders, but have been dismissed in 12–18 months after undergoing phonologically based therapy (Hodson, 1992; Hodson & Paden, 1983; Klein, in press; Monahan, 1986; Weiner, 1981; Young, 1983). In short, phonologically based intervention works. We have seen excellent results, as have hundreds if not thousands of speech-language pathologists across the country. And, of course, the true beneficiaries are the children with speech disorders, who no longer have to bear the onus of a handicapping condition during the bulk of their formative years.

4. It is now easier for us to prove that we, as speech-language pathologists, are really doing something. We have had a crisis of confidence in our field with regard to articulation therapy for many years. Perhaps it's been caused by all those children who have come back from Christmas break having progressed more in that 2 weeks without therapy than they have in the prior 4 months with therapy. Perhaps it's been caused by the 10-year-old who has received speech therapy for 6 years, but is still very difficult to understand. Perhaps it's even been caused by the child who has finally learned to produce the *s* sound, but every time he or she

tries to put it into a word (e.g., *sun*), it becomes *s-s-s-tun*. Whatever the reasons, for many clinicians articulation therapy has historically been a dreaded part of the profession—drills, boredom, excruciatingly slow progress. And when progress has occurred, we have often wondered whether we should take the credit for it—in the back of our minds questioning whether the child would've improved anyway just due to maturation.

Happily, with the use of a phonological framework, these questions and doubts can be put to rest. Improvement is rapid enough that a clear cause-effect relationship between intervention and improvement can be drawn. And once one has observed this rapid change in several clients across different ages, it becomes clear that simple maturation is no longer a viable alternate explanation for the improvement.

In order to illustrate these benefits most clearly, let's return for the last time to the sample of reduced phonology appearing at the beginning of Chapter 1. Table 2–3 compares the three analyses performed earlier with a phonological analysis of the same sample. The differences between these different forms of analysis stand out immediately. First, the quantity of errors decreases dramatically, from traditional to distinctive feature to phonological analysis. Compared to 39 errors given a traditional description and 12–15 errors given a distinctive feature analysis, a phonological analysis yields only 7 errors (two of which might be considered language errors). Second, perhaps more importantly, the consistency of errors *increases* greatly across the three analyses. What has been a totally inconsistent speech pattern when described traditionally now becomes totally consistent, given a phonological framework. As we'll see later, this shift to an emphasis on consistency rather than inconsistency will greatly alter our thoughts about therapy.

TABLE 2–3. Comparison of four analyses of severe articulation disorder.

Traditional	Place, Manner, Voice

Inconsistent substitution of:

d for *w, g, y, l, r, dj, th*(v), *z*	(initial)
d for *b, g, ng, l, r, v, z, th*(v)	(medial)
d for *b, ng*	(final)
h for *p, k, f, t, ch, s, sh, th*(u)	(initial)
*b for *v*	(all pos.)
n for *m*	(init., fin.)
n for *dj*	(med., fin.)
t for *p, m, f, sh, s*	(medial)
t for *k, f, sh, th*(u), *s*	(final)

Inconsistent omission of:

b	(initial)
n, th(u)	(medial)
p, l, r, z	(final)

Manner

– Stopping fricatives except initial voiceless and *h*.
* – Stopping glides and laterals in initial, medial.
– Stopping nasals in medial inconsistently.
* – Fricating voiceless stops.
– Nasalizing voiced affricates, medial and final.
– Stopping voiced affricates, initial.
* – Unstopping voiceless affricate, initial.

Place

* – Glottalizing voiceless stops and fricatives, initial.
* – Bilabializing voiced labiodentals.
– Alveolarizing velar stops, nasals, palatals.

Omissions

– Bilabial stop.
– Voiced alveolar nasals, fricatives, and laterals.

Chomsky-Halle D.F. (a la McReynolds/Engmann)	Phonological Process (Rule, Error, etc.) Analysis

	% incorrect
+ vocalic (no vowels tested)	100
– vocalic	0
+ consonantal	14
– consonantal	50
*+ high	80
– high	0
* + back	77
– back	0
+ low	0
– low	13
+ anterior	13
– anterior	64
+ coronal	13
– coronal	67
+ voice	3
– voice	0
* + continuant	82
– continuant	15
+ nasal	43
– nasal	5
* + strident	90
– strident	0

* – Alveolar assimilation
* – Deletion of unstressed syllable (3-syllable sequences)
* – "h" ing of initial voiceless consonants
* – Stopping of fricatives and releasing liquids and glides
* – Deletion of plural morphemes
* – Deletion of present progressive "ing"
* – Cluster reduction

*=consistent error

There are other differences between the three modes of analysis that might not be quite as obvious as the changes in the number of errors and the consistency of those errors. A summary of all of these differences appears in Table 2–4. As stated, the quantity of errors given a traditional description is very high; there are fewer errors given a distinctive feature analysis but fewer yet given a phonological framework. As also discussed, many traditional descriptions yield little or no consistency. Distinctive feature approaches yield high levels of consistency but much inconsistency typically remains. On the other hand, procedures for phonological analysis can result in total or almost total consistency if an appropriate analytical methodology is used.

A less obvious difference between the three types of analysis has to do with how the client's errors are described. A tradi-tional description yields only a list of sound errors. Indeed, the description is static; no real analysis of the source of the problem is being conducted. A distinctive feature description involves active analysis but the focus is on deficiency—what the child is *not* doing. A phonological description, on the other hand, while also dynamic, uses an efficiency model, which emphasizes what the child is doing.

Another difference has to do with how the three frameworks consider the role of the child in speech production. Arising from traditional methodologies has been the view of the child with speech-disorders as a passive speaker who makes errors; she is incompetent as she tries to match the adult model. Unsurprisingly, the therapy arising from traditional frameworks has usually revolved around the attempt to teach the adult model. Distinctive feature methodolo-

TABLE 2–4. Summary of differences between traditional, distinctive feature, and phonological analysis.

	Traditional	Distinctive Feature	Phonological Process Analysis
Quantity of errors	Very high	Less	Few
Consistency of errors	Little or none	Some, but still much inconsistency	Total (or close to)
Description of errors	Static; no analysis	Dynamic-deficiency model; analysis of what child is *not* doing	Dynamic-efficiency model; analysis of what child *is* doing
Role of child in production	Passive; incompetent attemptor of adult model; error-maker	Passive; incompetent attemptor of adult model; error-maker	Active; purposeful simplifier of adult model; creator of own system
Therapy	Teach adult model	Teach contrast between adult model and child production (emphasis on producing contrast)	Teach conception of difference between adult model and child production (emphasis on understanding contrast)

gies also view the child with speech-disorders as a passive error maker. Although the focus is on features rather than sounds, the child is still viewed as incompetent—this time an incompetent feature producer. Again unsurprisingly, the therapeutic emphasis has been one of teaching the child how to produce the features she lacks by having her learn the contrast between the adult model and her incorrect production. In contrast with these approaches, in a phonological framework, children are viewed as active, purposeful simplifiers of the adult model. Instead of being considered as error-makers, they are seen as creators of their own phonological systems; unfortunately (for us) their systems are at variance with the system we (the adult community) would like them to have. But the key is, they are not incompetent speakers randomly making stabs at correctly producing the words they want to say. Their systems are logical, rule-bound, and consistent, and we can discover these elements if we search deeply enough for them.

Finally, this altered view of the child's role in speech production ideally changes our conception of appropriate therapy. Rather than teaching the child *how* to produce a given sound or feature, a phonological approach to therapy tries to get the child to *understand* the contrast between her production and the production of the community. As will be explained more fully in a later chapter, the thesis is that once the child understands the rule-bound contrast between her production and the correct production, it becomes rather easy to stimulate this child to adopt this correct production.

As can be seen in Table 2–4, the three types of analysis are different from one another. However, it should be equally clear that the three are clearly related to one another. In fact, phonological analysis is a logical outgrowth of earlier models of articulation analysis.

In conclusion, it may be instructive to consider the following dictionary definition of the word *analysis*:

> Separating or breaking up of any whole into its parts, especially with an explanation of these parts, to find out their nature, function or interrelationship (Webster, 1976).

This chapter has attempted to show that, over the years, we have learned how to better separate the whole into its parts. We've developed a greater understanding of what these parts are (as illustrated in the Model of Parameters of Articulatory Constraint) and we are now capable of studying these parts in order to find out their nature, function, and interrelationship. In other words, we have finally learned how to do a complete articulation analysis.

✦ PART II ✦

Phonological Analysis

CHAPTER ◆ 3

The Tools of Our Trade

When parents first notice that their child is misarticulating certain sounds, their first move is often to sit in front of the child and try to show him or her how to produce the sounds correctly. Techniques like phonetic placement may have been formally described for speech pathologists by Van Riper and Irwin (1958), but parents discovered that technique long before the profession of Speech-Language Pathology ever existed. So then, what makes a speech-language pathologist any different from a well-meaning parent or teacher? An in-depth knowledge of communication and its disorders certainly helps. So does a broad background of experience with children having speech and language disorders. But what really separates any professional from a lay person is the former's knowledge of and facility with using the tools of his or her profession. For the lawyer, it means having knowledge of precedent, statutes, codes and rules of practice, and procedure, while having facility with the ability to analyze facts and apply them to the law. For the surgeon, it means having knowledge of anatomy and facility with using a scalpel, clamp, needle and thread, and even a laser. And for the speech pathologist working with children with speech disorders, it means knowledge of and facility with using phonetic transcription and the parameters of articulatory constraint as described in Chapter 2.

The problem is, as stated earlier, because traditional modes of articulation description and intervention make little or no use of these tools, many clinicians have forgotten how to use them, or at least feel very rusty. Hence this chapter. The purpose of this chapter is not to teach you everything you need to know about phonetics, place, manner, voicing, assimilation, and other areas of vital concern in the field of clinical phonology. There just isn't room available in a volume of this sort. Instead, it will be assumed that all of you will have learned this material at some point in your training and just need a refresher. For those of you who do feel the need for a more in-depth review, several additional resources will be listed at the end of this chapter.

The Use of Phonetics

In order to understand why phonetic transcription abilities are so important in phonological analysis, it may be instructive to explore why so many speech pathologists currently in the field are no longer using phonetics. Here is the story of P.T., a clinician who has been in the public schools for 10 years:

I, of course, learned phonetics in my M.A. program, but we never were forced to use it in clinical practicum. When I got out to the schools, I suddenly had a case-load of 60 and less than a month to complete my IE's (initial evaluations). Although most of these kids had artic. disorders, I didn't feel that I had the time to do phonetic transcription—after all, I wasn't too good at it and it just seemed easier to use the Goldman-Fristoe test form and then try to write in English what it seemed the child said. So if the picture was testing the *s* sound and the child said *th*, it was quicker and more natural to cross out the *s* and write *th*, rather than taking the time to try to remember the phonetic symbol. Before long, phonetics was a distant memory.

P.T. was then asked, "What about if a child had problems with vowels?" Her answer:

> Those were the times when I most felt that I *should've* used phonetics, but I couldn't remember the symbols. So I ended up again trying to write it in English. Most of the time this worked, although on occasion, when looking at it later, I couldn't understand what I had tried to write.

Some purists may say, "OK, so one clinician doesn't use phonetics. She's probably not very good anyway. Any *good* speech pathologist uses phonetics in his or her work." Not true. In fact, P.T. doesn't exist, per se, but is a composite of hundreds of clinicians surveyed from across the United States and Canada, working in schools, hospitals, clinics, and virtually every other setting imaginable. Many of these clinicians are excellent, according to their supervisors. In short, the fault lies not with the speech therapists who no longer use phonetics, but with the analytic/therapeutic frameworks they've been taught, which makes phonetic transcription superfluous in most cases. The key to why this is true lies embedded in the previous story when P.T. says, "So if the picture was testing the *s* sound . . . "

By their nature, traditional articulation tests encourage the clinician to concentrate on only one, or at most, two sounds at a time. This makes the clinician's listening task easier and indeed, given the limited scope of the listening task, phonetic transcription probably isn't necessary, unless the child's output is so bizarre that it cannot be written orthographically. In phonological analysis, on the other hand, all sounds in a given word are evaluated simultaneously; no sound is ever viewed in isolation from the other sounds in the word (vowels included). So a stimulus like *vacuum cleaner* (from the Goldman-Fristoe test form) necessitates transcription of 11 sounds sequentially. If the child misarticulates several of these sounds, it becomes virtually impossible to attempt to devise an appropriate orthographic representation; instead, phonetic transcription becomes the most accurate and reliable route to preserving the child's utterance, so that a phonological analysis can be performed.

A Compilation of Essential Phonetic Symbols for Clinicians

The list found in Table 3–1 includes the phonetic symbols that are needed most by clinicians working with American English speaking children and adults.

Most of you will probably recognize that these lists do not represent all of the sounds that can possibly be produced by the human articulatory mechanism. However, whereas the International Phonetic Alphabet (IPA) maintains symbols for just about any sound possible, it is not necessary for clinicians to learn all of these symbols. Instead, a working knowledge of the most commonly occurring symbols in normal and deviant American English phonology will usually suffice. Of course, although this makes our learning task easier, it creates problems if the child demonstrates an unusual error for which we do not have a standard symbol.

TABLE 3–1. Essential phonetic symbols for clinicians.

Consonants		Vowels	
Phonetic Symbol	Sample Word	Phonetic Symbol	Sample Word
p	pie	i	beet
b	bye	ɪ	bit
m	my	e (sometimes /eɪ/)	bait
w	why	ɛ	bet
f	fat	æ	bat
v	vat	u	boot
θ (voiceless)	thin	ʊ	book
ð (voiced)	this	o (sometimes /oʊ/)	boat
t	tie	ɔ	brought
d	die	a	top
s	sue	aɪ	type
z	zoo	aʊ	town
n	no	ɔɪ	toy
l	low	ɜ (stressed)	her
ʃ	ship	ɚ (unstressed)	other
ʒ	rouge	ʌ (stressed)	but
tʃ	chip	ə (unstressed)	about
dʒ	gyp	ɔr (sometimes /or/)	four
j	yet		
r	red		
k	kick		
g	gig		
ŋ	ring		
h	how		
ʔ (Glottal stop)	Not a phoneme in typical American English phonology		

But keep in mind, there is nothing sacred about the IPA symbols, except insofar as communication across professionals is enhanced. If you hear a sound that you don't have a symbol for, create a new symbol that will describe to you what the child is doing. Only make sure that the newly created symbol is clear enough that you will be able to look at your transcription later and recreate the child's production as well as describe what was happening. For example, when we first observed the "Buddy Hackett Rule," the symbol ← was created and placed over the sounds in question—specifying that the child was moving her lips and jaw to the left during production of those sounds. So while there are other accepted symbols that specify unusual phonological events (for example, ~ specifies nasality, according to the IPA), there is no requirement that you learn them, as long as two guidelines are followed:

1. Be able to describe and recreate the error when you look at your transcription after the initial assessment period.
2. Do not label anything a *distortion*. The term distortion communicates nothing but our inability to describe what is actually happening. Sometimes it will take several listenings, but a clear description of what the child is doing is always our final goal.

Relearning Phonetics

For those of you realizing that some relearning of phonetic transcription awaits you (in other words, many of you), don't despair. Hundreds if not thousands of clinicians who are now regularly using phonological procedures in their therapy were not too long ago in the same position you're in now. Nevertheless, there are some suggestions that might make the process easier.

Don't push yourself too hard to achieve 100% accuracy. It will come by itself eventually. At first, of course, you will make many errors in your transcription. But if you look at your early transcriptions carefully, you'll note that even then you will be about 70% accurate—and that level of accuracy is more than sufficient to perform the beginnings of a phonological analysis.

Don't push yourself too hard to achieve speed. As with accuracy, increased speed will come with time. Until then, there might be some short periods of uncomfortable (for you) silence while you are transcribing. Those periods will bother you more than the child; try to ignore them.

Don't be afraid to ask children to repeat themselves. At least initially, you will have to do this frequently. As long as you don't make a big thing out of it, most children will comply easily.

Don't try to transcribe every word during samples of conversation. It cannot be done, so don't even try. As we will see, if you transcribe 30 2- to 3-word phrases from out of the child's conversation, you will have enough conversational data to perform most of your analysis.

Try to avoid the use of your tape recorder, at least as much as possible. Although this will eliminate a security blanket many of you probably feel that you need at this point, not relying on your tape recorder will serve several purposes. First, live tran-

scription practice speeds up the phonetic relearning process much more than tape transcription. Most importantly, though, tape transcription is just not very accurate; fricatives especially tend to be distorted because of the narrow frequency response of most tape recorders and all consonants are subject to some distortion. In short, live transcription, even less than perfect live transcription, as a rule tends to be more reliable than tape transcription. For optimum accuracy, a tape recorder should be used only to check and verify your live transcription.

Set yourself a one-year goal for achieving sufficient transcription accuracy and speed. There is a tendency on the part of most clinicians to feel that they are not progressing quickly enough in the relearning process. Unfortunately, although these feelings are usually based on unrealistic expectations, they often create self-doubt, lack of confidence, and other roadblocks to eventual success. Setting a 1-year goal will help alleviate some of the pressure in the short term and allow you to concentrate on the learning itself, rather than on your feelings and doubts about it.

Practice, practice, practice. As is implied in all of these suggestions, the greatest indicator as to how well you'll be able to transcribe in the future is how much practice you're able to get. Force yourself to transcribe even when you don't need to. In fact, those are probably the best opportunities for practice because nobody's future is riding on your results. Create opportunities for additional practice away from your work setting, if possible—force yourself to transcribe a newpaper editorial daily, for instance, or administer a test to your children. Remember, the key is not just to transcribe disordered speech; transcription of correct speech is almost as valuable in improving your skills. The bottom line is, the more practice you can get, the more second-nature phonetic transcription will become.

Place, Manner, Voicing for Consonants

Knowledge of place, manner, and voicing is the other vital tool that most speech-language pathologists have to relearn in order to master phonological analysis. Unfortunately, this area is a bit more difficult from the relearning perspective because all opportunities for practice must be self-generated by the clinician. Figure 3–1 provides a summary of the place, manner, and voicing characteristics of 25 American English consonants. As can be seen, there are seven alternatives that exist in the placement parameter:

1. *Bilabials* (*p, b, m,* and *w*)—sound made with two lips. (Because production of *w* is constrained such that the tongue must remain in the high-back position for the vowel /μ/, it is sometimes called *labial-velar.*)

ENGLISH CONSONANT PHONEMES

Manner & Voicing			Bilabial	Labiodental	Interdental	Alveolar	Palatal	Velar	Glottal
Stops	Vl		P			t		K	ʔ
	Vd		b			d		g	
Affricates	Vl						tʃ		
	Vd						dʒ		
Fricatives	Vl		f		θ	s	ʃ		h
	Vd			v	ð	z	ʒ		
Lateral	Vd					l			
Nasals	Vd		m			n		ŋ	
Glides	Vd		w				j		
Liquids	Vd					l	r		

Figure 3–1. Place, manner, and voicing for American English consonants.

2. *Labiodentals* (*f* and *v*)—sounds produced with lower lip and upper teeth contact.
3. *Interdentals* (*th* voiced and voiceless)—sounds made with the tongue tip slightly protruded between the teeth.
4. *Alveolars* (*t*, *d*, *s*, *z*, *l*, and *n*)—sounds produced with contact occurring between the tongue and the alveolar ridge.
5. *Palatals* (*ch*, *dj*, *sh*, *zh*, *r*, and *y*)—sounds produced by contact or narrowing between the body of the tongue and the hard palate. (Although *y* is traditionally called *palatal*, the tongue is actually farther forward in the mouth for *y* than it is for the other *palatals*, and seems closer to the *alveolar* than the *palatal* position. For the sake of consistency with other sources, we've placed *y* with the *palatals* in Figure 3–1, but keep in mind the probable inaccuracy and we'll have more to say about it in later chapters.)
6. *Velars* (*k*, *g* and *ng*)—sounds made with contact between the back of the tongue and the velar, or soft-palate, area.
7. *Glottals* (*h* and the glottal stop)—sounds produced at the level of the vocal cords.

When categorizing the sounds according to the manner parameter, there are also several alternatives that exist in American English phonology:

1. *Stops* (*p*, *t*, *k*, *b*, *d*, *g* and the glottal stop)—sounds produced with a stoppage followed by an explosion of air.
2. *Fricatives* (*f*, *v*, *th* [voiced], *th* [voiceless], *s*, *z*, *sh*, *zh*, and *h*)—sounds made with a continuous flow of air rushing through a constriction in the oral or pharyngeal cavity.
3. *Affricatives* (*ch* and *dj*)—sounds combining qualities of both stops and fricatives. These sounds are produced with a brief air stoppage followed by a brief explosion of air.
4. *Nasals* (*m*, *n* and *ng*)—sounds made with complete oral closure but opening of the velopharyngeal port.
5. *Glides* (*w* and *y*)—sounds produced by changing the tongue position from one vowel position to another. The sound that results from this position change is considered a *glide*.
6. *Liquids* (*l* and *r*)—although these sounds have somewhat different manners of production, they are often grouped together and called liquids by clinical phonologists. Although the reasons for calling these sounds liquids are unknown to this author, both sounds are continuants like fricatives, but without the fricative-like turbulence caused by air rushing through a constriction. By the way, *l* is called a *lateral* in some systems and *r* has many other names, including *rhotic* (which means *r*-like), *retroflex*, and several derogatory names coined by frustrated clinicians.

The voicing parameter is easily memorized because there are seemingly only two alternatives. *Voiced* sounds are those that accompany vocal fold vibration and include *b*, *d*, *g*, *dj*, *v*, *th* (voiced), *z*, *zh*, *m*, *n*, *ng*, *w*, *y*, *l*, and *r*. *Voiceless* or *unvoiced* sounds are produced without vocal cord movement and include *p*, *t*, *k*, *ch*, *f*, *th* (voiceless), *s*, *sh*, and *h*. Finally, a third category of voicing exists in American English phonology. Whenever an alveolar stop (*t*, *d*) occurs in the medial position of a word at the beginning of an unstressed syllable, the resultant sound is not voiceless but neither is it truly voiced—it's somewhere in between. This *semi-voiced* sound is called a *flap* (phonetic symbol ɾ) by some, for example, when referring to the medial alveolar stop in the word *butter*. However, it should be noted that this semi-voiced sound also exists when *b* or *g* occur medially in words (e.g., *rubber* or *bigger*). This distinction of semi-voicedness is often unimportant—unless you are trying to teach a child to produce these medial sounds, at which time the distinction becomes quite important. For example, in the word *butter*, teaching the child to produce a voiceless *t* will make him sound

British rather than American. Teaching him to produce a voiced alveolar will make his speech sound strained and plodding. In fact, the child's speech will sound natural only if he learns to produce this semi-voiced sound.

Vowel Characteristics

Many clinicians ignore vowels completely, except in the most severe disorders exhibited by their clients. As we'll see in Chapter 7, this is unfortunate because vowels often provide us with important information that helps us to do a better analysis of the child's phonological system.

Voicing is not a factor in vowel production because all vowels (except those whispered) are voiced. However, the parameters of placement and manner remain relevant for vowel differentiation.

Figure 3–2 illustrates the vowel quadrilateral that differentiates vowels on the basis of two placement dimensions: *height of the tongue in the mouth* and *front to back positioning of the tongue*. The high vowels are /i/, /ɪ/, /µ/, and /ʊ/. The middle vowels are /e/, /ɛ/, /ɜ/, and /ɚ/, /ʌ/ and /ə/, /o/, and /ɔ/. The low vowels are /æ/ and /a/.

Using the front-back dimension, the front vowels are /i/, /ɪ/ /e/, /ɛ/, and /æ/; the central vowels are /ɜ/, /ɚ/, /ʌ/, and /ə/; and the back vowels are /µ/, /ʊ/, /o/, /ɔ/, and /a/.

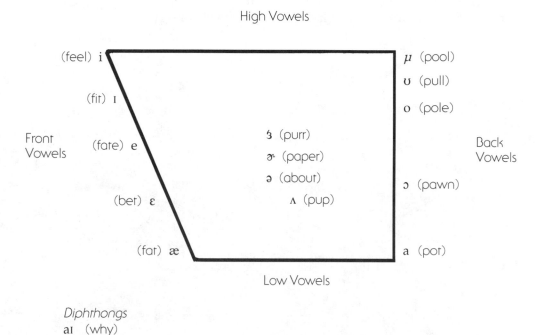

Figure 3–2. Vowel quadrilateral.

The manner characteristics related to vowels are *lip-roundedness* and *vowel duration*. (Although some investigators posit a *tense-lax* classification for vowels along the lines of the vowel duration category, the idea that some vowels are produced with more or less muscular tension has been called into question, e.g., see MacKay, 1987.) The *lip-rounded* vowels are /µ/, /ʊ/, /o/, /ɔ/, and /ɝ/ or /ɚ/. All other vowels are produced without lip-rounding. The *long* vowels are /i/, /µ/, /e/, /o/, /a/, /æ/, and /ɝ/. The *short* vowels are /ɪ/, /ɛ/, /ʊ/, and /ə/.

Relearning Place-Manner-Voicing Characteristics of Consonants and Vowels

Relearning and internalizing the place, manner, and voicing characteristics of the speech sounds will be very similar to memorizing multiplication facts—and just about as stimulating. But the payoff can be substantial, because the speed and ease with which one can perform a phonological analysis is highly related to one's knowledge of place, manner, and voicing. Further, the more a clinician has internalized this particular tool of the trade, the less he or she will tend to describe a child's error as a distortion, which is essentially meaningless.

In order to help in the relearning process, the first of several *Clinical Mastery Exercises* follows. Since breakdowns in learning how to do phonological analysis and intervention usually occur at this level, it would probably be beneficial to review this particular exercise daily, or at least several times over the next 2–4 weeks. Rest assured that once you have internalized the place, manner, and voicing characteristics of the speech sounds, the major part of your relearning battle is won.

Clinical Mastery Exercise #3–1
Review of Place-Manner-Voicing

A. For each of the following descriptions, write the sound or sounds that are being described. (Be careful! One description could refer to more than one sound).

<u>Sound(s)</u>

1. Voiceless labiodental fricative   _____
2. Voiced alveolar nasal   _____
3. Velar stop   _____
4. Voiced palatal fricative   _____
5. Labial glide   _____
6. Voiceless glottal fricative   _____
7. Affricate   _____
8. Palatal liquid   _____
9. Voiced stop   _____
10. Voiceless palatal fricative   _____
11. Voiced labiodental fricative   _____
12. Voiceless alveolar   _____
13. Voiced labial   _____
14. Voiced bilabial   _____
15. Voiceless interdental   _____

B. For each of the following consonants, describe the place-manner-voicing characteristics.

<u>Description</u>

1. g   _____
2. s   _____
3. tʃ   _____
4. w   _____
5. f   _____
6. ŋ   _____
7. l   _____
8. θ   _____
9. v   _____
10. n   _____

C. For each of the following vowels, check the appropriate boxes.

	High	Middle	Low	Front	Central	Back	Rounded	Unrounded
1. e								
2. ɪ								
3. ɔ								
4. ɝ								
5. æ								
6. µ								
7. o								
8. ʊ								
9. ʌ								
10. ɛ								

Assimilation and the Effects of Context

The final tool of the clinical phonologist's "trade" is a knowledge of assimilation and the effects of phonetic context on speech production. Traditionally, if a child said /gɔg/ for *dog* it was regarded as a *g/d* substitution, regardless of how he or she articulated other words. Now, if a child says /gɔg/ for *dog* but also produces the *d* correctly in words such as *daddy*, *dumb*, and *door*, the belief is that the child misarticulated the word not because of any inherent difficulty in producing the *d* sound, but because the final *g* caused the initial sound to move to the *g* position. In other words, the final *g* was a culprit (Weiner, 1982) in this case and "caused" the misarticulation. Without the culprit, the sound error would not have occurred.

In *assimilation*, then, one sound takes on the features of another sound, the culprit. Assimilation can occur when a sound early in the word affects a sound later in the word (*progressive assimilation*, e.g., /dɔd/ for *dog*) or when a sound toward the end of the word affects an earlier sound (*regressive assimilation*, e.g., /lɛlo/ for *yellow*). The good news is, from a practical perspective, it's not important to worry about the different kinds of assimilation. Although regressive assimilation seems to occur most often in children who are developing normally (Edwards & Shriberg, 1983), in children with speech disorders assimilation seems to occur most of the time in both directions; that is, whether the culprit is at the beginning or the end of a word, the assimilation will take place in a child who has an assimilation rule. So although division of assimilation into its different types is a fine academic exercise, it is probably not important from a therapeutic perspective. On the other hand, it is valuable to realize that assimilation, while most often occurring within single words, can also occur across words. So a culprit in one word *can* affect the production of a sound in another word.

Traditionally trained clinicians tend to have particular problems in differentiating between placement and assimilation errors. Yet the ability to make this distinction is a vital prerequisite to the development of appropriate therapy. Because of its importance, much more will be said about assimilation in subsequent chapters.

The Tools of Our Trade Revisited

Once you have become adept at phonetic transcription, once you've internalized the parameters of place, manner, and voicing, and once you've learned the distinction between placement and assimilaton errors, you have all the background necessary to be able to perform a generic phonological analysis in a reasonably short period of time. Part II of this book is dedicated to teaching you how to perform that analysis, while providing you with a brief overview of other procedures currently available. So read on . . . you're well on your way to mastering phonological analysis and intervention.

Additional Resources for Phonetics, Place, Manner, Voicing

Calvert, D. R. (1992). *Descriptive phonetics* (2nd ed.). New York: Thieme.

Calvert, D. R., & Calvert, C. (1986). *Descriptive phonetics transcription workbook* (2nd ed.). New York: Thieme.

Edwards, M. L. (1986). *Introduction to applied phonetics*. Boston: College-Hill Press.

Van Riper, C. G., & Smith, D. (1992). *An introduction to general American phonetics* (3rd ed.). Prospect Heights, IL: Waveland.

CHAPTER ◆ 4

Overview of Phonological Evaluation

A time of transition is always difficult, especially for those caught in the middle of the transition. Unfortunately, we all qualify for this lamentable position today. Although it seems quite clear that articulation assessment in the year 2020 will be very different from what it was in 1970, it is difficult to predict the exact nature of all the changes to come. What is certain is the fact that speech pathologists engaged in evaluation of articulation are probably never again going to be mostly concerned with determining lists of sounds misarticulated by their clients. But what will be considered important by the speech pathologists of the future? Although it's impossible to tell with precision, there are some factors that can begin to provide us with some clues:

Our major goal as clinicians will continue to be the stimulation of behavior change—in this case, articulation improvement. The first step in changing any behavior is being able to describe that behavior completely and precisely. Since the "tools of our trade" allow us to do so, they will become increasingly important in the articulatory evaluation of the future. Likewise, since determination of phonological rules seems to be the most precise yet parsimonious mode of explaining a client's phonological system, the evaluation of the future will undoubtedly increasingly revolve around a determination of these rules (although it

is highly possible and even probable that the precise description of these rules will be different from our current understanding).

Along the road into the future, we will all be limited by our past learning. Both Winitz (1969) and Mowrer (1982) labeled this phenomenon *negative transfer* when describing it in children with speech-disorders. Unfortunately, even as adults, clinicians, and/or test developers, we are not immune to this form of interference with acquiring new information. So it is neither surprising nor unexpected that clinicians first learning about phonological approaches have a tendency to "regress" to a traditional framework when faced with ambiguity that is not immediately resolvable. (We'll discuss this issue in more detail in Chapter 14.) Likewise, it's not particularly startling that several of the newer formal phonological assessment devices now available still recommend that clinicians undertake a traditional sound analysis in addition to a phonological rule analysis— even though there is good reason to question whether there's any value in obtaining lists of sounds that the child does and does not articulate correctly.

In short, we are all limited by our past learning. Even those of us who believe strongly in phonological approaches to speech intervention and are writing and speaking on the subject were originally trained according to a traditional perspective. It most likely remains for those clinicians being trained today, without traditional biases, to bring us fully into the age of clinical phonology.

But even if we are all being brought somewhat reluctantly into the future, where does that leave us today? With new ideas nervously coexisting alongside some traditional holdovers; with some phonology tests also focusing on the child's production of sounds; and with clinicians nervously trying to adjust to the schizophrenia created by these inconsistencies. In Chapter 2, it was suggested that development of the newer tests of phonology on the market might represent an unfortunate detour in our long road toward a complete understanding of speech disorders. In the remainder of this chapter, we will find out why, and try to present a workable alternative.

Two Modes of Analysis

Since 1979, several assessment tools have been published in the area of phonological analysis. Despite some superficial differences between these tests (which we will discuss in Chapter 10), they are identical to one another in one important respect: All start off with a predetermined list of phonological rules to be investigated. The children are presented with specially selected stimuli (pictures or objects) designed to allow the examiner to determine whether these predefined rules exist. Because the examiner has already begun with a framework of predefined rules and then goes to the child's productions to see how the output interacts with his or her framework, one can say that this examiner is proceeding from the whole (the framework of rules) to the parts (the child's productions). In science, this type of problem solving is called *deductive reasoning*; borrowing from the field of economics, a good term for this type of evaluation might be *macroanalysis*, where the speech is evaluated in terms of whole systems of predetermined rules.

Now, there is nothing inherently unsound about deductive reasoning. Certainly it is one of our primary modes of problem solving. But there's one large downside to deductive reasoning: The accuracy of any conclusions we make depends heavily on the soundness and completeness of our predefined framework. Here, unfortunately, the macroanalytic tests of phonology fall short. Consider, for example, the *Natural Process Analysis (NPA)* (Shriberg & Kwiatkowski, 1980). The predefined framework in this test consists of only eight possible rules. If a given child's phonological system doesn't match this narrow framework (and remember how many possibilities for errors there are), two things will result:

1. Insufficient/inadequate description of the child's rule system.
2. Much seeming inconsistency in the rules that are found.

Each of the formal tests of phonology currently available have the same problems, albeit to lesser extents. Even the *Assessment of Phonological Processes-Revised (APP-R)* (Hodson, 1986), which allows for the evaluation of more possible rules than any other formal test, only looks at 40 possibilities.

In short, deductive reasoning is not the best way to undertake an accurate phonological analysis because the necessary predefined framework, even if it could be determined, is much too large. Happily, we have available to us another mode of problem solving that allows for the accuracy and consistency we need. *Inductive reasoning* is reasoning from the part to the whole and forms the basis of the scientific method. In the case of articulation analysis, we would be using this type of reasoning if we started not from the framework of a test, but from the child's utterances themselves. If we took those utterances, observed their characteristics and only then generated a statement of general principles or laws (i.e., phonological rules), then we would be using inductive reasoning. A good term for this type of analysis might be *microanalysis*, although the term *generative analysis* has been around for many years and was used by linguists long before the macroanalytic tests of phonology were published.

The use of microanalysis or generative analysis in the evaluation of phonology has several advantages over macroanalytic, or formal test procedures. First, microanalysis allows for improved precision and greater accuracy in describing an individual's rule system. Because there is no predefined framework of rules, all sound errors are considered and then explained in some way that helps to define the person's unique rule system. Rules that look inconsistent through macroanalytic methods suddenly can be seen as consistent when inductive methods are used. Microanalysis allows for the determination of limited and idiosyncratic rules, two special types of rules that are not considered in formal devices. Finally, once the parameters of articulatory constraint are internalized, generative analysis is decidedly faster than administration of formal tests of phonology.

There is one question that may be occurring to you at this point. If phonological microanalysis is more accurate, more precise, and potentially faster than the formal tests currently on the market; if knowledge of generative analytical procedures has been around for many years, then why hasn't it filtered down to clinicians in the field? Actually, there are two reasons: first, our old friends place, manner, and voicing are once again at the heart of the matter. Knowledge of place, manner and voicing is an absolutely essential prerequisite to undertaking a microanalysis of phonology. Without this knowledge, a generative analysis just cannot be done. As such, it's not at all surprising that the tests that have been developed—the macroanalytic tests —have been designed to eliminate any need for knowledge of place, manner, and voicing; hence the earlier suggestion that development of these tests might represent an unfortunate detour from the road on which we should be traveling.

A second reason that generative or microanalysis hasn't filtered down to working clinicians is that, by its nature, inductive reasoning is difficult to teach. And although the need for microanalytic skills has been noted in the literature (e.g., Camarata & Gandour, 1984; Leonard, 1985), no previous attempt has been made to teach these skills in a systematic way.

The Next Step

At this point, you have all the background you need. Now the fun starts. The remainder of Part II will be dedicated to teaching you how to do a generative analysis of phonology, and Chapter 10 will summarize the formal tests of phonology currently available. You will notice that much space is devoted to teaching you how to do the analysis. That's because it's the most important part of the process. As you progress through the practice exercises, you will of course see your evaluation skills improve. But more importantly, and perhaps not as obviously, your entire way of thinking about speech sounds and their interrelationships is about to change subtly. And this will prepare you for the chapters on therapy to follow. So please resist the temptation to go right to the therapy chapters now; you will get a lot more out of them *after* you learn to do a generative analysis.

CHAPTER ◆ 5

Microanalysis of Phonology, Part 1: Elementary Generative Analysis

The underlying thesis of a phonological approach to studying deviant articulation is that the client has developed a set of phonological rules which simplifies his or her speech and sets it apart from community norms. The purpose of phonological assessment is to ascertain these rules in as comprehensive a fashion as possible. Unfortunately, current formal tests of phonology on the market help to illuminate only a part of the phonological puzzle. Because they rely on macroanalysis, or deductive reasoning, accuracy and precision are sacrificed for the expedient of beginning with a predetermined set of phonological rules.

Shifting to generative analysis, or inductive reasoning, on the other hand, allows the clinician to overcome these problems and precisely identify *all* of the rules contributing to the speech disorder. The purpose of this and the next four chapters is to teach you how to perform a generative analysis of a speech sample. As you will see, becoming proficient at generative analysis will take practice and dedication —mostly in relearning the tools of the trade as described in Chapter 3—but happily, your payoff will begin almost immediately, when you have your first realization that you are not looking at your client's disordered speech in exactly the same way as you might have before.

The Generic 6-Step Procedure

Inductive reasoning is particularly difficult to teach because the mental operations that one person will perform to induce an answer (go from parts to the whole) might differ greatly from the mental operations another person would perform, even while coming up with the same answer. As you might imagine, then, there is no one consummate way to perform a generative analysis. Nevertheless, all modes of generative analysis require at least the following:

- Knowledge of the parameters of articulatory constraint and all alternatives available in each parameter.
- Ability to devise hypotheses about individual utterances, and systematically test those hypotheses against the data presented by the speech sample as a whole.
- Ability to problem-solve if seemingly ambiguous situations arise.

The greatest difficulty for the new learner, of course, lies in the fact that generative analysis requires that all of this knowledge and skill be demonstrated almost simultaneously. However, like most new learning, the task becomes easier if it is broken down into its component parts. The 6-step generic procedure for phonological analysis (see Generic Worksheet) is an

PROCEDURE FOR PHONOLOGICAL ANALYSIS — GENERIC WORKSHEET

I. Take one error and choose possible parameters

ERROR:
ANALYSIS: Manner?   ⟶

              Voicing?   ⟶

              Placement? ⟶

              Context?   ⟶

              Structure?   ⟶

              Linguistic?   ⟶

              Semantic?   ⟶

> If unclear as to whether placement or context, perform Parameter Confusion Test (See Form). Otherwise go to Step II.

II. Make initial conclusion re: rule by describing the difference between target and client production.

_____ PARAMETER

Description: _____

Rule: _____

III. Perform Consistency Check (See Consistency Check Form)

IV. Describe rule in Final Form

Rule: _____

V. Go to phonological rule summary, find all words for which rule is operating, and note.

VI. Perform final check

— Make sure all changes in target word can be explained by rule. If so, check the word off. If not, leave until next analysis.

attempt to do just that. Once again, it is important to keep in mind that this procedure may not be the only way to do a generative analysis. In fact, many of you will undoubtedly begin looking for shortcuts once you begin to understand the method. It is important that you avoid this temptation. The procedure you are about to learn is the culmination of several years of development and revision and has been successfully used to help hundreds if not thousands of clinicians across the country master the intricacies of phonological microanalysis, even if they have had little previous experience with phonology. So it is important that, at least initially, you stick as close as possible to the published procedure. Then, after a few more chapters, as you become more familiar with generative analysis, suggestions will be given as to shortcuts that can be taken to speed up the process.

Let us first summarize each of the steps in the generic 6-step procedure.

I. Take one error and choose possible parameters. The clinician selects one misarticulated word from the speech sample and asks herself each of the following questions concerning the word:

- Has a manner problem caused the speech error?
- Is it a voicing problem that has resulted in the error?
- Could a placement problem be the cause of the error?
- Could context have created conditions for the error to occur?
- Is a structural problem the source of the misarticulation?
- Is the error tied to a linguistic problem?
- Is the misarticulation due to a semantic difficulty?

The clinician should answer these questions with six *noes* and one *yes*, thus specifying the parameter of difficulty for the client. Once the parameter of difficulty is specified, Step 2 can be commenced. On occasion, the clinician will be uncertain as to whether the violated parameter is placement or context; in this situation, a *placement-context parameter confusion test* will be undertaken.

II. Make initial conclusion re: rule by describing the difference between the target and the client's production. In this step, the clinician provides a dynamic description, using place-manner-voicing terminology, of the contrast between the target and the client's incorrect production. From that description, a label is created which becomes the client's phonological rule. Note that the label for the rule is secondary in importance to the description; the clinician only formulates the label after a thorough analysis of the phonological behavior has been undertaken. Thus, the clinician is proceeding from the part (the client's speech behaviors) to the whole (a rule that describes those behaviors), rather than in the opposite direction, as is the case for the macroanalytic formal tests of phonology.

III. Perform consistency check. The purpose of this step is to find out whether the rule found in Step 2 is consistently demonstrated across other applicable words in the client's speech sample. A separate form is used which allows the clinician to devise lists of *yes* and *no* words (words in which the rule does and does not occur). If the rule, as labeled in Step 2, does not occur across all applicable words in the client's speech, a new rule is then devised which accounts for the seeming inconsistency.

IV. Describe rule in final form. After explaining any seeming inconsistency in Step 3, the newly devised rule is now listed here.

V. Go to phonological rule summary, find all words for which rule is operating, and note. The phonological rule summary is the form upon which the gloss (client's speech sample) is recorded. (See Phonological Rule Summary Form.) The clinician now returns to each applicable word from the sample and enters the rule found in Steps 1–4 in the appropriate column.

PHONOLOGICAL RULE SUMMARY

Client: _____

Check	Target Word	Client Production	Rule(s) Operating

VI. Perform final check. For this final step, the clinician returns to each word for which a rule has been entered, studies the word, and determines whether the listed rule completely explains the client's error. If so, the word is checked off in the appropriate column. If not, the word is returned to at a later time.

The 6 steps are repeated until all of the words in the client's speech sample have been checked off. By then, the clinician will have a list of rules that characterizes the client's deficient speech.

At this point, many of you may have noticed that the procedure actually involves only a few steps of real analysis. Much of it is just organization and book-keeping. In fact, you will find that the more familiar you become with the formal procedure, the less you will need the various worksheets that help guide the analytical process. This underlines the fact that in learning how to do generative analysis, you are not mastering a new test; instead, you are learning a different way of thinking about articulation.

Working with the Generic 6-Step Procedure: Child #001

Before we attempt an entire speech sample, let us see how the procedure would work with a single word. Child #001 says /tʌn/ for *sun*. The completed abbreviated Generic Worksheet illustrates the first two steps of a correctly completed worksheet for this child. In order to help you learn how to go about filling out the worksheet, let us review the first two steps point by point, question by question. Follow along with the completed worksheet for Child #001, which follows.

Child #001—Review

I. *Take one error and choose possible parameters.*
   A. Fill in the error being analyzed (in this case, *sun* becomes /tʌn/ or in shorthand, *sun* → /tʌn/).
   B. Ask question: Is manner the parameter being violated in *sun* → /tʌn/? (Answer: Since /s/ is a fricative and /t/ is a stop, the answer is *yes*—fill in on worksheet.)
   C. Ask question: Is a voicing problem causing *sun* to go to /tʌn/? (Answer: *No*. Fill in on worksheet.)
   D. Ask question: Could a placement problem be causing *sun* → /tʌn/? (Answer: *No*. Since /s/ and /t/ both have the same placement, alveolar, one can hardly label this a placement problem.)
   E. Ask question: Could a context problem be causing *sun* → /tʌn/? (Answer: *No*. The context /n/ is an alveolar, as are both *s*, the target, and /t/, the error. Clearly /n/ couldn't have caused /s/ to change to /t/.)
   F. Ask question: Could a structural difficulty be causing *sun* → /tʌn/? (Answer: *No*. Both *sun* and /tʌn/ have a consonant-vowel-consonant [CVC] syllable structure. That is certainly not the problem.)
   G. Ask question: Might a linguistic problem be causing *sun* → /tʌn/? (Answer: *Unlikely*. *Sun* is a noun, one of the most basic linguistic categories. It is unlikely that Child #001 has a problem with nouns that has created the misarticulation.)
   H. Ask question: Could a semantic problem have caused *sun* → /tʌn/? (Answer: Again *unlikely*. *Sun* is a very early lexical item and it is doubtful that this is the cause for the error.)
   I. Since there is one *yes* and all the remaining parameters are *no* or *unlikely*, we have found the parameter responsible for the error. Because there is no confusion between placement and context, there is no need to perform a Parameter Confusion Test. It is now time to move on to Step 2.
II. *Make initial conclusion re: rule by describing the difference between target and client production.*
   A. Fill in the violated parameter, as per Step 1 (in this case, manner).
   B. Describe what the client is doing: In this case, a fricative is turning into a stop.

PROCEDURE FOR PHONOLOGICAL ANALYSIS — GENERIC WORKSHEET

I. Take one error and choose possible parameters

    ERROR: _sun_ ⟶ /tʌn/

    ANALYSIS:
        Manner? ⟶ _Yes_
        Voicing? ⟶ _No_
        Placement? ⟶ _No_
        Context? ⟶ _No_
        Structure? ⟶ _No_
        Linguistic? ⟶ _Unlikely_
        Semantic? ⟶ _Unlikely_

> If unclear as to whether placement or context, perform Parameter Confusion Test (See Form). Otherwise go to Step II.

II. Make initial conclusion re: rule by describing the difference between target and client production.

    Manner **PARAMETER**

        Description: _Fricative turning into a stop_

        Rule: _Stopping of Fricatives_

C. Label the rule: The conventional label for this rule is "Stopping of Fricatives." However, it is important to realize that there is nothing magical about the conventional label. It might just as easily be called "Defricativization," for example. In short, knowledge of the conventional labels for different rules is much less important than is a thorough knowledge of what exactly is happening in the mouth of the client. Once the latter is accomplished, naming the rule is easy. That is why no attempt is made to describe even the most common rules until later in the book.

Because we have only been provided with one word for Child #001, we cannot perform Steps 3–6 of the procedure. If we did have a complete speech sample, however, we would next perform a consistency check, where we would go to each word in the sample having a fricative, see if it was stopped, and record our results on the Consistency Check Form.

Working with the Generic 6-Step Procedure: Child #002

Child #002 will give you an opportunity to try the first two steps of the procedure on your own. Child #002 says /tau/ for *cow*. Now, try to fill in the first two steps of the worksheet on the next page without reading the answer on page 58 or looking at the completed worksheet on page 61. (Complete worksheet for Child #002 now, prior to reading any further.)

PROCEDURE FOR PHONOLOGICAL ANALYSIS — GENERIC WORKSHEET

I. Take one error and choose possible parameters

      ERROR:

      ANALYSIS: Manner? ————▶

                Voicing? ————▶

                Placement? ————▶

                Context? ————▶

                Structure? ————▶

                Linguistic? ————▶

                Semantic? ————▶

> If unclear as to whether placement or context, perform Parameter Confusion Test (See Form). Otherwise go to Step II.

II. Make initial conclusion re: rule by describing the difference between target and client production.

      _____ PARAMETER

          Description: _____

          Rule: _____

Child #002—Review

I. *Take one error and choose possible parameters.*
   A. Fill in the error being analyzed (*cow* → /taʊ/).
   B. Ask question: Has a problem with manner caused *cow* to become /taʊ/? (Answer: *No.* Both the *k* in *cow* and the *t* in /taʊ/ are stops, so there is no manner error.)
   C. Ask question: Has a voicing problem caused *cow* → /taʊ/? (Answer: *No.* Both productions are voiceless; thus, voicing is not a factor here.)
   D. Ask question: Could a placement problem have caused the error? (Answer: *Yes.* The placement for *cow* is velar; the placement for /taʊ/ is alveolar. Clearly, in the absence of any other hypothesis, placement is the violated parameter here.)
   E. Ask question: Could the context of the word have caused the error? (Answer: *No.* Because there is no other consonant present in the word, no contextual factor exists that could have changed the velar in *cow* to the alveolar in /taʊ/.)
   F. Ask question: Might a structural problem have caused the error? (Answer: *No.* The structure of both *cow* and /taʊ/ is identical—they are both CV words.[5]
   G. Ask question: Could a linguistic problem have caused *cow* to become /taʊ/? (Answer: *Unlikely.* Again, *cow* is a noun, one of the earliest classes of words to develop linguistically.)
   H. Ask question: Has a semantic difficulty caused the error? (Answer: Again, *unlikely.* *Cow* is a very early lexical item in most children, making it doubtful that the semantic parameter is the cause of the phonological problem.)
   I. Since there is only one *yes* and the remaining parameters are *no* or *unlikely*, it is clear that the placement parameter is responsible for the error. Because there is no confusion between placement and context, there is no need to perform a Parameter Confusion Test. Instead, we move on to Step 2.

II. *Make initial conclusion re: rule by describing the difference between target and client production.*
   A. Fill in the violated parameter, as per Step 1 (in this instance, placement).
   B. Describe what the client is doing: In this case, a velar is moving forward in the mouth and becoming an alveolar.
   C. Label the rule: The conventional label for this rule is "Fronting of Velars." Once again, however, there is nothing inherently superior in the conventional term, and terms like "Alveolarization of Velars,"

---

[5]Clinicians first learning this procedure often commit early errors in their attempts to determine the syllable structure of words. Specifically, the orthographic spelling of a word sometimes confuses the attempt to determine syllable structure. In *cow*, for example, the syllable structure is CV despite the spelling, which might imply CVC. The avoidance of errors of this type is a vital prerequisite to an accurate phonological analysis.

"Apicalization of Velars," or even "Develarization" might convey a similar message. To repeat, knowledge of conventional terminology for the various phonological rules is less important than is a thorough knowledge by the clinician of what is happening in the client's mouth. So, if you came up with a different term for Child #002's error, that is fine as long as you adequately described what was happening. You will easily learn the conventional terminology at a later time.

As was the case with our first example, we cannot perform Steps 3–6 of the procedure for Child #002, because we have been provided with only one word. If we had had additional words, we would next perform a consistency check, to see if all velars in the sample were indeed being fronted to alveolars.

PROCEDURE FOR PHONOLOGICAL ANALYSIS — GENERIC WORKSHEET

I. Take one error and choose possible parameters

ERROR: _cow_ → /taʊ/
ANALYSIS:
- Manner? ⟶ *No*
- Voicing? ⟶ *No*
- Placement? ⟶ *Yes*
- Context? ⟶ *No*
- Structure? ⟶ *No*
- Linguistic? ⟶ *Unlikely*
- Semantic? ⟶ *Unlikely*

> If unclear as to whether placement or context, perform Parameter Confusion Test (See Form). Otherwise go to Step II.

II. Make initial conclusion re: rule by describing the difference between target and client production.

Placement **PARAMETER**

Description: _Velar moving to alveolar position_

Rule: _Fronting of Velars_

Clinical Mastery Exercises in Generative Phonological Analysis

A series of *clinical mastery exercises* has been developed to help you master the intricacies of generative analysis. As you will see, the exercises are highly structured, presenting challenges of slowly increasing difficulty. The early exercises have been manufactured as teaching tools to help illustrate various features of the analytical process; later exercises incorporate speech samples from real clients and are characteristic of the most challenging phonological analyses you will have to confront in your own caseloads.

The presentation format for these *clinical mastery exercises* will be identical across all levels of difficulty. Each exercise will begin with an introduction presented on a left page. On the right page facing that introduction, the speech sample for that client will appear on an otherwise blank phonological rule summary form. Following that, several pages of blank worksheets will appear, corresponding to the work that has to be done in order to perform a generative analysis for the given client. After the blank pages, a description of each step involved in analyzing the sample will be provided. Embedded within this description will be any necessary explanation of new information arising from the issues being discussed. Finally, a second phonological rule summary will appear, this one correctly filled out for the client that has just been presented.

How should you proceed? First, try to go through the steps on your own, without reading the solution. Only go to the solution if you feel you have correctly finished the analysis or if you get stuck at any point and feel unable to continue. In the latter case, try to return to working on your own as soon as possible. Second, as part of the initial step for every new rule, you will be asking yourself a series of questions designed to identify the parameter being violated as a result of the client's error. As much as possible, try to ask and answer those questions prior to reading the answers provided for you in the text. This suggestion is given because familiarity with these parameters is a principal prerequisite for generative analysis; only by answering

the questions on your own will this familiarity come. If necessary, feel free to make a copy of the place-manner-voicing chart that appeared in Figure 3–1 and use it as a "cheat sheet" for as long as you need it. Regardless, go to the written answer *only* as a last resort. Finally, even if you think you have correctly analyzed the sample, read *all* of the textual information presented in the solution. This is because all new learning will be presented first within the text of the solutions to the analyses. Also, you will discover that on a few occasions, you have been modestly "tricked," in the interests of new learning. You will discover the "trick" only by reading the text in its entirety.

There are a few other suggestions and comments which should enhance the learning process:

- Use a pencil or erasable pen while filling out the worksheets initially. This will accomplish two purposes. First, it will allow you to make mistakes and correct them without cluttering the worksheet. More importantly, it will allow you to erase all of your previous work and begin the analysis anew, if you wish to review a particular exercise before going on. In fact, it is a good idea not to go on to a more difficult exercise until earlier exercises have been mastered.

- Each blank worksheet requiring completion for a given analysis has been properly filled out in Appendix A. This is meant to supplement the step-by-step explanations appearing in the text, and will also allow you to check yourself, in an interim manner, after each form has been completed.

- As clinicians begin learning the analytical procedure, they often have questions concerning why something has been done in a particular way. In the attempt to anticipate and address some of these questions which typically arise during the early learning process, the text of the solution will be periodically interrupted with italicized questions and answers to those questions. It is hoped that this will help to stimulate a true workshop atmosphere, even though the learning is occurring through a book.

Clinical Mastery Exercise—Flora Duh

Introduction

The purpose of this initial exercise is to give you practice in going through the entire 6-step procedure. Because the speech sample is quite limited and only one rule is working, you may have an impulse to try to discover the rule without having to execute each step in the procedure. You are urged to resist this impulse. At this point, especially, the solution is much less important than the process leading to that solution. Again, there is one rule working and your job is finished when you have checked off every word in Flora's summary sheet.

Worksheets required for Flora Duh
- Phonological Rule Summary
- Generic 6-step procedure
- Consistency Check Form

The initial step in the analysis is to go to the first word of the sample (in this case, *key*) and perform the 6-step generic procedure, in order to determine the first (and in this instance only) rule.

Why the first word? Wouldn't the choice of any word yield the same result?

Yes, but stick to choosing the first word in the sample for awhile. Later on, you will learn how to scan a speech sample to identify ideal test words, but until then, these exercises have been constructed such that by progressing in a logical top to bottom sequence, learning will be optimized.

(Solution on page 67)

PHONOLOGICAL RULE SUMMARY

Client: _FLORA DUH_

Check	Target Word	Client Production	Rule(s) Operating
	key	ti	
	cup	tʌp	
	two	tu	(correct)
	gum	dʌm	
	pick	pɪt	
	top	tap	(correct)
	cake	tet	
	go	do	
	cow	taʊ	
	big	bɪd	

PROCEDURE FOR PHONOLOGICAL ANALYSIS — GENERIC WORKSHEET

I. Take one error and choose possible parameters

ERROR:
ANALYSIS: Manner? ⟶

Voicing? ⟶

Placement? ⟶

Context? ⟶

Structure? ⟶

Linguistic? ⟶

Semantic? ⟶

> If unclear as to whether placement or context, perform Parameter Confusion Test (See Form). Otherwise go to Step II.

II. Make initial conclusion re: rule by describing the difference between target and client production.

_____ PARAMETER

Description: _____

Rule: _____

III. Perform Consistency Check (See Consistency Check Form)

IV. Describe rule in Final Form

Rule: _____

V. Go to phonological rule summary, find all words for which rule is operating, and note.

VI. Perform final check

— Make sure all changes in target word can be explained by rule. If so, check the word off. If not, leave until next analysis.

CONSISTENCY CHECKLIST

Initial Rule Description: _____

Rule Operating (Yes)	Rule Not Operating (No)

Check for Consistency	Yes Words	No Words	Sig. Diff.
1. Phonetic Context			
— List vowel preceding			
— List vowel following			
— List consonant preceding			
— List consonant following			
— List other sig. non-adjacent sounds			
2. Position			
— List I, M, F for initial medial, final			
3. Intra-class Variability			
— List correct/incorrect sounds, search for intra-class patterns			
4. Syllable Structure/ Word Length			
— List syllable structures			
5. Part of Speech/Morphological Endings			
— List grammatical categories			
6. Syllable Stress			
— List U, S for unstressed, stressed			
7. Syllable Boundary			
— List words/Draw line between syllable boundaries; Note differences			

Note other factors: Elicitation mode, situational context, overlearned words, etc.

Final Rule Description: _____

Solution

I. *Take one error and choose possible parameters.*
   A. Fill in the error being analyzed (*key* → /ti/).
   B. Ask question: Has a problem with manner caused *key* to become /ti/? (Answer: *No*. Both the /k/ in *key* and the /t/ in /ti/ are stops, so there is no manner error.)
   C. Ask question: Has a voicing problem caused *key* → /ti/? (Answer: *No*. Both productions are voiceless; thus voicing is not a factor here.)
   D. Ask question: Could a placement problem have caused the error? (Answer: *Yes*. The placement for *key* is velar; the placement for /ti/ is alveolar. In the absence of any other hypothesis, placement is the violated parameter.)
   E. Ask question: Could the context of the word have caused the error? (Answer: *No*. Because there is no other consonant present in the word, no contextual factor exists that would have changed *key* to /ti/.)
   F. Ask question: Might a structural problem have precipitated the error? (Answer: *No. Key* and /ti/ both have CV syllable structures.)
   G. Ask question: Could a linguistic problem have caused *key* to become /ti/? (Answer: *Unlikely. Key* is a noun, one of the earliest classes of words to develop linguistically.)
   H. Ask question: Has a semantic difficulty caused the error? (Answer: Again, *unlikely. Key* is an early lexical item.)
   I. Because there is only one *yes* and the remaining parameters are *no* or *unlikely*, it is clear that the placement parameter is responsible for the error. Because there is no confusion between placement and context, there is no need to perform a Parameter Confusion Test. Instead, we move on to Step 2.

II. *Make initial conclusion re: rule by describing the difference between target and client production.*
   A. Fill in the violated parameter, as per Step 1 (in this case, placement).
   B. Describe what the client is doing: A velar is moving forward in the mouth and becoming an alveolar.
   C. Label the rule: The conventional label for this rule is "Fronting of Velars," although any term that describes the same phenomenon to you and other clinicians is acceptable.

III. *Perform Consistency Check.*
   A. Go to Consistency Checklist and put the word analyzed in Steps 1 and 2 into the *yes* column. In other words, the rule (Fronting of Velars) is operating for that test word (*key*).
   B. Find the next word in the sample in which Fronting of Velars could occur (in this case, *cup*). Ask yourself: Does it occur? If so, put word into *yes* column; if not, put it into *no* column. (Answer: *Yes*. Fronting of Velars occurs in *cup*, so word is placed in *yes* column.)

C. Find the next word in the sample in which Fronting of Velars could occur (i.e., *gum*). Does it occur? (Answer: *Yes*. Place the word in *yes* column.)

D. Repeat Step B or C until all words with the possibility of Fronting of Velars have been exhausted. By the end of this step, all words in the speech sample having the possibility of the rule being tested should be listed in either the *yes* or *no* columns of the Consistency Checklist.

E. In the case of Flora, all words with velars belong in the *yes* column (i.e., *key, cup, gum, pick, cake, cake, go, cow*, and *big*). All of these words exhibit Fronting of Velars.

Why is the word cake *listed twice in the list of* yes *words?*

Because there are two opportunities for Fronting of Velars in the word *cake*. Because all word positions must be included in the analysis, *cake* is listed twice in the *yes* column.

F. Fill in the final rule description on the bottom line of the Consistency Checklist. In this case, because all words were found to have the rule operating, the final description is identical to the initial description—Fronting of Velars. (A correctly completed Consistency Checklist for Flora appears in Appendix A.)

IV. *Describe rule in final form.*

A. Transfer the final rule description (in this instance, Fronting of Velars) from the bottom of the Consistency Checklist to the appropriate space on the generic worksheet.

V. *Go to phonological rule summary, find all words for which rule is operating, and note.*

A. On the phonological rule summary, go to each word exhibiting Fronting of Velars and record that rule in the appropriate column.

VI. *Perform final check.*

A. Return to the first word listed on the phonological rule summary (i.e., *key*). Ask question: Does Fronting of Velars totally explain *key* → /ti/? (Answer: *Yes*. The only thing happening in that word is the fact that a velar sound is becoming alveolar.) Because the answer is *yes*, check off the word in the appropriate column. (If the answer had been *no*, we would have had to return to the word at a later time, to determine what other rules were working.)

B. One by one, return to each of the other words determined to have Fronting of Velars. Using the same previous question, decide whether the client's production of each word has been totally explained by the Fronting of Velars rule. Because the answer is *yes* for all of the words in Flora's sample, each of the words is given a check in the left-hand column.

C. Because all misarticulated words have now been checked off, Flora's analysis is complete. (See correctly completed phonological rule summary for Flora on page 69.)

PHONOLOGICAL RULE SUMMARY

Client: _FLORA DUH_

Check	Target Word	Client Production	Rule(s) Operating
✔	key	ti	Fronting of Velars
✔	cup	tʌp	FV
✔	two	tu	(correct)
✔	gum	dʌm	FV
✔	pick	pɪt	FV
✔	top	tap	(correct)
✔	cake	tet	FV; FV
✔	go	do	FV
✔	cow	tav	FV
✔	big	bɪd	FV

Discussion

Well, how did you do with the Flora Duh exercise? Obviously, if you were able to go through the 6-step procedure without consulting the written solution, you are well on your way to mastering generative analysis. Even if you did need to consult the solution once or several times, that is normal at this stage. The question is, if you were asked to repeat this exercise again *now*, step-by-step, could you do it? If so, you are ready for the next exercise. If not, why not try Flora once again before going on? You will be glad you did.

Clinical Mastery Exercise—Raoul Schwartz

Introduction

In many ways, this exercise is quite similar to the previous one. Raoul's speech sample is very limited and there is only one phonological rule working in his speech. Or might there be two? Well, that will be determined shortly. One word of advice: Be careful with Step 6 . . . . A small challenge awaits you.

Worksheets required for Raoul Schwartz
- Phonological Rule Summary
- Generic 6-step procedure
- Consistency Check Form

Once again, the analysis begins by going to the first word of the speech sample (i.e., *sun*) and performing the 6-step generic procedure, in order to determine the first rule.

(Solution on page 75)

PHONOLOGICAL RULE SUMMARY

Client: _RAOUL SCHWARTZ_

Check	Target Word	Client Production	Rule(s) Operating
	sun	tʌn	
	zoo	du	
	nose	nod	
	thin	tɪn	
	suit	tut	
	miss	mɪt	
	sheep	tip	
	fight	paɪt	
	very	bɛrt	
	five	paɪb	

PROCEDURE FOR PHONOLOGICAL ANALYSIS — GENERIC WORKSHEET

I. Take one error and choose possible parameters

        ERROR:
        ANALYSIS: **Manner?** ————▶

                   Voicing? ————▶

                   Placement? ————▶

                   Context? ————▶

                   Structure? ————▶

                   Linguistic? ————▶

                   Semantic? ————▶

> If unclear as to whether placement or context, perform Parameter Confusion Test (See Form). Otherwise go to Step II.

II. Make initial conclusion re: rule by describing the difference between target and client production.

       ————————— **PARAMETER**

         Description: _____

         Rule: _____

III. Perform Consistency Check (See Consistency Check Form)

IV. Describe rule in Final Form

         Rule: _____

V. Go to phonological rule summary, find all words for which rule is operating, and note.

VI. Perform final check

        — Make sure all changes in target word can be explained by rule. If so, check the word off. If not, leave until next analysis.

CONSISTENCY CHECKLIST

Initial Rule Description: _____

Rule Operating (Yes)	Rule Not Operating (No)

Check for Consistency	Yes Words	No Words	Sig. Diff.
1. **Phonetic Context**			
— List vowel preceding			
— List vowel following			
— List consonant preceding			
— List consonant following			
— List other sig. non-adjacent sounds			
2. **Position**			
— List I, M, F for initial medial, final			
3. **Intra-class Variability**			
— List correct/incorrect sounds, search for intra-class patterns			
4. **Syllable Structure/ Word Length**			
— List syllable structures			
5. **Part of Speech/Morphological Endings**			
— List grammatical categories			
6. **Syllable Stress**			
— List U, S for unstressed, stressed			
7. **Syllable Boundary** — List words/Draw line between syllable boundaries; Note differences			

Note other factors: Elicitation mode, situational context, overlearned words, etc.

Final Rule Description: _____

Solution

   I. *Take one error and choose possible parameters.*

     A. Fill in the error being analyzed (*sun* → /tʌn/).

     B. Ask question: Has a problem with manner caused *sun* to become /tʌn/? (Answer: *Yes*. The *s* in *sun* is a fricative whereas the *t* in /tʌn/ is a stop. The manner parameter is being violated here.)

     C. Ask question: Has a voicing problem caused *sun* → /tʌn/? (Answer: *No*. Both /s/ and /t/ are voiceless.)

     D. Ask question: Could a placement problem have caused the error? (Answer: *No*. The placement for the /s/ in *sun* is alveolar; likewise, the placement for /t/ in /tʌn/ is alveolar. Thus, placement is not where the error lies.)

     E. Ask question: Could the context within the word have precipitated the error? (Answer: *No*. The other consonant in the word is *n*, which is also an alveolar. In short, there is nothing in the nature of *n* which could have caused *s* → /t/, resulting in /tʌn/.)

     F. Ask question: Might a structural problem have caused the error? (Answer: *No*. Both *sun* and /tʌn/ have identical CVC syllable structures. This is not the factor.)

     G. Ask question: Could a linguistic problem have caused *sun* → /tʌn/? (Answer: *Unlikely*, with *sun* being a noun.)

     H. Ask question: Might a semantic difficulty have caused the error? (Answer: *Unlikely*, given the low vocabulary level of the word.)

     I. Because there is only one *yes* and the remaining parameters are *no* or *unlikely*, it is concluded that the manner parameter is responsible for the error. Because there is no ambiguity as to whether placement or context is responsible for the error, there is no need to perform a Parameter Confusion Test. Instead, we move on to Step 2.

  II. *Make initial conclusion re: rule by describing the difference between target and client production.*

     A. Fill in the violated parameter, as per Step 1 (in this case, manner).

     B. Describe what the client is doing: A stop is being turned into a fricative.

     C. Label the rule: The conventional label for this rule is "Stopping of Fricatives," although any term that describes the same phenomenon to you and other clinicians is equally acceptable.

  III. *Perform Consistency Check.*

     A. Go to Consistency Checklist and put the word analyzed in Steps 1 and 2 (i.e., *sun*) into the *yes* column, indicating that the rule (Stopping of Fricatives) is operating for that test word.

     B. Go to the next word in the sample that could demonstrate Stopping of Fricatives (i.e., *zoo*). Does it? If so, put word into the *yes* column; if not, place it into the *no* column. (Answer: *Yes*, Stopping of Fricatives occurs in *zoo*, so word is placed into *yes* column.)

    C. Repeat Step B until all words with the possibility of Stopping of Fricatives have been listed in the *yes* and *no* columns of the Consistency Checklist, as appropriate.

    D. In the case of Raoul, all words with fricatives are stopped; thus, all belong in the *yes* column (including *nose, thin, suit, miss, sheep, fight, very, five,* and *five*).

    E. Fill in the final rule description on the bottom line of the Consistency Checklist. In this case, because all words exhibit the rule, the final description is identical to our initial description—Stopping of Fricatives. (See Appendix A for correctly completed Consistency Checklist for Raoul.)

IV. *Describe rule in final form.*

    A. Transfer the final rule description (in this case, Stopping of Fricatives) from the bottom of the Consistency Checklist to the appropriate space on the generic worksheet.

V. *Go to phonological rule summary, find all words for which rule is operating, and note.*

    A. On the phonological rule summary, go to each word exhibiting Stopping of Fricatives and record that rule in the appropriate column. Make sure to record the rule twice for the word *five* (because the rule occurs twice in that word).

VI. *Perform final check.*

    A. Return to the first word listed on the phonological rule summary (i.e., *sun*). Ask question: Does Stopping of Fricatives totally explain the error? (Answer: *Yes.* The only thing happening in that word is the fact that a fricative is becoming a stop. All other parameters—place, voicing, structure, etc.—are unchanged from *sun* to /tʌn/.) Since the answer is *yes*, check off the word in the appropriate column.

    B. Ask the same question with *zoo.* (Answer: *Yes.* Check off the word.)

    C. Ask the same question with *nose.* (Answer: *Yes.* The error can be totally explained by Stopping of Fricatives. Check it off.)

    D. Ask the same question with *thin.* (Answer: *Uncertain.* The *th* in *thin* is an interdental whereas the *t* in /tɪn/ is an alveolar. Thus, there is a placement change in addition to the manner error. It seems as if something else is going on and the word cannot yet be checked off.)

    E. Ask the same question with *suit.* (Answer: *Yes.* Check the word off.)

    F. Ask the same question with *miss.* (Answer: *Yes.* Check it off.)

    G. Ask the same question with *sheep.* (Answer: *Uncertain.* The same problem exists as with the word *thin.* The *sh* in *sheep* is a palatal whereas the *t* in /tip/ is an alveolar. Thus, there seems to be a placement change in addition to the manner error. The word cannot yet be checked off.)

    H. Ask the same question with *fight, very,* and *five.* (Answer: *Uncertain.* None of the words can yet be checked off. In addition to the fricative being stopped, in all three words a labiodental (*f* or *v*) is becoming a bilabial (*p* or *b*).

Normally, at this point, the next step would be to perform another 6-step generic procedure, determine another rule and then see whether the remaining words could be checked off. But before we do that, let us look at the nonchecked words again. For example, *thin* → /tɪn/. Certainly Stopping of Fricatives is occurring, as we have already demonstrated. But is there also a placement error on the part of Raoul? After all, *th* is an interdental whereas *t* is an alveolar. Well, probably not. To understand why, consider the sound that Raoul would have to produce for *th* if he didn't change the placement to the alveolar position. He would have to produce an interdental stop. But there *is* no interdental stop in American English phonology. And if you now try to produce an interdental stop to yourself, you will see how difficult it is to articulate—and you will realize why Raoul would go instead to the nearest naturally occurring stop in American English—the alveolar stop. Because *t* is the closest natural stopping place for /ə/ in our phonological system, it is unsurprising that Raoul stops /ə/ in that position and it cannot be considered an additional placement error.

The concept of *natural stopping places* is a very important one in phonological analysis and will be discussed more fully in the next section, but let us first try to finish our analysis of Raoul. Since we now have explained *thin* → /tɪn/ just by stopping of fricatives, we can now check off that word. What about *sheep* → /tip/? Once again, there is no naturally occurring palatal stop in American English phonology and if you attempt to make such a sound to yourself now, you will see why Raoul goes to the alveolar. Given our phonological system, production of a palatal stop is very difficult and Raoul instead goes to the nearest natural stopping place. The words *fight, very*, and *five* present similar problems. There is no labiodental stop in American English phonology and given our phonological system, it would be a very difficult sound to produce. So Raoul goes to the nearest natural stopping place—the labial position in this case—and produces *p* for *f* and *b* for *v*. Once again, even though placement is changing modestly in these words, this placement change is only an artifact of the stopping rule.

Now that we can completely explain the errors in *thin, sheep, fight, very*, and *five* by combining Stopping of Fricatives with our knowledge of natural stopping places, we can check off each of these words for the phonological rule summary. Raoul's analysis is now complete. See the correctly completed phonological rule summary for Raoul on page 78.

PHONOLOGICAL RULE SUMMARY

Client: _RAOUL SCHWARTZ_

Check	Target Word	Client Production	Rule(s) Operating
✔	sun	tʌn	Stopping of Fricatives
✔	zoo	du	SF
✔	nose	nod	SF
✔	thin	tɪn	SF
✔	suit	tut	SF
✔	miss	mɪt	SF
✔	sheep	tip	SF
✔	fight	paɪt	SF
✔	very	bɛrt	SF
✔	five	paɪb	SF; SF (Occurs twice in word)

78

Natural Stopping Places

If a client has Stopping of Fricatives, all *s* sounds in his or her speech will change into /t/ and all *z* sounds will become /d/. It is easy to see why this would occur: *s* is a voiceless alveolar; if it is stopped, it makes sense that it would become /t/, also a voiceless alveolar. Likewise, *z* is a voiced alveolar; it is logical that if stopped, it would change into /d/, also a voiced alveolar. In fact, /t/ and /d/ are called the *homorganic* (made in the same place) stops for *s* and *z*.

Unfortunately, no homorganic stops exist in American English phonology for the other fricatives /f/, /v/, /θ/, /ð/, /ʃ/, and /ʒ/. This presents a dilemma for the client with Stopping of Fricatives. Does he try to produce a homorganic stop that is unnatural within his phonological system (for example does he try to produce a labiodental, interdental, or palatal stop) or does he search for a substitute that is less accurate from the perspective of placement but is more natural to the phonology of his community? In most cases, the client with speech disorders takes the latter course and thus, the concept of natural stopping places becomes important for the clinician.

The following list summarizes the natural stopping places for the six relevant fricatives in American English phonology:

Fricative		Natural Stopping Place
θ	⟶	t
ð	⟶	d
ʃ	⟶	t
ʒ	⟶	d
f	⟶	p
v	⟶	b

In each case, the client substitutes the stop that is closest in placement to the target fricative but is still natural within the speech community's phonological system.

Should this modest placement change be considered a placement error, in addition to the Stopping of Fricatives? In the absence of other placement errors, no; only the lack of a homorganic stop for the deviant fricative has caused the placement change here. One would expect the appropriate placement to return once the Stopping of Fricatives has been eliminated (as, indeed, it does in most instances).

Two other issues must be considered prior to concluding this discussion. First, because what is natural for a given child depends on the speech model in his or her community, one might expect that a child from a different speech community might demonstrate different natural stopping places. In reality, this seems to be true. For example, many English-speaking French-Canadian children with Stopping of Fricatives exhibit /k/ and /g/ as the natural stops for the palatal fricative /ʃ/ and /ʒ/ (rather than the /t/ and /d/ exhibited by American-English-speaking children). One can hypothesize that this difference is related to the fact that the French language has many more palatal and velar sounds than does English. As such, the velar position may well be a more natural alternative than the alveolar position for children who speak both French and English. In short, although you should learn and internalize the customary natural stopping places for your American-English-speaking clients, you should always be aware of the fact that a different phonological environment could result in distinctive natural stopping places.

Finally, just as there are natural stopping places for certain fricatives, there are *natural fricative places* for certain stops. For example, /p/ and /b/ do not have homorganic fricatives. As such, if the child has a rule turning stops into fricatives, /p/ will become /f/ and /b/ will become /v/. Although the concept of natural fricative places is used in phonological analysis much less frequently than natural stopping places, we will later see that it is valuable to include the concept as part of our analytical framework.

Working with the Parameter Confusion Test: Child #003

The first step of the 6-step analytical procedure requires that we take one of the client's errors and choose the parameter involved in the error. Thus far, we have had no difficulty in doing this; after systematically evaluating each of the parameters, we have been able to determine the correct parameter being violated without any real uncertainty or confusion. Unfortunately, it is not always so easy. For example, consider Child #003, who has the following words in her repertoire:

Target	Client Production
bed	/dɛd/
bee	/bi/

Let us attempt to complete Step 1 of the generic procedure for bed → /dɛd/. If you would like, follow along with the abbreviated Generic Worksheet.

Child #003—Review

Generic Worksheet

I. *Take one error and choose possible parameters.*
   A. Fill in the error being analyzed (in this case, *bed* → /dɛd/).
   B. Ask question: Is manner the parameter being violated when *bed* changes to /dɛd/? (Answer: *No.* Both /b/ and /d/ are stops.)
   C. Ask question: Is a voicing problem causing *bed* to go to /dɛd/? (Answer: *No.* Both words contain voiced sounds.)
   D. Ask question: Could a placement problem be causing *bed* → /dɛd/? (Answer: Although your initial reaction might be to say *yes*, the best we can realistically answer at this point is *maybe*. Yes, the client might have made the error because she has a problem producing a sound having a labial placement (in other words, the /b/ in *bed*). But there is another possible hypothesis: Maybe the final alveolar is really the guilty party. Maybe this final alveolar is a culprit causing the /b/ in *bed* to shift to the alveolar position. Maybe it is not a placement error after all. To clarify further, let us ask our next question.)
   E. Ask question: Could the context of the word have caused the error? (Answer: Again, *maybe*. It is possible that assimilation from the final alveolar has caused the /b/ to shift to a /d/.)
   F. Ask question: Is the structure of the word creating the error? (Answer: *No.* The structure of both *bed* and /dɛd/ is CVC.)
   G. Ask question: Has a linguistic problem caused *bed* to become /dɛd/? (Answer: *Unlikely.*)
   H. Ask question: Has a semantic difficulty caused the error? (Answer: *Unlikely.* *Bed* is a very low-level lexical item.)

PROCEDURE FOR PHONOLOGICAL ANALYSIS — GENERIC WORKSHEET

I. <u>Take one error and choose possible parameters</u>

ERROR: bed ⟶ /dɛd/

ANALYSIS:
Manner?	⟶	No
Voicing?	⟶	No
Placement?	⟶	Maybe
Context?	⟶	Maybe
Structure?	⟶	No
Linguistic?	⟶	Unlikely
Semantic?	⟶	Unlikely

> If unclear as to whether placement or context, perform Parameter Confusion Test (See Form). Otherwise go to Step II.

Inconveniently, our analysis has left us not with one *yes* but with two *maybes*. In other words, we are confused as to whether placement or context is the parameter responsible for the child's error; we need to perform a Parameter Confusion Test.

Parameter Confusion Test

For Child #003, resolving the confusion is not too difficult. Follow along as we go through the steps of a Parameter Confusion Test (see the completed form on the next page):

    A. Note the target word on the line indicated (i.e., *bed*).

    B. Note the client's production (i.e., /dɛd/).

    C. Choose test word. This is the most important step of the Parameter Confusion Test. You want to choose a word from the client's speech sample in which there is no chance for assimilation to occur. In other words, you want a word with no culprit. (For this child, you have been provided with the test word: *bee* → /bi/.)

Why did you choose bee *as the test word? Don't you instead need a test word having the same syllable structure as the target* (bed)*? The word* bee *has a different syllable structure!*

Although it is probably ideal if your test word has the same syllable structure as the target, we find that on a practical level, it really does not make a difference. And there is a positive payoff. Because we are willing to choose test words having different syllable structures than the target word, our search for test words becomes easier.

    D. Does the error being investigated still occur in the test word, even though the culprit has been removed? If the answer is *yes*, you have a placement error; even though there is no longer an opportunity for assimilation to occur, the client still makes the error. If the answer is *no*, you have a situation whereby getting rid of the culprit has also gotten rid of the error. So the culprit *is* the cause of the problem after all, and the error is due to context, or assimilation. (In Child #003, the answer is *no*. When the culprit is eliminated, the error disappears. So Child #003 has an assimilation error.)

    E. Now we can return to Step 1 of the 6-step generic procedure. We can cross out the *maybe* after placement and change it to a *no*. Likewise, we can cross out the *maybe* for context and now write *yes*. (See correctly altered Step 1 in Appendix A.) If we were proceeding further with this analysis, we would now go on to Step 2 and attempt to define and label the rule. However, as the purpose here has only been to teach you how to perform a Parameter Confusion Test, we will discontinue the analysis for Child #003, and present you with another opportunity to resolve a parameter confusion.

PLACEMENT CONTEXT. PARAMETER CONFUSION CHECK

Target Word: *bed*

Client Production: /dɛd/

Choose Test Word:
   (Word in which there's no culprit; i.e no   *bee → /bi/*
      chance for assimilation to occur).

Error Still Occur? _____ Yes

                    ✓ No

   Yes = Placement error; even though chance for assimilation has been
         removed, error still occurs.

   No = Assimilation error; error disappears when culprit is removed.

Return to Step 1 - Generic Worksheet

Working with the Parameter Confusion Test: Child #004

Child #004 has the following words in his repertoire:

Target	Client Production
cat	/tæt/
key	/ti/

Use the blank worksheets provided on pages 86 and 88 to finish Step 1 of the generic procedure for Child #004. Try this one on your own, if possible, prior to reading the answer.

Child #004—Review

Generic Worksheet

I. *Take one error and choose possible parameters.*
    A. Fill in the error being analyzed (in this case, cat → /tæt/).
    B. Ask question: Is manner the parameter being violated when *cat* changes to /tæt/? (Answer: *No*. Both words contain stops.)
    C. Ask question: Is a voicing problem causing cat to become /tæt/? (Answer: *No*. Both words have voiceless sounds.)
    D. Ask question: Could a placement problem be causing *cat* → /tæt/? (Answer: *Maybe*. Although the client may have a problem with the velar placement for the /k/ sound, another hypothesis is that the final alveolar is a culprit, causing the /k/ sound to become /t/.)
    E. Ask question: Might the context of the word have caused the error? (Answer: Again, *maybe*. It is possible (though not assured) that assimilation from the final alveolar has caused the sound change.)
    F. Ask question: Is the structure of the word creating the error? (Answer: *No*.)
    G. Ask question: Has a linguistic problem caused *cat* to become /tæt/? (Answer: *Unlikely*.)
    H. Ask question: Has a semantic problem caused the error? (Answer: *Unlikely*.)

Once again, our analysis has left us with two *maybes* rather than the *yes* we were looking for. Because we are confused as to whether placement or context is the parameter responsible for the child's error, we must perform a Parameter Confusion Test.

PROCEDURE FOR PHONOLOGICAL ANALYSIS — GENERIC WORKSHEET

I. **Take one error and choose possible parameters**

        ERROR:

        ANALYSIS: Manner?   ⟶

                     Voicing?   ⟶

                     Placement? ⟶

                     Context?   ⟶

                     Structure? ⟶

                     Linguistic? ⟶

                     Semantic? ⟶

> If unclear as to whether placement or context, perform Parameter Confusion Test (See Form). Otherwise go to Step II.

Parameter Confusion Test for Child #004.

    A. Note the target word on the line indicated (i.e., *cat*).

    B. Note the client's production (i.e., /tæt/).

    C. Choose test word. Once again, you would normally at this point go to the speech sample and find a word in which there is no chance for assimilation to occur. In other words, you want a word that has a /k/ sound, but no alveolar. In this case, you have already been provided with this word: *key*.

    D. Does the error still occur? (Answer: *Yes*. As *key* becomes /ti/, the error still occurs even after the chance for assimilation has been eliminated. Thus, it is not context but placement that is the cause of the client's error.)

    E. Now return to Step 1 of the 6-step generic procedure. Cross out the *maybe* after placement and write *yes*. Then cross off the *maybe* after context and indicate *no*. To proceed further with this analysis, you would now go on to Step 2, secure in your knowledge that the placement parameter has been violated.

Refer to Appendix A for correctly filled-out worksheets for Child #004.

Discussion

To review briefly, anytime you are unsure whether placement or context is the parameter responsible for the client's error, you must perform a parameter confusion test. At this point, you might be wondering whether other types of confusions ever occur; for example, is there ever a confusion between manner and context? Technically speaking, yes; other types of confusions can occur. However, in practical terms, they happen so rarely that we can ignore them at this stage of the analysis. And, as you will see, the Consistency Check will resolve any lingering confusions we have about the true nature of the phonological rule that we are identifying. So at this point, the only time you should use the word *maybe* for Step 1 of the analysis is when you are confused between the placement and context parameters.

PLACEMENT CONTEXT. PARAMETER CONFUSION CHECK

Target Word: _____

Client Production: _____

Choose Test Word: _____
    (Word in which there's no culprit; i.e no
      chance for assimilation to occur).

Error Still Occur? _____Yes

                _____No

   Yes = Placement error; even though chance for assimilation has been
       removed, error still occurs.

   No = Assimilation error; error disappears when culprit is removed.

Return to Step 1 – Generic Worksheet

Clinical Mastery Exercise—Bob Alou

Introduction

This next exercise gives you practice in completing a Parameter Confusion Test as part of a full analysis. Try to complete it on your own first and then turn to the solution on page 94 to check your work. There is only one rule working.

Worksheets required for Bob Alou
- Phonological Rule Summary
- Generic 6-step procedure
- Parameter Confusion Test worksheet
- Consistency Check Form

(Solution on page 94)

PHONOLOGICAL RULE SUMMARY

Client: _Bob Alov_

Check	Target Word	Client Production	Rule(s) Operating
	talk	tɔk	(correct)
	pot	pap	
	big	bɪb	
	cat	kæt	(correct)
	cup	pʌp	
	soup	fup	
	sick	sɪk	(correct)
	cow	kav	(correct)
	two	tu	(correct)
	pig	pɪb	

PROCEDURE FOR PHONOLOGICAL ANALYSIS — GENERIC WORKSHEET

I. **Take one error and choose possible parameters**

   ERROR:
   ANALYSIS: **Manner?** ————▶

         Voicing? ————▶

         Placement? ————▶

         Context? ————▶

         Structure? ————▶

         Linguistic? ————▶

         Semantic? ————▶

> If unclear as to whether placement or context, perform Parameter Confusion Test (See Form). Otherwise go to Step II.

II. **Make initial conclusion re: rule by describing the difference between target and client production.**

     _____ **PARAMETER**

       Description:_____

       Rule:_____

III. **Perform Consistency Check (See Consistency Check Form)**

IV. **Describe rule in Final Form**

       Rule:_____

V. **Go to phonological rule summary, find all words for which rule is operating, and note.**

VI. **Perform final check**

       — Make sure all changes in target word can be explained by rule. If so, check the word off. If not, leave until next analysis.

PLACEMENT CONTEXT. PARAMETER CONFUSION CHECK

<u>Target Word:</u> _____

<u>Client Production:</u> _____

<u>Choose Test Word:</u> _____
    (Word in which there's no culprit; i.e no
      chance for assimilation to occur).

<u>Error Still Occur?</u> _____Yes

                _____No

    <u>Yes</u> = Placement error; even though chance for assimilation has been
           removed, error still occurs.

    <u>No</u> = Assimilation error; error disappears when culprit is removed.

<u>Return to Step 1 – Generic Worksheet</u>

CONSISTENCY CHECKLIST

Initial Rule Description: _____

Rule Operating (Yes)	Rule Not Operating (No)

Check for Consistency	Yes Words	No Words	Sig. Diff.
1. **Phonetic Context**			
— List vowel preceding			
— List vowel following			
— List consonant preceding			
— List consonant following			
— List other sig. non-adjacent sounds			
2. **Position**			
— List I, M, F for initial medial, final			
3. **Intra-class Variability**			
— List correct/incorrect sounds, search for intra-class patterns			
4. **Syllable Structure/ Word Length**			
— List syllable structures			
5. **Part of Speech/Morphological Endings**			
— List grammatical categories			
6. **Syllable Stress**			
— List U, S for unstressed, stressed			
7. **Syllable Boundary**			
— List words/Draw line between syllable boundaries; Note differences			

Note other factors: Elicitation mode, situational context, overlearned words, etc.

Final Rule Description: _____

Solution

Normally, we would begin the analysis by going to the first word in the speech sample. However, in Bob's case, the first word is articulated correctly, so we proceed to the second word, *pot*. As usual, we then perform a 6-step generic procedure, in order to determine the first (and in this case, only) rule.

I. *Take one error and choose possible parameters.*
    A. Fill in the error being analyzed (*pot* → /pap/).
    B. Ask question: Is *pot* becoming /pap/ because of manner? (Answer: *No.* The manner remains the same from the target to Bob's production.)
    C. Ask question: Has a problem with voicing caused *pot* → /pap/? (Answer: *No.* Both the target and Bob's production are voiceless.)
    D. Ask question: Could a placement problem have caused the error? (Answer: *Maybe.* Perhaps Bob has a problem whereby he can't produce alveolars and changes them all to labials. But there is another hypothesis.)
    E. Ask question: Might the context within the word have induced the error? (Answer: *Maybe.* Perhaps the initial labial sound is a culprit that is causing the final alveolar to shift to the labial position.)
    F. Ask question: Is there a structural problem that has caused *pot* to become /pap/? (Answer: *No.* Both *pot* and /pap/ have identical CVC structures.)
    G. Ask question: Could a linguistic problem be the cause of the error? (Answer: *Unlikely.*)
    H. Ask question: Might a semantic difficulty have caused *pot* → /pap/? (Answer: *Unlikely.*)
    I. Because we have two *maybes* rather than one *yes*, we must perform a Parameter Confusion Test, in order to determine the parameter being violated.

I-a. *Parameter Confusion Test.*
    A. Note the target word on the line indicated (i.e., *pot*).
    B. Note the client's production (i.e., /pap/).
    C. Choose test word. We want a word that contains the sound error being focused upon (i.e., /t/, or an alveolar) but doesn't contain a culprit (i.e., a labial). In other words, we want to eliminate the chance for assimilation to occur. (There are several words in Bob's sample that meet this requirement, including *talk, cat, sick*, and *two*. In this case, we will pick *talk*, since it is first on the list.)
    D. Does the error still occur in the test word? (Answer: *No.* When the chance for assimilation has been removed, Bob produces an alveolar correctly. Thus, the *p* in *pot* is indeed a culprit and the error is one of context, not placement.)
    E. Return to Step 1 of the 6-step generic procedure. Cross out the *maybe* after placement and write *no*. Then cross out the *maybe* after context and write *yes*. Now we can proceed to Step 2. (Refer to Appendix A for correctly completed Parameter Confusion Test worksheet for Bob.)

Why can you choose test words like talk *or* sick? *In* talk, *the alveolar is in a different position than it is in the target* (pot). *In* sick, *not only is the alveolar in a different position, but it is also a different alveolar! Won't these factors invalidate the results of the parameter confusion test?*

No. In almost all cases, assimilation, if it exists, occurs in all members of a class (for example, alveolars). So an /s/ can test for assimilation just as well as a /t/ can, in this instance. Further, in almost all cases, assimilation occurs in either direction. So even though the target (*pot*) has /t/ in the final position, we can still test for assimilation with an alveolar in the initial position (as in *talk* and *sick*). This flexibility in our choice of test words helps to speed the process of performing the Parameter Confusion Test, because in most cases it allows us to use words we have already gathered in our initial speech sample, without having to go back to the client and gather more speech output.

You said "in almost all cases . . ." What about the occasions where a client has a limited assimilation rule whereby the error will be masked if you choose a test word with a different sound or position than the target?

All limited rules will be identified by means of the consistency check.

II. *Make initial conclusion re: rule by describing the difference between target and client production.*
   A. Fill in the violated parameter, as per Step 1 (in this case, context).
   B. Describe what the client is doing: Whenever there is a labial in a word, other sounds in the word go to the labial position.
   C. Label the rule: The conventional label for this rule is "Labial Assimilation." Once again, however, any other term describing the same phenomenon for you and other clinicians is acceptable.

Why is the rule called labial assimilation rather than bilabial assimilation? After all, p *is a bilabial.*

Labiodentals and bilabials tend to act as a single class when it comes to assimilation. Thus, labial assimilation is the rule that occurs most frequently. Bilabial assimilation, on the other hand, is a more limited rule that occurs rarely, and will be picked up by means of the consistency check if necessary. This leads to a good rule of thumb: When defining and labeling rules, make them as general as possible initially; any limitations that exist will be easily determined during the consistency check.

III. *Perform Consistency Check.*

    A. Go to Consistency Checklist and place the word analyzed in Steps 1 and 2 (*pot*) into the *yes* column, indicating that the rule (Labial Assimilation) is operating for that word.

    B. Go to the next word in the sample in which there is a possibility of Labial Assimilation (i.e., *big*). Does labial assimilation occur? If so, put the word into the *yes* column; if not, place it in the *no* column. (Answer: *Yes.* Labial Assimilation occurs when *big* → /bɪb/.)

    C. Repeat Step B until all words with the possibility of Labial Assimilation have been listed in either the *yes* or *no* column of the Consistency Checklist, as appropriate. (In Bob's case, the remaining words *cup, soup,* and *pig* all have the possibility of Labial Assimilation; because they all do indeed demonstrate Labial Assimilation, all belong in the *yes* column.)

Why would soup → /fup/ *be called Labial Assimilation?*

The easy answer is that the /f/ in /fup/ is indeed a labial; thus, an alveolar (s) is changing to a labial (f) because of the labial elsewhere in the word (i.e., Labial Assimilation). A better question might be "Why does *soup* change to /fup/ rather than /pup/, which would look more like the child's other words?" The answer to this question relates to the discussion earlier in this chapter on Natural Fricative Places. Because the /s/ in *soup* is a fricative, unless there is another rule working at the same time, it should retain its fricative nature even after the assimilation takes place. (If /s/ had instead become /p/, not only would labial assimilation be taking place, but a fricative would be stopped at the same time.) Because /f/ is the natural labial fricative, that is the sound that replaces the /s/ when Labial Assimilation occurs.

    D. Fill in the final rule description on the bottom line of the Consistency Checklist. (In this case, as all words exhibit the rule, the final description is identical to our initial description—Labial Assimilation; see Appendix A for correctly completed Consistency Checklist for Bob.)

IV. *Describe rule in final form.*

    A. Transfer the final rule description (in this case, Labial Assimilation) from the bottom of the Consistency Checklist to the appropriate space on the generic worksheet.

V. *Go to phonological rule summary, find all words for which rule is operating, and note.*

    A. On the phonological rule summary, go to each word exhibiting Labial Assimilation and record that rule in the appropriate column.

VI. *Perform final check.*
   A. Return to the first error listed on the phonological rule summary (i.e., *pot*). Ask question: Does Labial Assimilation totally explain the error? (Answer: *Yes.*) As the answer is *yes*, check off the word in the appropriate column.
   B. Ask the same question with *big*. (Answer: *Yes*. Check off the word.)
   C. Ask the same question with *cup*. (Answer: *Yes*. Check off the word.)
   D. Ask the same question about *soup*. (Answer: *Yes. Soup* → /fup/ can totally be explained by Labial Assimilation along with our knowledge of Natural Fricative Places.)
   E. Ask the same question about *pig*. (Answer: *Yes*. Check off the word.)
   F. Because all misarticulated words have now been checked off, Bob's analysis is complete. (See the correctly completed phonological rule summary for Bob on page 98.)

PHONOLOGICAL RULE SUMMARY

Client: _Bob Alou_

Check	Target Word	Client Production	Rule(s) Operating
—	talk	tɔk	(correct)
✓	pot	pap	Labial Assimilation
✓	big	bɪb	LA
—	cat	kæt	(correct)
✓	cup	pʌp	LA
✓	soup	fup	LA
—	sick	sɪk	(correct)
—	cow	kaʊ	(correct)
—	two	tu	(correct)
✓	pig	pɪb	LA

Discussion

You have now reached the end of the section on elementary generative analysis. As you will see as you proceed into the next chapter, we have only scratched the surface of the challenge called phonological analysis. But there is some good news. First, you have been exposed to all of the different worksheets that you will need to complete even an advanced level analysis. In fact, before long, as the process becomes more internalized, we will explore ways of using fewer forms. Second, by now you should have enough familiarity with the 6-step generic procedure so that the process will begin to get faster. (As well it should; if you regularly took as long as we have been taking to analyze every rule exhibited by a given client, you would never get to therapy.)

Because familiarity with the material presented in this chapter is a prerequisite to being successful at higher levels, it is important that you not move on at this time unless you feel you have mostly mastered what has been presented thus far. To help you in determining whether to move on at this point, ask yourself the following questions:

1. Do I have a general familiarity with the generic 6-step procedure and worksheet?

2. Do I have sufficient knowledge of the Parameters of Articulatory Constraint to be able to successfully complete Step 1 of the 6-step procedure for a given error?

3. Can I correctly complete a consistency check for a given rule that *is* consistent?

4. Am I able to determine whether a given rule completely explains the client's error or misarticulated word?

5. Do I understand the concepts of Natural Stopping Places and Natural Fricative Places?

6. Am I able to indicate the Natural Stopping and Fricative Places of the applicable speech sounds?

7. Do I understand why parameter confusions occur?

8. Can I successfully perform a Parameter Confusion Test, including being able to choose a test word?

If you can answer at least a weak *yes* to each of the above questions, you are now ready to go on to the next chapter. However, if your answer is *no* to any of the questions listed, you are urged to review the relevant section(s) of this chapter before proceeding further. Either way, congratulations! You are well on your way to mastering phonological analysis.

CHAPTER 6

Microanalysis of Phonology, Part 2: Intermediate Generative Analysis

So far, we have learned how to perform a generative analysis with clients who have one rule in their phonological systems. Unfortunately, very few clients referred to us have the good manners to demonstrate only one phonological rule. (Six or more rules is more the norm and as many as 10–12 rules is very possible for unintelligible clients.) If this makes you feel as if you are still only at the base of a very large mountain that needs to be climbed, try not to despair. As you will see, the process actually becomes easier the more familiar you become with it. More importantly, any time you invest in learning the procedure now will be repaid several times over in the future, in the time you will save with your clients. So stick with it for a while longer; as stated at the conclusion of the last chapter, you are well on your way!

The major purpose of this chapter is to present you with increasingly more difficult speech samples needing analysis. Each of the clients will have more than one rule working and several additional challenges will be incorporated along the way. As usual, you are urged to attempt each practice exercise on your own prior to studying the solution.

Clinical Mastery Exercise—Sissy Sassafrasser

Introduction

Sissy's speech sample introduces several new elements. First, there are two phonological rules to be identified. These rules do not interact with one another; in other words, each sound error in a given word can be explained by one rule only. However, for the first time, there may be two rules occurring in a single word if there is more than one sound error in the word. In these instances, be careful that you do not check off a word in Step 6 until all of the errors in the word have been explained. One more hint: As usual, begin your analysis with the first word listed in the sample and continue in an orderly manner until both rules have been deciphered.

Worksheets required for Sissy Sassafrasser (in correct order of use)
- Phonological rule summary
- Generic 6-step procedure
- Consistency Check Form
- Generic 6-step procedure
- Parameter Confusion Test
- Consistency Check Form

(Solution on page 109)

PHONOLOGICAL RULE SUMMARY

Client: _Sissy Sassafrasser_

Check	Target Word	Client Production	Rule(s) Operating
	soup	tup	
	sick	tɪt	
	feet	pit	
	sock	tat	
	shoe	tu	
	walk	wat	
	dog	dɔd	
	gas	dæt	
	big	bɪd	

PROCEDURE FOR PHONOLOGICAL ANALYSIS — GENERIC WORKSHEET

I. Take one error and choose possible parameters

      ERROR:

      ANALYSIS: **Manner?** ⟶

                     Voicing? ⟶

                     Placement? ⟶

                     Context? ⟶

                     Structure? ⟶

                     Linguistic? ⟶

                     Semantic? ⟶

> If unclear as to whether placement or context, perform Parameter Confusion Test (See Form). Otherwise go to Step II.

II. Make initial conclusion re: rule by describing the difference between target and client production.

      _____ **PARAMETER**

          Description: _____

          Rule: _____

III. Perform Consistency Check (See Consistency Check Form)

IV. Describe rule in Final Form

          Rule: _____

V. Go to phonological rule summary, find all words for which rule is operating, and note.

VI. Perform final check

               — Make sure all changes in target word can be explained by rule. If so, check the word off. If not, leave until next analysis.

CONSISTENCY CHECKLIST

Initial Rule Description: _____

Rule Operating **(Yes)**	Rule Not Operating **(No)**

Check for Consistency	**Yes** Words	**No** Words	Sig. Diff.
1. **Phonetic Context**			
— List vowel preceding			
— List vowel following			
— List consonant preceding			
— List consonant following			
— List other sig. non-adjacent sounds			
2. **Position**			
— List I, M, F for initial medial, final			
3. **Intra-class Variability**			
— List correct/incorrect sounds, search for intra-class patterns			
4. **Syllable Structure/ Word Length**			
— List syllable structures			
5. **Part of Speech/Morphological Endings**			
— List grammatical categories			
6. **Syllable Stress**			
— List U, S for unstressed, stressed			
7. **Syllable Boundary**			
— List words/Draw line between syllable boundaries; Note differences			

Note other factors: Elicitation mode, situational context, overlearned words, etc.

Final Rule Description: _____

PROCEDURE FOR PHONOLOGICAL ANALYSIS — GENERIC WORKSHEET

I. Take one error and choose possible parameters

        ERROR:
        ANALYSIS: Manner? ———————➤

                       Voicing? ———————➤

                       Placement? ———————➤

                       Context? ———————➤

                       Structure? ———————➤

                       Linguistic? ———————➤

                       Semantic? ———————➤

> If unclear as to whether placement or context, perform Parameter Confusion Test (See Form). Otherwise go to Step II.

II. Make initial conclusion re: rule by describing the difference between target and client production.

            _____ PARAMETER

                Description: _____

                Rule: _____

III. Perform Consistency Check (See Consistency Check Form)

IV. Describe rule in Final Form

                Rule: _____

V. Go to phonological rule summary, find all words for which rule is operating, and note.

VI. Perform final check

               — Make sure all changes in target word can be explained by rule. If so, check the word off. If not, leave until next analysis.

PLACEMENT CONTEXT PARAMETER CONFUSION CHECK

Target Word: _____

Client Production: _____

Choose Test Word: _____
   (Word in which there's no culprit; i.e no
     chance for assimilation to occur).

Error Still Occur? _____Yes

             _____No

    Yes = Placement error; even though chance for assimilation has been
         removed, error still occurs.

    No = Assimilation error; error disappears when culprit is removed.

Return to Step 1 - Generic Worksheet

CONSISTENCY CHECKLIST

Initial Rule Description: _____

Rule Operating **(Yes)**	Rule Not Operating **(No)**

Check for Consistency	Yes Words	No Words	Sig. Diff.
1. Phonetic Context			
— List vowel preceding			
— List vowel following			
— List consonant preceding			
— List consonant following			
— List other sig. non-adjacent sounds			
2. Position			
— List I, M, F for initial medial, final			
3. Intra-class Variability			
— List correct/incorrect sounds, search for intra-class patterns			
4. Syllable Structure/ Word Length			
— List syllable structures			
5. Part of Speech/Morphological Endings			
— List grammatical categories			
6. Syllable Stress			
— List U, S for unstressed, stressed			
7. Syllable Boundary			
— List words/Draw line between syllable boundaries; Note differences			

Note other factors: Elicitation mode, situational context, overlearned words, etc.

Final Rule Description: _____

Solution

As usual, we begin the analysis by going to the first word in the speech sample (i.e., *soup*) and performing the 6-step generic procedure. This will help us to identify the first rule.

I. *Take one error and choose possible parameters.*

    A. Fill in the error being analyzed (*soup* → /tup/).

    B. Ask question: Is manner the parameter that is violated when *soup* becomes /tup/? (Answer: *Yes*. There is definitely a manner problem here; a fricative is becoming a stop.)

    C. Ask question: Is there a voicing problem that is causing or contributing to the error? (Answer: *No*. Both the target and Sissy's production are voiceless.)

    D. Ask question: Has a placement problem caused *soup* → /tup/? (Answer: *No*. Both the /s/ in *soup* and the /t/ in /tup/ are alveolars; placement is not a factor.)

    E. Ask question: Might the context within the word have stimulated the error? (Answer: *No*. The only context in the word is the labial /p/; as the /s/ has not changed to the labial position, context is not a factor here.)

Wait a minute. Why isn't context a maybe? *After all, the /p/ is a stop and the /s/ changes from a fricative to a stop. Why can't you hypothesize that the* p *is a culprit causing some sort of "stop assimilation" rather than assuming that the error is caused due to a problem with manner?*

Remember, at this level, we are interested in confusions between placement and context only. Although technically confusions between manner and context, perhaps resulting in a "stop assimilation," can occur, these happen rarely. For this reason, we have decided to concentrate only on placement-context confusions at this level; if indeed a rule like "stop assimilation" occurs, we will discover it during the consistency check anyway.

    F. Ask question: Has a structural problem caused *soup* to become /tup/? (Answer: *No*. Both the target and Sissy's production have a CVC syllable structure.)

    G. Ask question: Could a linguistic problem be the cause of the error? (Answer: *Unlikely*.)

    H. Ask question: Might a semantic difficulty have caused the error? (Answer: *Unlikely*.)

    I. Because there is only one *yes* and the remaining parameters are *no* or *unlikely*, it is clear that the manner parameter is the one being violated by the error. Since there is no need for a Parameter Confusion Test, we move on to Step 2.

II. *Make initial conclusion re: rule by describing the difference between target and client production.*

    A. Fill in the violated parameter, as per Step 1 (in this case, manner).

    B. Describe what the client is doing: A fricative is turning into a stop.

    C. Label the rule: Stopping of Fricatives.

III. *Perform Consistency Check.*

    A. Go to Consistency Checklist and put the word analyzed in Steps 1 and 2 into the *yes* column, indicating that the rule (Stopping of Fricatives) is working for that word (*soup*).

    B. Find the next word in the sample in which Stopping of Fricatives could occur (in this case, the /s/ in *sick*). Ask yourself: Does it occur? If so, put word into *yes* column; if not, put it into the *no* column. (Answer: *Yes*, Stopping of Fricatives occurs in *sick*, so the word is placed in the *yes* column.)

    C. Repeat Step B for all words in which Stopping of Fricatives is a possibility (i.e., *feet, sock, shoe, gas*).

    D. In the case of Sissy, because all possible words exhibit Stopping of Fricatives, they are all put into the *yes* column.

    E. Fill in the final rule description on the bottom line of the Consistency Checklist. In this case, because all words were found to have the rule operating, the label Stopping of Fricatives is unchanged. (See Appendix A for correctly completed Consistency Checklist.)

IV. *Describe rule in final form.*

    A. Transfer the final rule description (in this case, Stopping of Fricatives) from the bottom of the Consistency Checklist to the appropriate space on the generic worksheet.

V. *Go to phonological rule summary, find all words for which rule is operating, and note.*

    A. On the phonological rule summary, go to each word exhibiting Stopping of Fricatives and record that rule in the appropriate column.

VI. *Perform final check.*

    A. Return to the first word listed on the phonological rule summary (i.e., *soup*). Ask question: Does Stopping of Fricatives totally explain the error? If so, check off the word in the appropriate column. If not, skip the word with the intention of returning to it later. (Answer: *Yes*. The word should be checked off.)

    B. Go to the second word in the list determined to have Stopping of Fricatives (i.e., *sick*). Ask question: Does Stopping of Fricatives totally explain the error? (Answer: *No*. The word should be skipped for now. By the way, if only Stopping of Fricatives was working, what would *sick* have become? [Answer: /tik/.] Since it becomes /tɪt/, you know something else is going on.)

   C. One by one, return to each of the remaining words determined to have Stopping of Fricatives. Using the previous question, determine whether a given word should be checked off or skipped. (Answer: *Feet* and *shoe* should be checked off, *sock* and *gas* must be skipped.)

Although we have now determined one of Sissy's rules, several words from her speech sample remain unchecked. So our next step is to return to the next error on the list (i.e., *sick*) and go through the process again. (We are now focusing on the second error in the word *sick*.)

   I. *Take one error and choose possible parameters.*
      A. Fill in the error being analyzed (*sick* → /tɪt/, with a focus on the /k/ → /t/).
      B. Ask question: Has a manner problem caused the /k/ in *sick* to become /t/? (Answer: *No*. Both sounds are stops.)
      C. Ask question: Is there a voicing problem which has caused the error? (Answer: *No*. Both the target and the error are voiceless.)
      D. Ask question: Has a placement problem caused *sick* → /tɪt/? (Answer: *Maybe*. Perhaps Sissy has a problem whereby she does not produce any velars and changes them all to alveolars. But there is another hypothesis.)
      E. Ask question: Might the context within the word have created the conditions for the error? (Answer: *Maybe*. The initial sound in *sick* is an alveolar; perhaps that alveolar is a culprit that is causing the shift of the final sound to the alveolar position.)
      F. Ask question: Is there a structural problem that has caused *sick* → /tɪt/? (Answer: *No*. Both *sick* and /tɪt/ have CVC structures.)
      G. Ask question: Might a linguistic problem be the cause of the error? (Answer: *Unlikely*.)
      H. Ask question: Could a semantic difficulty have caused *sick* to become /tɪt/? (Answer: *Unlikely*. Children learn very early what *sick* means.)
      I. Because we have two *maybes* rather than one *yes*, we must perform a Parameter Confusion Test.
   I-a. *Parameter Confusion Test.*
      A. On the appropriate form, note the target word on the line indicated (i.e., *sick*).
      B. Note the client's production (i.e., /tɪt/).
      C. Choose test word. An appropriate test word will contain a velar but will not contain an alveolar, thus eliminating the chance for assimilation. (Sissy only has two words in her sample that meet this requirement—*walk* and *big*.)
      D. Does the error still occur? (Answer: *Yes*. Even when the chance for assimilation has been removed, the velar still turns into an alveolar. So the problem is not one of context, but of placement.

> *Why can't words like* dog *or* gas *be chosen as test words?*
>
> Because although *dog* and *gas* have velars, they both have alveolars (the *d* in *dog* and the *s* in *gas*). Thus, you have not eliminated the chance for assimilation if you use either of those words.

    E. Return to Step 1 of the 6-step generic procedure. Cross out the *maybe* after placement and write *yes*. Then cross out the *maybe* after context and write *no*. Now we can proceed with Step 2. (Refer to Appendix A for correctly completed Parameter Confusion Test worksheet for Sissy.)

  II. *Make initial conclusion re: rule by describing the difference between target and client production.*
    A. Fill in the violated parameter, as per Step 1 (in this case, placement).
    B. Describe what the client is doing: All velar sounds are shifting forward in the mouth to the alveolar position.
    C. Label the rule: Fronting of Velars.

 III. *Perform Consistency Check.*
    A. Go to Consistency Checklist and place the word analyzed in Steps 1 and 2 (*sick*) into the *yes* column, indicating that the rule (Fronting of Velars) is operating for that word.
    B. Find the next word in the sample with a velar (i.e., *sock*). Is the velar fronted to the alveolar position? If so, put the word into the *yes* column; if not, put it in the *no* column. (Answer: *Yes.*)
    C. Repeat Step B until all remaining words with velars have been evaluated and listed in either the *yes* or *no* column of the Consistency Checklist. (In Sissy's case, the words *walk, dog, gas,* and *big* all demonstrate Fronting of Velars and all belong in the *yes* column.)
    D. Fill in the final rule description on the bottom line of the Consistency Checklist (i.e., Fronting of Velars; see Appendix A for completed Checklist).

 IV. *Describe rule in final form.*
    A. Transfer the final rule description (i.e., Fronting of Velars) from the bottom of the Consistency Checklist to the appropriate space on the generic worksheet.

  V. *Go to phonological rule summary, find all words for which rule is operating, and note.*
    A. On the phonological rule summary, go to each word having Fronting of Velars and record that rule in the appropriate column.

 VI. *Perform final check.*
    A. Return to first unchecked error listed on the phonological rule summary (i.e., *sick*). Ask question: Is the error now totally explained by

the rules listed? (Answer: *Yes*.) In order to prove this to yourself, fill in the blanks below, which illustrate the interim steps.

Target	Fronting of Velars	Stopping of Fricatives
sick ⟶	/ / ⟶	/ /

You see that after the second rule, you have reached an utterance matching Sissy's output on the phonological rule summary. [See Appendix A for interim utterances.] The word can now be checked off.

B. Ask the same question with the next unchecked word (i.e., *sock*). (Answer: *Yes*.) Fill in the interim steps below:

Target	Fronting of Velars	Stopping of Fricatives
sock ⟶	/ / ⟶	/ /

C. Ask the same question with *walk*. (Answer: *Yes*. Check off the word.)
D. Ask the same question with *dog*. (Answer: *Yes*. Check off the word.)
E. Ask the same question with *gas*. (Answer: *Yes*.) Check off the word and fill in the interim steps below:

Target	Fronting of Velars	Stopping of Fricatives
gas ⟶	/ / ⟶	/ /

F. Ask the same question with *big*. (Answer: *Yes*. Check off the word.)
G. Because all misarticulated words have now been checked off, Sissy's analysis is complete. (See completed phonological rule summary on page 114.)

PHONOLOGICAL RULE SUMMARY

Client: _Sissy Sassafrasser_

Check	Target Word	Client Production	Rule(s) Operating
✓	soup	tup	Stopping of Fricatives
✓	sick	tɪt	Stopping of Fricatives; Fronting of Velars
✓	feet	pit	SF
✓	sock	tɑt	SF; FV
✓	shoe	tu	SF
✓	walk	wat	FV
✓	dog	dɔd	FV
✓	gas	dæt	SF; FV
✓	big	bɪd	FV

Discussion

Now that we know that Sissy has two rules—Stopping of Fricatives and Fronting of Velars—we can predict what she will say, given any comparable word containing fricatives or velars. For example, we know that for the word *cat*, Sissy will say /tæt/. The word *shock* will go through /ʃat/ (Fronting of Velars) before resulting in /tat/ (Stopping of Fricatives). (Or it may go through /tak/ [Stopping of Fricatives] before resulting in /tat/ [Fronting of Velars]; the rules can be applied in any order, yet the result will be the same.)

This concept of prediction is a very important one in phonological analysis. Because we can predict a client's output once we know his or her rule system, it allows us as clinicians to obtain smaller speech samples than we might otherwise need. Also, the realization that we can predict what a client will say without yet having heard him or her say it, takes some of the mystery out of articulation disorders and helps to enforce the notion that children are orderly, not random, in their misarticulations. A clear appreciation for this latter fact, of course, will be an important prerequisite for the successful implementation of phonological approaches to therapy.

The following words will provide you with practice, not only in prediction, but with being able to manipulate rules. Using Sissy's rule system, try to predict what she will say for each of the words presented (answer appears in Appendix A).

1. *take* ⟶
2. *cash* ⟶
3. *fig* ⟶
4. *thick* ⟶
5. *calf* ⟶
6. *fog* ⟶
7. *scissor* ⟶

Golden Words and Embedded Rules

In each of the four phonological analyses we have completed thus far, one factor has helped to make our job easier: Each error that we have seen has been caused by only one rule. So with Sissy, who said /tup/ for *soup*, /s/ ⟶ /t/ could be explained by one rule—Stopping of Fricatives. Likewise, when *sick* ⟶ /tɪt/, even though it had two errors, each could be explained by a single rule: the /s/ ⟶ /t/ because of Stopping of Fricatives and the /k/ ⟶ /t/ due to Fronting of Velars.

Words that have errors that are caused by a single phonological rule have been labeled *golden words* (Klein, 1987). The term has been developed to underscore the value of these words during the analytic process. Think of it . . . A given child with speech disorders may have six to eight rules that account for all of his or her errors; if you can find only three to five golden words, half of your analytical work is completed very easily. Unfortunately, much of the time, a single sound error is caused by several rules interacting with one another. The examples to follow will provide practice in analyzing interacting, or as we call them, embedded rules.

Working with Embedded Rules: Child #005

Child #005 says /to/ for *go*. As Step 1 of the generic 6-step procedure is completed next, you will notice a difference between this error and the errors evaluated previously. (See correctly completed form on page 115.)

Child #005—Review

    I. *Take one error and choose possible parameters.*
      A. Fill in the error being analyzed (*go* → /to/).
      B. Ask question: Is manner the parameter that is violated when *go* becomes /to/? (Answer: *No*. Both /g/ and /t/ are stops.)
      C. Ask question: Is a voicing problem causing *go* → /to/? (Answer: *Yes*. The /g/ in *go* is voiced whereas the /t/ in /to/ is voiceless.)
      D. Ask question: Is a placement problem causing *go* to become /to/? (Answer: *Yes*. The /g/ in *go* is a velar whereas the /t/ in /to/ is an alveolar.)
      E. Ask question: Might the context of the word have caused the error? (Answer: Given the lack of other consonants in the word, *no*.)
      F. Ask question: Structure? (Answer: *No*.)
      G. Ask question: Linguistic? (Answer: *Unlikely*.)
      H. Ask question: Semantic? (Answer: *Unlikely*.)

As you can see, the analysis has resulted in two responses of *yes*; in other words at least two rules are working simultaneously in Child #005's production of *go*. This is an example of *embedded rules* (or, as Edwards, 1984, calls them, *interacting rules*).

What should you do about embedded rules when you come across them during an analysis? *Ignore them* (at least initially) and go on to another word in the sample (which will hopefully be a golden word). Remember, our goal is to make the analytical process as clinically efficient—and easy for us as possible. Nothing is quite so frustrating clinically as trying to analyze a single word that has five deeply embedded rules working together, so that the client's production doesn't even begin to resemble the target. Yet those same five rules can be easily identified with a fraction of the time and frustration just by searching the speech sample for golden words. So to review, if after you finish Step 1 of the generic procedure, you find yourself with two *yes* responses, skip the word and go on to the next word in the speech sample.

One more factor should be considered before moving on. It is possible that you were able to figure out the two rules in *go* → /to/. If so, great! It means that you are a step ahead in the learning process at this point. Should you still skip the "two-*yes*" words when you come to them? Absolutely! Keep in mind, the previous example was, by design, unusually simple. At this point, your long-term learning will be best served by skipping words with embedded rules and looking for golden words instead.

PROCEDURE FOR PHONOLOGICAL ANALYSIS — GENERIC WORKSHEET

I. **Take one error and choose possible parameters**

      ERROR: $go \longrightarrow /tol/$

      ANALYSIS: **Manner?**   ⟶ *No*

                     Voicing?   ⟶ *Yes*

                     Placement?   ⟶ *Yes*

                     Context?   ⟶ *No*

                     Structure?   ⟶ *No*

                     Linguistic?   ⟶ *Unlikely*

                     Semantic?   ⟶ *Unlikely*

> **If unclear as to whether placement or context, perform Parameter Confusion Test (See Form). Otherwise go to Step II.**

117

Working with Embedded Rules: Child #006

For another example of embedded or interacting rules, consider Child #006, who says /tu/ for *zoo*. Once again, Step 1 of the generic 6-step procedure will now be performed. (See abbreviated generic worksheet.)

Child #006—Review

I. *Take one error and choose possible parameters.*
   A. Fill in the error being analyzed (*zoo* → /tu/).
   B. Ask question: Has a problem with manner caused *zoo* to become /tu/? (Answer: *Yes*. A fricative is replaced by a stop.)
   C. Ask question: Is there a voicing problem which has caused *zoo* →/tu/? (Answer: *Yes*. The /z/ in *zoo* is voiced; the /t/ in /tu/ is voiceless.)
   D. Ask question: Placement? (Answer: *No*. Both /z/ and /t/ are alveolars.)
   E. Ask question: Context? (Answer: *No*.)
   F. Ask question: Structure? (Answer: *No*.)
   G. Ask question: Linguistic? (Answer: *Unlikely*.)
   H. Ask question: Semantic? (Answer: *Unlikely*.)

In the case of Child #006, the two responses of *yes* indicate the existence of at least two rules embedded in the one sound error. Again, the advice is to skip this word and go on to another word in the speech sample.

PROCEDURE FOR PHONOLOGICAL ANALYSIS — GENERIC WORKSHEET

I. **Take one error and choose possible parameters**

      ERROR: zoo —➞ /tu/

      ANALYSIS: **Manner?** ————➞ Yes

                  Voicing? ————➞ Yes

                  Placement? ————➞ No

                  Context? ————➞ No

                  Structure? ————➞ No

                  Linguistic? ————➞ Unlikely

                  Semantic? ————➞ Unlikely

> If unclear as to whether placement or context, perform Parameter Confusion Test (See Form). Otherwise go to Step II.

Clinical Mastery Exercise—Farrell Zeiscreem #1

Introduction

Farrell's speech sample will provide you with some practice at analyzing words that have embedded rules. There are two rules working in Farrell's phonological system and in at least some cases, these rules are embedded. Try it yourself first on the worksheets provided before reading the following solution. And remember . . . if you come across a word with two *yes* responses, skip it and go on to the next word.

Worksheets required for Farrell #1 (in correct order of use)
- Phonological rule summary
- Generic 6-step procedure
- Generic 6-step procedure
- Consistency Check Form
- Generic 6-step procedure
- Generic 6-step procedure
- Parameter Confusion Test
- Consistency Check Form

(Solution on page 129)

PHONOLOGICAL RULE SUMMARY

Client: FARRELL ZEISCREEM #1

Check	Target Word	Client Production	Rule(s) Operating
	save	ses	
	dig	tɪt	
	pig	pɪk	
	sick	sɪt	
	peek	pik	
	boat	tot	
	do	tu	
	zoo	su	
	bad	tæt	

PROCEDURE FOR PHONOLOGICAL ANALYSIS — GENERIC WORKSHEET

I. **Take one error and choose possible parameters**

      ERROR:

      ANALYSIS: **Manner?**   ⟶

                  Voicing?   ⟶

                  Placement? ⟶

                  Context?   ⟶

                  Structure? ⟶

                  Linguistic? ⟶

                  Semantic? ⟶

> If unclear as to whether placement or context, perform Parameter Confusion Test (See Form). Otherwise go to Step II.

II. **Make initial conclusion re: rule by describing the difference between target and client production.**

    _____ **PARAMETER**

        Description: _____

        Rule: _____

III. **Perform Consistency Check (See Consistency Check Form)**

IV. **Describe rule in Final Form**

        Rule: _____

V. **Go to phonological rule summary, find all words for which rule is operating, and note.**

VI. **Perform final check**

        — Make sure all changes in target word can be explained by rule. If so, check the word off. If not, leave until next analysis.

PROCEDURE FOR PHONOLOGICAL ANALYSIS — GENERIC WORKSHEET

I. **Take one error and choose possible parameters**

   ERROR:
   ANALYSIS: Manner? ──────▶

   Voicing? ──────▶

   Placement? ──────▶

   Context? ──────▶

   Structure? ──────▶

   Linguistic? ──────▶

   Semantic? ──────▶

   > If unclear as to whether placement or context, perform Parameter Confusion Test (See Form). Otherwise go to Step II.

II. **Make initial conclusion re: rule by describing the difference between target and client production.**

   _____ PARAMETER

   Description: _____

   Rule: _____

III. **Perform Consistency Check (See Consistency Check Form)**

IV. **Describe rule in Final Form**

   Rule: _____

V. **Go to phonological rule summary, find all words for which rule is operating, and note.**

VI. **Perform final check**

   — Make sure all changes in target word can be explained by rule. If so, check the word off. If not, leave until next analysis.

CONSISTENCY CHECKLIST

Initial Rule Description: _____

Rule Operating **(Yes)**	Rule Not Operating **(No)**

Check for Consistency	**Yes** Words	**No** Words	Sig. Diff.
1. **Phonetic Context**			
— List vowel preceding			
— List vowel following			
— List consonant preceding			
— List consonant following			
— List other sig. non-adjacent sounds			
2. **Position**			
— List I, M, F for initial medial, final			
3. **Intra-class Variability**			
— List correct/incorrect sounds, search for intra-class patterns			
4. **Syllable Structure/ Word Length**			
— List syllable structures			
5. **Part of Speech/Morphological Endings**			
— List grammatical categories			
6. **Syllable Stress**			
— List U, S for unstressed, stressed			
7. **Syllable Boundary** — List words/Draw line between syllable boundaries; Note differences			

Note other factors: Elicitation mode, situational context, overlearned words, etc.

Final Rule Description: _____

PROCEDURE FOR PHONOLOGICAL ANALYSIS — GENERIC WORKSHEET

I. **Take one error and choose possible parameters**

      ERROR:

      ANALYSIS: **Manner?** ———▶

                Voicing? ———▶

                Placement? ———▶

                Context? ———▶

                Structure? ———▶

                Linguistic? ———▶

                Semantic? ———▶

> If unclear as to whether placement or context, perform Parameter Confusion Test (See Form). Otherwise go to Step II.

II. **Make initial conclusion re: rule by describing the difference between target and client production.**

      ————————— **PARAMETER**

          Description: _____

          Rule: _____

III. **Perform Consistency Check (See Consistency Check Form)**

IV. **Describe rule in Final Form**

          Rule: _____

V. **Go to phonological rule summary, find all words for which rule is operating, and note.**

VI. **Perform final check**

          — Make sure all changes in target word can be explained by rule. If so, check the word off. If not, leave until next analysis.

PROCEDURE FOR PHONOLOGICAL ANALYSIS — GENERIC WORKSHEET

I. <u>Take one error and choose possible parameters</u>

        ERROR:
        ANALYSIS: Manner?   ————►

                     Voicing?   ————►

                     Placement? ————►

                     Context?   ————►

                     Structure? ————►

                     Linguistic? ————►

                     Semantic? ————►

> If unclear as to whether placement or context, perform Parameter Confusion Test (See Form). Otherwise go to Step II.

II. <u>Make initial conclusion re: rule by describing the difference between target and client production.</u>

           ————————— PARAMETER

             Description: _____

             Rule: _____

III. <u>Perform Consistency Check (See Consistency Check Form)</u>

IV. <u>Describe rule in Final Form</u>

             Rule: _____

V. <u>Go to phonological rule summary, find all words for which rule is operating, and note.</u>

VI. <u>Perform final check</u>

           — Make sure all changes in target word can be explained by rule. If so, check the word off. If not, leave until next analysis.

PLACEMENT CONTEXT. PARAMETER CONFUSION CHECK

Target Word: _____

Client Production: _____

Choose Test Word: _____
   (Word in which there's no culprit; i.e no
     chance for assimilation to occur).

Error Still Occur? _____ Yes

                _____ No

   Yes = Placement error; even though chance for assimilation has been
       removed, error still occurs.

   No = Assimilation error; error disappears when culprit is removed.

Return to Step 1 — Generic Worksheet

CONSISTENCY CHECKLIST

Initial Rule Description: _____

Rule Operating **(Yes)**	Rule Not Operating **(No)**

Check for Consistency	**Yes** Words	**No** Words	Sig. Diff.
1. **Phonetic Context**			
— List vowel preceding			
— List vowel following			
— List consonant preceding			
— List consonant following			
— List other sig. non-adjacent sounds			
2. **Position**			
— List I, M, F for initial medial, final			
3. **Intra-class Variability**			
— List correct/incorrect sounds, search for intra-class patterns			
4. **Syllable Structure/ Word Length**			
— List syllable structures			
5. **Part of Speech/Morphological Endings**			
— List grammatical categories			
6. **Syllable Stress**			
— List U, S for unstressed, stressed			
7. **Syllable Boundary** — List words/Draw line between syllable boundaries; Note differences			

Note other factors: Elicitation mode, situational context, overlearned words, etc.

Final Rule Description: _____

Solution

Once again, the analysis begins by taking the first word in Farrell's speech sample (i.e., *save*) and performing the 6-step generic procedure.

I. *Take one error and choose possible parameters.*
   A. Fill in the error being analyzed (*save* → /ses/).
   B. Ask question: Is manner the cause of the error when *save* → /ses/? (Answer: *No*. Both /v/ and /s/ are fricatives.)
   C. Ask question: Is there a voicing problem that has helped cause *save* → /ses/? (Answer: *Yes*. The /v/ in *save* is voiced whereas the /s/ in /ses/ is voiceless.)
   D. Ask question: Has a placement problem helped cause *save* to become /ses/? (Answer: *Maybe*. Perhaps Farrell has a problem with production of labiodentals whereby those sounds all retreat to the alveolar position. However, there is another hypothesis.)
   E. Ask question: Might the context in the word have caused the /v/ in *save* to go to the alveolar position? (Answer: *Maybe*. Perhaps the initial /s/ is an alveolar culprit that is causing the other sound in the word to go to the alveolar position.)
   F. Ask question: Has a structural problem caused *save* → /ses/? (Answer: *No*. Both the target and Farrell's production were CVC.)
   G. Ask question: Could a linguistic problem have created the conditions for *save* → /ses/? (Answer: *Unlikely*. The word *save* is a verb, again an early developing linguistic category.)
   H. Ask question: Might a semantic problem have created the conditions for *save* to become /ses/? (Answer: *Maybe*. Perhaps Farrell does not know the lexical item, a fairly high-level word, and his utterance reflects an attempt to produce a word with which he really has no experience.)

What a mess! There is one *yes* and three *maybes* (or at least two if you do not accept the possibility of a problem with the semantic parameter). Clearly, this translates into at least two embedded rules, so it is best that we skip the word for now and instead go on to the next error: the /d/ in *dig*.

I. *Take one error and choose possible parameters.*
   A. Fill in the error being analyzed (*dig* → /tɪt/ with a focus on the initial sound).
   B. Ask question: Is manner the parameter being violated when the *d* in *dig* becomes /t/? (Answer: *No*. Both sounds are stops.)
   C. Ask question: Is there a voicing problem that has caused the error? (Answer: *Yes*. The *d* in *dig* is voiced whereas the /t/ in /tɪt/ is voiceless.)
   D. Ask question: Placement? (Answer: *No*. Both are alveolars.)
   E. Ask question: Context? (Answer: *No*.)

    F. Ask question: Structure? (Answer: *No.*)

    G. Ask question: Linguistic? (Answer: *Unlikely.*)

    H. Ask question: Semantic? (Answer: *Unlikely.*)

    I. Because we have one *yes* and no confusion, we can now proceed to Step 2.

II. *Make initial conclusion re: rule by describing the difference between target and client production.*

    A. Fill in the violated parameter, as per Step 1 (in this case, voicing).

    B. Describe what the client is doing: A voiced consonant is becoming unvoiced.

    C. Label the rule: Devoicing of Consonants (although, once again, any other label that communicates essentially the same thing is acceptable).

III. *Perform Consistency Check.*

    A. Go to Consistency Checklist and put the word analyzed in Steps 1 and 2 into the *yes* column, indicating that the rule (Devoicing of Consonants) is working for that word. You may also want to circle the /d/ to remind yourself of the sound that has been focused upon.

    B. Find the first word in the sample in which Devoicing of Consonants could occur (i.e., the/ v/ in *save*). Ask yourself: Does it occur? If so, put word into *yes* column; if not, put it in the *no* column. (Answer: *Yes.* Devoicing of Consonants occurs in *save*, so the word is placed in the *yes* column.)

    C. Repeat Step B for all other words that have the possibility for Devoicing of Consonants (i.e., the /g/ in *dig* and *pig;* the /b/ in *boat* and *bad;* the /d/ in *dig, do,* and *bad;* and the /z/ in *zoo.*

    D. In Farrell's case, all voiced sounds are indeed devoiced. Thus, all words are put into the *yes* column. The *g* in *dig* is circled to indicate the error being focused upon. *Bad* is written twice with the /b/ circled in one and the /d/ in the other.

    E. Fill in the final rule description on the bottom line of the Consistency Checklist. In this case, as all words were found to have the rule operating, the label Devoicing of Consonants is unchanged. (See Appendix A for completed checklist.)

IV. *Describe rule in final form.*

    A. Transfer the final rule description (in this case, Devoicing of Consonants) from the bottom of the Consistency Checklist to the appropriate space on the generic worksheet.

V. *Go to phonological rule summary, find all words for which rule is operating, and note.*

    A. On the phonological rule summary, go to each word exhibiting Devoicing of Consonants and record that rule in the appropriate column.

VI. *Perform final check.*

    A. Return to the first word listed on the phonological rule summary (i.e., *save*). Ask question: Does Devoicing of Consonants totally explain the error? If so, check off the word in the appropriate column. If not, skip the word with the intention of returning to it later. (Answer: *No*. With only Devoicing of Consonants *save* would become /sef/; because this is not what Farrell is saying, we skip the word and will return to it later.)

B. Go to the second word on the list determined to have Devoicing of Consonants (i.e., *dig*). Ask question: Does Devoicing of Consonants totally explain the error? (Answer: *No*. The word should be skipped for now.)

C. Return to each of the remaining words determined to have Devoicing of Consonants. Using the same question, determine whether a given word should be checked off or skipped. (Answer: *pig*, *do*, and *zoo* should be checked off; *boat* and *bad* should be skipped.)

We have now determined one of Farrell's rules; however, several words from the sample have not yet been checked off. Thus, our next step is to return to the next error on the list (i.e., the /g/ in *dig*) and go through the process again.

I. *Take one error and choose possible parameters.*
   A. Fill in the error being analyzed (*dig* → /tɪt/, with the focus on the final /g/ going to /t/).
   B. Ask question: Has a problem with manner caused the /g/ in *dig* to change to /t/? (Answer: *No*. Both sounds are stops.)
   C. Ask question: Voicing? (Answer: *Yes*. The /g/ in *dig* is voiced; the /t/ in /tɪt/ is voiceless.)
   D. Ask question: Placement? (Answer: *Maybe*. Perhaps Farrell has a problem whereby he cannot produce a sound in the velar position. However, there is another explanation.)
   E. Ask question: Context? (Answer: *Maybe*. Perhaps Farrell does not have a problem with velars after all. Instead, it is possible that the initial alveolar is a culprit causing the final sound to also move to the alveolar position.)

Actually, we might as well stop here, without even going through the remaining parameters. With a *yes* and two *maybes*, we know that there are at least two rules working in this word! So it makes sense at this point to go on to the next word with an error. (As *pig* → /pɪk/ has now been explained, our next word will be *sick*.)

I. *Take one error and choose possible parameters.*
   A. Fill in the error being analyzed (i.e., *sick* → /sɪt/).
   B. Ask question: Manner? (Answer: *No*.)
   C. Ask question: Voicing? (Answer: *No*.)
   D. Ask question: Placement? (Answer: *Maybe*. It could be that because Farrell cannot produce any velar position sounds, the /k/ in *sick* became /t/. However, there is an alternative explanation.)

E. Ask question: Context? (Answer: *Maybe*. The other possibility is that the initial /s/ sound is an alveolar culprit causing the final sound to shift to the alveolar position.)

F. Ask question: Structure? (Answer: *No*. Both *sick* and /sɪt/ have identical CVC syllable structures.)

G. Ask question: Linguistic? (Answer: *Unlikely*.)

H. Ask question: Semantic? (Answer: *Unlikely*.)

I. Because we have two *maybes* rather than one *yes*, we must perform a Parameter Confusion Test.

I-a. *Parameter Confusion Test.*

A. On the appropriate form, note the target word on the line indicated (i.e., *sick*).

B. Note the client's production (i.e., /sɪt/).

C. Choose test word. An appropriate test word will contain a velar but will not contain an alveolar, thus eliminating the chance for assimilation. (Farrell has two words that meet this requirement: *pig* and *peek*; we will choose *pig*.)

D. Does the error still occur? (Answer: *No*. Although the word *pig* demonstrates a voicing error, the velar remains a velar when the culprit is eliminated. So context is indeed the problem when *sick* → /sɪt/.)

E. Return to Step 1 of the 6-step generic procedure. Cross out the *maybe* after placement and write *no*. Then cross out the *maybe* after context and write *yes*. Now we can proceed with Step 2. (A completed Parameter Confusion Test for Farrell appears in Appendix A.)

II. *Make initial conclusion re: rule by describing the difference between target and client production.*

A. Fill in the violated parameter, as per Step 1 (in this case, context).

B. Describe what the client is doing: Whenever there is an alveolar in the word, other sounds in the word go to the alveolar position.

C. Label the rule: Alveolar Assimilation.

III. *Perform Consistency Check.*

A. Go to Consistency Checklist and place the word analyzed in Steps 1 and 2 (*sick*) into the *yes* column, indicating that the rule (Alveolar Assimilation) is operating for that word.

B. One by one, go to the remaining words in the sample for which Alveolar Assimilation is a possibility. Does the rule occur? If so, put the given word into the *yes* column; if not, place it in the *no* column. (Answers: Alveolar Assimilation occurs in *save, dig, boat,* and *bad*, all of the words having the possibility of the rule. Each of those words should go into the *yes* column.)

C. Fill in the final rule description on the bottom line of the Consistency Checklist (i.e., Alveolar Assimilation; see Appendix A for completed Checklist).

IV. *Describe rule in final form.*
   A. Transfer the final rule description (i.e., Alveolar Assimilation) from the bottom of the Consistency Checklist to the appropriate space on the generic worksheet.
 V. *Go to phonological rule summary, find all words for which rule is operating, and note.*
   A. On the phonological rule summary, go to each word with Alveolar Assimilation, as determined in the previous steps, and record that rule in the appropriate column.
VI. *Perform final check.*
   A. Return to the first unchecked error (i.e., *save*). Ask question: Is the error now totally explained by the rules listed? (Answer: *Yes. Save* goes to /sef/ because of Devoicing of Consonants and /sef/ →/ses/ due to Alveolar Assimilation. Or you can proceed in the opposite direction should you choose, with *save* → /sez/ [Alveolar Assimilation] and /sez/ → /ses/ [Devoicing of Consonants]. The word can now be checked off.)
   B. Ask the same question with the next unchecked word (i.e., *dig*). (Answer: *Yes. Dig* → /tɪk/ [Devoicing of Consonants] and then /tɪk/ → /tɪt/ [Alveolar Assimilation].) Check it off.
   C. Ask the same question with *sick*. (Answer: *Yes.* Check off the word.)
   D. Ask the same question with *boat*. (Answer: *Yes. Boat* becomes /pot/ due to Devoicing of Consonants and /pot/ → /tot/ after Alveolar Assimilation.)
   E. Ask the same question with *bad*. (Answer: *Yes. Bad* → /pæt/ as a result of Devoicing of Consonants and /pæt/ → /tæt/ due to Alveolar Assimilation.)
   F. Because all misarticulated words have now been checked off, Farrell's analysis is complete. (See completed phonological rule summary on page 134.)

PHONOLOGICAL RULE SUMMARY

Client: _Farrell Zeiscreem #1_

Check	Target Word	Client Production	Rule(s) Operating
	save	ses	Devoicing of Consonants; AA
	dig	tɪt	DC; DC; AA
	pig	pɪk	DC
	sick	sɪt	Alveolar Assimilation (correct)
	peek	pik	
	boat	tot	DC; AA
	do	tu	DC
	zoo	su	DC
	bad	tæt	DC; DC; AA

Discussion

In the previous example, Farrell was found to exhibit two rules—Devoicing of Consonants and Alveolar Assimilation. As you saw, in a number of words, these rules were embedded. However, these words did not really create much of a problem for us because we were able to find golden words for each of the rules and then all we had to do was recognize the existence of these rules in the embedded words.

There is another factor that has facilitated our analyses up until this point: We have performed several consistency checks, but we have been lucky. Not only have our rules seemed consistent, but they also have been consistent. Sadly, this is not always the case. The next practice exercise presents another Farrell. As you will see, this Farrell is very similar to the child we have just analyzed. However, you will notice a few subtle differences.

Clinical Mastery Exercise—Farrell Zeiscreem #2

Introduction

This Farrell will also have two rules working. Once again, in at least some words, these rules will be embedded. But as you come to the Consistency Check for the first rule, you will observe a decided difference between this Farrell and Farrell #1. Just for the additional practice, why not work out the first steps again for yourself. Then see if you can solve the seeming inconsistency on your own, prior to reading the solution below.

Worksheets required for Farrell #2 (in correct order of use)
- Phonological rule summary
- Generic 6-step procedure
- Generic 6-step procedure
- Consistency Check Form

(Solution on page 141)

PHONOLOGICAL RULE SUMMARY

Client: _Farrell Zeiscreem #2_

Check	Target Word	Client Production	Rule(s) Operating
	save	ses	
	dig	dɪt	
	pig	pɪk	
	sick	sɪt	
	peek	pik	
	boat	dot	
	do	du	
	zoo	zu	
	bad	dæt	

PROCEDURE FOR PHONOLOGICAL ANALYSIS — GENERIC WORKSHEET

I. Take one error and choose possible parameters

ERROR:
ANALYSIS: Manner? ————➤
Voicing? ————➤
Placement? ————➤
Context? ————➤
Structure? ————➤
Linguistic? ————➤
Semantic? ————➤

> If unclear as to whether placement or context, perform Parameter Confusion Test (See Form). Otherwise go to Step II.

II. Make initial conclusion re: rule by describing the difference between target and client production.

_____ PARAMETER

Description: _____

Rule: _____

III. Perform Consistency Check (See Consistency Check Form)

IV. Describe rule in Final Form

Rule: _____

V. Go to phonological rule summary, find all words for which rule is operating, and note.

VI. Perform final check

— Make sure all changes in target word can be explained by rule. If so, check the word off. If not, leave until next analysis.

PROCEDURE FOR PHONOLOGICAL ANALYSIS — GENERIC WORKSHEET

I. Take one error and choose possible parameters

        ERROR:

        ANALYSIS: **Manner?**   ⟶

                      Voicing?   ⟶

                      Placement?   ⟶

                      Context?   ⟶

                      Structure?   ⟶

                      Linguistic?   ⟶

                      Semantic?   ⟶

> If unclear as to whether placement or context, perform Parameter Confusion Test (See Form). Otherwise go to Step II.

II. Make initial conclusion re: rule by describing the difference between target and client production.

        _____ **PARAMETER**

            Description: _____

            Rule: _____

III. Perform Consistency Check (See Consistency Check Form)

IV. Describe rule in Final Form

            Rule: _____

V. Go to phonological rule summary, find all words for which rule is operating, and note.

VI. Perform final check

                — Make sure all changes in target word can be explained by rule. If so, check the word off. If not, leave until next analysis.

CONSISTENCY CHECKLIST

Initial Rule Description: _____

Rule Operating **(Yes)**	Rule Not Operating **(No)**

Check for **Consistency**	**Yes** Words	**No** Words	Sig. Diff.
1. **Phonetic Context**			
— List vowel preceding			
— List vowel following			
— List consonant preceding			
— List consonant following			
— List other sig. non-adjacent sounds			
2. **Position**			
— List I, M, F for initial medial, final			
3. **Intra-class Variability**			
— List correct/incorrect sounds, search for intra-class patterns			
4. **Syllable Structure/ Word Length**			
— List syllable structures			
5. **Part of Speech/Morphological Endings**			
— List grammatical categories			
6. **Syllable Stress**			
— List U, S for unstressed, stressed			
7. **Syllable Boundary**			
— List words/Draw line between syllable boundaries; Note differences			

Note other factors: Elicitation mode, situational context, overlearned words, etc.

Final Rule Description: _____

Solution

Normally, we would begin the analysis by taking the first misarticulated word in Farrell #2's speech sample (i.e., *save*) and performing the generic procedure. However, we saw in Farrell #1 that the word *save* had one *yes* and three *maybes*, causing us to skip the word. Because *save* still becomes /ses/ in Farrell #2, our result would be the same and we might as well go right on to the second error: the /g/ in *dig*.

    I. *Take one error and choose possible parameters.*
      A. Fill in the error being analyzed (*dig* → /dɪt/).
      B. Ask question: Manner? (Answer: *No.*)
      C. Ask question: Voicing? (Answer: *Yes.*)
      D. Ask question: Placement? (Answer: *Maybe.* The velar /g/ may be going to the alveolar position because Farrell cannot produce any sounds having the velar placement. However, there is another hypothesis.)
      E. Ask question: Context? (Answer: *Maybe.* Perhaps the initial alveolar is serving as a culprit to move the /g/ in *dig* to the alveolar position.)

Once again, we may as well stop at this point, with one *yes* and two *maybes*. There are at least two embedded errors in that final sound and it is best that we skip this word and proceed to the next error (i.e., *pig*).

    I. *Take one error and choose possible parameters.*
      A. Fill in the error being analyzed (*pig* → /pɪk/).
      B. Ask question: Manner? (Answer: *No.*)
      C. Ask question: Voicing? (Answer: *Yes*; the /g/ in *pig* is voiced whereas the /k/ in /pɪk/ is voiceless.)
      D. Ask question: Placement? (Answer: *No.*)
      E. Ask question: Context? (Answer: *No.*)
      F. Ask question: Structure? (Answer: *No.*)
      G. Ask question: Linguistic? (Answer: *Unlikely.*)
      H. Ask question: Semantic? (Answer: *Unlikely.*)
      I. Because there is only one *yes*, we are ready to go on to Step 2.
   II. *Make initial conclusion re: rule by describing the difference between target and client production.*
      A. Fill in the violated parameter, as per Step 1 (in this case, voicing).
      B. Describe what the client is doing: A voiced consonant is becoming unvoiced.
      C. Label the rule: Devoicing of Consonants.
  III. *Perform Consistency Check.*
      A. Go to Consistency Checklist and place the word analyzed in Steps 1 and 2 into the *yes* column, indicating that the rule (Devoicing of Consonants) is working for that word.

B. Go back to Farrell's gloss (speech sample) and find the first word in which Devoicing of Consonants could occur (i.e., *save*). Ask yourself: Does it occur? If so, put word into the *yes* column; if not, put it in the *no* column. (Answer: *Yes*. Devoicing of Consonants occurs in *save* so the word is placed in the *yes* column.)

C. Repeat Step B for the /d/ in *dig*. (Answer: *No*. For the first time, we have come across a sound that could be subject to the Devoicing rule but is not. Thus, the word should be placed in the *no* column, with the /d/ circled to specify the sound being considered.)

D. Repeat Step B for the /g/ in *dig*. (Answer: *Yes*. Word should be placed in the *yes* column with the /g/ circled to specify the sound being considered.)

E. Repeat Step B with *boat*. (Answer: *No*. Put word in the *no* column.)

F. Repeat Step B with *do*. (Answer: *No*. Word goes in *no* column.)

G. Repeat Step B with *zoo*. (Answer: *No*. Put in *no* column.)

H. Repeat Step B with the /b/ in *bad*. (Answer: *No*. Put in *no* column and circle the /b/.)

I. Repeat Step B with the /d/ in *bad*. (Answer: *Yes*. Put in *yes* column and circle the /d/ sound.)

For the first time, we have a seeming inconsistency, with four words in the *yes* column and five words designated *no*. But if you circle all of the sounds being studied, a pattern begins to emerge. (If you were unable to complete Farrell #2 on your own, go now to the completed Consistency Checklist in Appendix A, look at the two columns and see if you can decipher the pattern.) This pattern is very easily seen, especially after studying the two columns of words for a few moments. Voiced sounds become voiceless when they are in the final position of a word. However, when they occur in the initial word position, these voiced sounds retain their voicing (i.e., do not change). Given this newly discovered pattern, we can now alter the label for the rule from Devoicing of Consonants to a more accurate Devoicing of Final Consonants. This new rule description should be placed on the bottom line of the Consistency Checklist. Now, to continue with our analysis . . .

IV. *Describe rule in final form.*
   A. Transfer the final rule description (in this case, Devoicing of Final Consonants) from the bottom of the Consistency Checklist to the appropriate space on the generic worksheet.

V. *Go to phonological rule summary, find all words for which rule is operating, and note.*
   A. On the phonological rule summary, go to each word exhibiting Devoicing of Final Consonants and record that rule in the appropriate column.

VI. *Perform final check.*
   A. Return to the first word that has been studied (i.e., *save*). Ask question: Does Devoicing of Final Consonants totally explain the error? If

PHONOLOGICAL RULE SUMMARY

Client: _FARRELL ZEISCREEM #2_

Check	Target Word	Client Production	Rule(s) Operating
✓	save	ses	FCD; AA
✓	dig	dɪt	FCD; AA
✓	pig	pɪk	Final Consonant Devoicing
✓	sick	sɪt	Alveolar Assimilation
✓	peek	pik	(correct)
✓	boat	dot	AA
✓	do	du	(correct)
✓	zoo	zu	(correct)
✓	bad	dæt	FCD; AA

so, check off the word. If not, skip the word with the intention of returning to it later. (Answer: *No*. Something else is going on when *save* → /ses/ besides Final Consonant Devoicing, so the word is skipped for now.)

B. Go to the remaining words studied and repeat Step A. (Answers: *pig* should be checked off; *dig* and *bad* should be skipped at this point.)

Determination of Farrell #2's first rule is now complete. There is no need for us to repeat the steps involved in determination of Farrell's second rule, as the remainder of Farrell #2's words are identical to those seen in Farrell #1 and the result would be the same—Alveolar Assimilation. So this Farrell's two rules are Devoicing of Final Consonants and Alveolar Assimilation. (See completed phonological rule summary for Farrell #2 on page 143.)

Discussion

Farrell #2 demonstrated a rule that, at first glance, seemed inconsistent. However, after putting the words in the appropriate *yes* and *no* columns and studying them for a while, we were able to decipher some consistency in the seemingly inconsistent data. What began as inconsistent Devoicing of Consonants became consistent Devoicing of Final Consonants when the words were organized in a systematic fashion.

Devoicing of Final Consonants is what is known as a *limited rule*. A limited rule is just as consistent as any other rule the client may demonstrate. However, some form of limitation exists (in the case of Farrell #2, a limitation by position in the word).

The good news is, limited rule is the last bit of new terminology you will need to know in order to perform a phonological analysis. But there is some bad news to go with the good. Unfortunately, we have only begun to scratch the surface in our study of limited rules. In fact, the concept of limited rules has been seriously underinvestigated in the field of speech-language pathology. Yet the concept is a vitally important one, because limited rules are the major contributors to what looks like inconsistency in our client's speech. Most of what we call inconsistent, isn't. It is just that we have not yet found the limitation that the client is using. This is one of the reasons why our Consistency Check is so important; it organizes our data so that we can determine the consistency in speech that at first glance seems inconsistent.

Much more will be presented on the topic of inconsistency in the next chapter. However, prior to ending this section on intermediate generative analysis, it would be beneficial to undertake one more practice exercise.

Clinical Mastery Exercise—Parsippany Ugg

Introduction

This practice exercise is a good one to help evaluate how well you are doing. There are two rules working in Parsippany's phonological system, and although these rules may be embedded in some words, there are enough golden words provided to help you find the rules with little problem. As you have been urged before, try not to cut corners at this stage, even if you feel you know a way to speed up the process. In other words, begin with the initial word in the speech sample, ask yourself the appropriate questions in Step 1, and finish all steps in the analysis prior to going to the second rule. If you can complete this exercise with few or no problems, you will be ready for advanced generative analysis, and some time-saving procedures that will help ease the workload.

Worksheets required for Parsippany (in correct order of use)
- Phonological rule summary
- Generic 6-step procedure
- Generic 6-step procedure
- Parameter Confusion Test
- Consistency Check Form
- Generic 6-step procedure
- Consistency Check Form

(Solution on page 153)

PHONOLOGICAL RULE SUMMARY

Client: _PARSIPPANY UGG_

Check	Target Word	Client Production	Rule(s) Operating
	soup	pup	(correct)
	cat	kæt	
	cup	pʌp	
	fake	pep	
	talk	tɔk	(correct)
	sick	tɪk	
	sheep	pip	
	shake	tek	

PROCEDURE FOR PHONOLOGICAL ANALYSIS — GENERIC WORKSHEET

I. **Take one error and choose possible parameters**

        ERROR:

        ANALYSIS: Manner? ————▶

                      Voicing? ————▶

                      Placement? ———▶   ┌─────────────────────┐

                      Context? ————▶   │ If unclear as to whether │

                      Structure? ———▶   │ placement or context, │

                      Linguistic? ——▶   │ perform Parameter Confu- │

                      Semantic? ———▶   │ sion Test (See Form). │

                                            │ Otherwise go to Step II. │

                                            └─────────────────────┘

II. **Make initial conclusion re: rule by describing the difference between target and client production.**

        _____ **PARAMETER**

                Description: _____

                Rule: _____

III. **Perform Consistency Check (See Consistency Check Form)**

IV. **Describe rule in Final Form**

                Rule: _____

V. **Go to phonological rule summary, find all words for which rule is operating, and note.**

VI. **Perform final check**

                — Make sure all changes in target word can be explained by rule. If so, check the word off. If not, leave until next analysis.

<u>PROCEDURE FOR PHONOLOGICAL ANALYSIS — GENERIC WORKSHEET</u>

I. <u>Take one error and choose possible parameters</u>

ERROR:
ANALYSIS: Manner? ———————▶

Voicing? ———————▶

Placement? ————————▶

Context? ————————▶

Structure? ————————▶

Linguistic? ————————▶

Semantic? ————————▶

> If unclear as to whether placement or context, perform Parameter Confusion Test (See Form). Otherwise go to Step II.

II. <u>Make initial conclusion re: rule by describing the difference between target and client production.</u>

_____ PARAMETER

Description: _____

Rule: _____

III. <u>Perform Consistency Check (See Consistency Check Form)</u>

IV. <u>Describe rule in Final Form</u>

Rule: _____

V. <u>Go to phonological rule summary, find all words for which rule is operating, and note.</u>

VI. <u>Perform final check</u>

— Make sure all changes in target word can be explained by rule. If so, check the word off. If not, leave until next analysis.

PLACEMENT CONTEXT. PARAMETER CONFUSION CHECK

Target Word: _____

Client Production: _____

Choose Test Word: _____
   (Word in which there's no culprit; i.e no
     chance for assimilation to occur).

Error Still Occur? _____Yes

               _____No

   Yes = Placement error; even though chance for assimilation has been
        removed, error still occurs.

   No = Assimilation error; error disappears when culprit is removed.

Return to Step 1 – Generic Worksheet

CONSISTENCY CHECKLIST

Initial Rule Description: _____

Rule Operating **(Yes)**	Rule Not Operating **(No)**

Check for Consistency	**Yes** Words	**No** Words	Sig. Diff.
1. **Phonetic Context**			
— List vowel preceding			
— List vowel following			
— List consonant preceding			
— List consonant following			
— List other sig. non-adjacent sounds			
2. **Position**			
— List I, M, F for initial medial, final			
3. **Intra-class Variability**			
— List correct/incorrect sounds, search for intra-class patterns			
4. **Syllable Structure/ Word Length**			
— List syllable structures			
5. **Part of Speech/Morphological Endings**			
— List grammatical categories			
6. **Syllable Stress**			
— List U, S for unstressed, stressed			
7. **Syllable Boundary**			
— List words/Draw line between syllable boundaries; Note differences			

Note other factors: Elicitation mode, situational context, overlearned words, etc.

Final Rule Description: _____

PROCEDURE FOR PHONOLOGICAL ANALYSIS — GENERIC WORKSHEET

I. Take one error and choose possible parameters

ERROR:
ANALYSIS: Manner? ————▶

Voicing? ————▶

Placement? ————▶

Context? ————▶

Structure? ————▶

Linguistic? ————▶

Semantic? ————▶

> If unclear as to whether placement or context, perform Parameter Confusion Test (See Form). Otherwise go to Step II.

II. Make initial conclusion re: rule by describing the difference between target and client production.

_____ PARAMETER

Description: _____

Rule: _____

III. Perform Consistency Check (See Consistency Check Form)

IV. Describe rule in Final Form

Rule: _____

V. Go to phonological rule summary, find all words for which rule is operating, and note.

VI. Perform final check

— Make sure all changes in target word can be explained by rule. If so, check the word off. If not, leave until next analysis.

CONSISTENCY CHECKLIST

Initial Rule Description: _____

Rule Operating **(Yes)**	Rule Not Operating **(No)**

Check for Consistency	**Yes** Words	**No** Words	Sig. Diff.
1. **Phonetic Context**			
— List vowel preceding			
— List vowel following			
— List consonant preceding			
— List consonant following			
— List other sig. non-adjacent sounds			
2. **Position**			
— List I, M, F for initial medial, final			
3. **Intra-class Variability**			
— List correct/incorrect sounds, search for intra-class patterns			
4. **Syllable Structure/ Word Length**			
— List syllable structures			
5. **Part of Speech/Morphological Endings**			
— List grammatical categories			
6. **Syllable Stress**			
— List U, S for unstressed, stressed			
7. **Syllable Boundary**			
— List words/Draw line between syllable boundaries; Note differences			

Note other factors: Elicitation mode, situational context, overlearned words, etc.

Final Rule Description: _____

Solution

I. *Take one error and choose possible parameters.*
   A. Fill in the error being analyzed (*soup* → /pup/).
   B. Ask question: Manner? (Answer: *Yes*. The /s/ in *soup* is a fricative whereas the /p/ in /pup/ is a stop.)
   C. Ask question: Voicing? (Answer: *No*.)
   D. Ask question: Placement? (Answer: *Maybe*. Perhaps Parsippany has a problem whereby she cannot produce sounds having an alveolar placement and changes all of these sound to labials. However, there is another explanation.)
   E. Ask question: Context? (Answer: *Maybe*. Perhaps the final /p/ in *soup* is a labial culprit, causing the initial sound to move to the labial position; maybe Parsippany has no problem with the production of alveolars after all.)

With one *yes* and two *maybes* there is no need to continue this first step. There are at least two rules working and as per our guidelines, we will now go on to Parsippany's second error and re-attempt an analysis.

I. *Take one error and choose possible parameters.*
   A. Fill in the error being analyzed (*cup* → /pʌp/).
   B. Ask question: Manner? (Answer: *No*.)
   C. Ask question: Voicing? (Answer: *No*.)
   D. Ask question: Placement? (Answer: *Maybe*. It could be that Parsippany has an inability to produce sounds having a velar placement and changes them all to labials. However, there is an alternative explanation.)
   E. Ask question: Context? (Answer: *Maybe*. Perhaps the first sound in *cup* is moving to the labial position only because of a labial culprit at the end of the word. Perhaps it is an assimilation rather than a placement problem.)
   F. Ask question: Structure? (Answer: *No*.)
   G. Ask question: Linguistic? (Answer: *Unlikely*.)
   H. Ask question: Semantic? (Answer: *Unlikely*.)
   I. Because we have two *maybes*, our next step is to undertake a Parameter Confusion Test.
I-a. *Parameter Confusion Test.*
   A. On the appropriate form, note the target word on the line indicated (i.e., *cup*).
   B. Indicate the client's production on the next line (i.e., /pʌp/).
   C. Choose test word. An appropriate test word will contain a velar but will not have a labial culprit. (There are several possibilities for test words, including *cat, talk, sick,* or *shake*. We cannot choose *fake* because the /f/ is a labial. For our purposes, we will choose the word *talk*.)

    D. Does the error still occur? (Answer: *No.* When the culprit [i.e., the chance for assimilation] has been eliminated, the velar is produced with the correct placement. So the problem with *cup* → /pʌp/ is one of assimilation, not placement.)

    E. Return to Step 1 of the 6-step procedure. Cross out the *maybe* after placement and write *no.* Then cross out the *maybe* after context and indicate *yes.* Now we can proceed with Step 2. (See Appendix A for completed Parameter Confusion Test worksheet.)

  II. *Make initial conclusion re: rule by describing the difference between target and client production.*

    A. Fill in the violated parameter, as per Step 1 (i.e., context).

    B. Describe what the client is doing: When there is a labial in a word, other sounds in the word go to the labial position.

    C. Label the rule: Labial Assimilation.

  III. *Perform Consistency Check.*

    A. Go to the Consistency Checklist and place the word analyzed in Steps 1 and 2 (*cup*) into the *yes* column.

    B. One by one, go to each word in the sample having the possibility for labial assimilation (*soup, fake, sheep*).

Why does fake *have the possibility for Labial Assimilation?*

Because the *f* in *fake* is a labial, specifically a labiodental.

    Does labial assimilation take place in these words? If so, put the word in the *yes* column; if not, put it in the *no* column. (Answer: *Yes* for all three words; each of the words with a possible culprit exhibits Labial Assimilation.)

    C. Fill in the final rule description (i.e., Labial Assimilation) on the bottom line of the Consistency Checklist. (See Appendix A for completed checklist.)

  IV. *Describe rule in final form.*

    A. Transfer the final rule description from the bottom of the Consistency Checklist to the appropriate space on the generic worksheet.

  V. *Go to phonological rule summary, find all words for which rule is operating, and note.*

    A. On the rule summary sheet, go to each word having Labial Assimilation and record that rule in the appropriate column.

  VI. *Perform final check.*

    A. Return to the first error listed on the phonological rule summary (i.e., *soup*). Ask question: Is the error now totally explained by the rule listed? (Answer: *No.* If only Labial Assimilation was working, *soup* would become /fup/, not /pup/, as it does. Skip the word for now and return to it later.)

    B. Ask the same question with the next word analyzed (i.e., *cup*). (Answer: *Yes*. Check the word off.)

    C. Ask the same question with *fake*. (Answer: *No*. If only Labial Assimilation was working, *fake* would have become /fep/. Skip the word.)

    D. Ask the same question with *sheep*. (Answer: *No*. Skip the word for now.)

Having determined the first of Parsippany's rules, our next step is to go on to the next error in the speech sample (i.e., the *f* in *fake*) and repeat the process.

  I. *Take one error and choose possible parameters.*

    A. Fill in the error being analyzed (*fake* → /pep/, with the focus on the initial /f/ becoming /p/).

    B. Ask question: Manner? (Answer: *Yes*. The /f/ in *fake* is a fricative whereas the /p/ in /pep/ is a stop.)

    C. Ask question: Voicing? (Answer: *No*.)

    D. Ask question: Placement? (Answer: *No*. Remember, /p/ is the natural stopping place for /f/.)

    E. Ask question: Context? (Answer: *No*.)

    F. Ask question: Structure? (Answer: *No*.)

    G. Ask question: Linguistic? (Answer: *Unlikely*.)

    H. Ask question: Semantic? (Answer: *Unlikely*.)

    I. Because we have one *yes* and no confusion, we can go on to Step 2.

  II. *Make initial conclusion re: rule by describing the difference between target and client production.*

    A. Fill in the violated parameter, as per Step 1 (in this case, manner).

    B. Describe what the client is doing: A fricative is becoming a stop.

    C. Label the rule: Stopping of Fricatives.

  III. *Perform Consistency Check.*

    A. Go to Consistency Checklist and put the word analyzed in Steps 1 and 2 into the *yes* column. You may also want to circle the /f/ in *fake* to indicate the sound that has been analyzed.

    B. One by one, evaluate the other words in the speech sample that have a possibility for Stopping of Fricatives (*soup, sick, sheep, shake*). Does Stopping of Fricatives occur? If so, put the given word into the *yes* column; if not, put it in the *no* column. (Answer: *Yes* for all four words.)

    C. Fill in the final rule description (i.e., Stopping of Fricatives) on the bottom line of the Consistency Checklist. (See Appendix A for completed checklist.)

  IV. *Describe rule in final form.*

    A. Transfer the final rule description from the bottom of the Consistency Checklist to the appropriate space on the generic worksheet.

  V. *Go to phonological rule summary, find all words for which rule is operating, and note.*

    A. On the rule summary sheet, go to the five words exhibiting Stopping of Fricatives and record the rule in the appropriate column.

VI. *Perform final check.*

A. Return once again to the first error listed on the phonological rule summary (i.e., *soup*). Ask question: Is the error now totally explained by the two rules listed? (Answer: *Yes. Soup* becomes /tʉp/ as a result of Stopping of Fricatives, and then /tʉp/ becomes /pʉp/ after Labial Assimilation. Or if you go in the other direction, *soup* → /fʉp/ [Labial Assimilation] and /fʉp/ → /pʉp/ [Stopping of Fricatives].)

B. Ask the same question with the next unchecked word that has been analyzed (i.e., *fake*). (Answer: *Yes. Fake* → /pek/ [Stopping of Fricatives] and /pek/ → /pep/ [Labial Assimilation].)

C. Ask the same question with *sick*. (Answer: *Yes.* Check off the word.)

D. Ask the same question with *sheep*. (Answer: *Yes. Sheep* becomes /fip/ [Labial Assimilation] and /fip/ → /pip/ [Stopping of Fricatives].)

E. Ask the same question with *shake*. (Answer: *Yes.* Check off the word.)

F. Because all misarticulated words have been checked off, Parsippany's analysis is now complete. (See completed phonological rule summary on page 157.)

PHONOLOGICAL RULE SUMMARY

Client: _PARSIPPANY UGG_

Check	Target Word	Client Production	Rule(s) Operating
✔	soup	pup	labial assimilation; stopping of fricatives (correct)
✔	cat	kæt	labial assimilation
✔	cup	pʌp	l.a.; stopping of fricatives (correct)
✔	fake	pep	
✔	talk	tɔk	s.f.
✔	sick	tɪk	s.f.
✔	sheep	pip	l.a.; s.f.
✔	shake	tek	s.f.

Practice in Prediction

As explained earlier in this chapter, now that we know Parsippany's rule system, we can predict how she will articulate words not included in her original speech sample. The following 10 words will provide you with additional practice in prediction. For each word, factor in the two rules previously determined (Labial Assimilation, Stopping of Fricatives) in order to arrive at a projection of what Parsippany would say (answers appear in Appendix A).

1. *shop* $\longrightarrow$
2. *five* $\longrightarrow$
3. *fog* $\longrightarrow$
4. *sash* $\longrightarrow$ (be careful!)
5. *push* $\longrightarrow$
6. *vase* $\longrightarrow$
7. *calf* $\longrightarrow$
8. *bath* $\longrightarrow$
9. *fish* $\longrightarrow$
10. *sofa* $\longrightarrow$ (be careful!)

Discussion

This concludes our discussion of intermediate generative analysis. If, at this point, you are feeling secure in the material presented thus far, feel free to skip this section and go directly to Chapter 7. If, on the other hand, you are feeling a bit overwhelmed, you are not unusual. In fact, you have now reached what many clinicians consider to be the toughest point in the learning process. Why is this the case? There are many reasons. First, although you have learned just enough to be able to complete a phonological analysis of a client having two rules, you possibly feel that you are not as adept or quick with the procedure as you would like. At the same time, you have probably now begun to realize just how much practice lies ahead before you do indeed feel comfortable with generative phonological analysis. Finally, because the difficulty of the practice exercises has increased so gradually, you may not have a clear sense of how much you have learned thus far. This last problem is easily remedied: go back to Flora or Raoul in the last chapter and try to complete those exercises again. Surely you will be amazed at how easy these exercises are for you at this point. As for the other problems, try to realize that you are on the same road that hundreds if not thousands of clinicians have navigated in the past. And believe it or not, the end of the road is closer than you think.

CHAPTER ◆ 7

The Question of Inconsistency in Speech Sound Production

Imagine the following situation: Yolanda, a 4-year-old girl with mostly unintelligible speech, is being evaluated for the first time. As the clinician shows her the first item from the *Goldman-Fristoe Test of Articulation* (i.e., *house*), Yolanda says something that sounds like /da/. The clinician tentatively marks down a /d/ for /h/ substitution (initial position) and an omission of /s/ (final position). However, she is uncertain whether she has heard Yolanda correctly, so she says, "Tell me again. What did you call this?" This time, Yolanda replies /tat/.

In traditional speech evaluation, the existence, and perhaps even the inevitability, of inconsistency on the part of the client has always been accepted. Even today, many phonologically oriented investigators have reconciled themselves to the belief that clients are frequently inconsistent in their output. For example, Hodson and Paden (1983), in their assessment procedure for phonological disorders, recommended that clinicians calculate percentages of occurrence for each of the phonological rules exhibited by their clients. Further, in four examples of real children provided by Hodson and Paden (1983), only 10 of the 36 rules exhibited by the children achieve a 100% level of occurrence (or consistency). It is quite clear that inconsistency is expected and accepted as part of this assessment procedure.

But even if the existence of inconsistency of speech sound production has been accepted by many clinicians and test authors alike, the question of what to do about that inconsistency has remained an enigma. For example, do we treat inconsistency as something positive, as Van Riper (1972) did? In fact, one of his primary therapeutic techniques, the *key word approach*, was based on the idea that inconsistent correct production of an error sound was a positive sign for therapy (Van Riper, 1972). Or do we regard inconsistency as a negative factor, indicative of a deviant organism? For example, one of the primary defining characteristics of childhood apraxia, a disorder thought by many to result from a deviant organism, is inconsistency of speech sound production (e.g., see Robin, 1992; Hall, 1992).

Fortunately, recent evidence has accumulated (e.g., see Camarata & Gandour, 1984; Leonard, 1985; Leonard & Brown, 1984; Leonard & Leonard, 1985) which indicates that we may not have to do anything about inconsistency after all . . . because it may not exist. In fact, it seems more and more likely that any inconsistency we think we see is instead an artifact created by our own inability to find the consistent pattern.

A Few Examples

Child #007, J.B., says /kʌp/ for *cup* but /pɪt/ for *pick*. Inconsistent? Maybe . . . after all he does say the /k/ correctly in *cup* yet substitutes the /t/ for the /k/ in *pick*. However, a two-word sample is hardly sufficient to allow for any definitive conclusions, so let us study the larger speech sample below:

Target	Child #007 Response
cup	/kʌp/
pick	/pɪt/
cat	/kæt/
car	/kaʊ/
rake	/wet/
sick	/tɪt/
cold	/kot/
cake	/ket/
book	/bʊt/
walk	/wɔt/
back	/bæt/

Is J.B.'s speech still inconsistent? It certainly seems to be. For example, the /k/ sound is correct in *cup, cat, car,* and *cold* but is incorrect in *pick, rake, sick, book, walk,* and *back*. In *cake*, one of the /k/ sounds is produced correctly, one incorrectly. You can hardly get more inconsistent than that—depending, of course, on what you choose to call "inconsistent." To illustrate, let us arrange these same words in a different fashion. This time, we shall separate the words with misarticulated /k/ sounds from those with correct /k/ production.

Incorrect /k/ production	Correct /k/ production
pi(ck)	(c)up
ra(ke)	(c)at
si(ck)	(c)ar
ca(ke)	(c)old
bo(ok)	(c)ake
wa(lk)	
ba(ck)	

At this point, the pattern is so obvious that many of you may be wondering about the point of this particular exercise. But stick with it for a few more minutes. One clinician miqht describe J.B. as having inconsistent production of the /k/ sound. But it is probably more accurate to refer to J.B as consistent—because he does indeed demonstrate a consistent rule: Whenever /k/ is in the initial position, he will produce the sound correctly; when it is in the final position, the /k/ will be switched to a /t/ sound. In this case, J.B. has a consistent, but limited rule, as was first described in the last chapter.

You may still be thinking "So what?" Child #008 should help to clarify the issue. As you will see, Child #008 also has speech which seems to be inconsistent. Let us study the gloss:

Target	Child #008 Response
book	/bʊk/
cap	/tæp/
keep	/tip/
deck	/dɛt/
joke	/dok/
back	/bæt/
cool	/kμo/
coke	/kok/
wake	/wet/
sock	/tak/
bike	/baɪt/
caught	/kɔt/

Once again, Child #008 seems to be inconsistent in his /t/ for /k/ substitution. But separating the words into columns of correct and incorrect production again allows us to study the words more closely. See if you can figure out the difference between words in the correct column and those in the incorrect column on the next page.

Incorrect /k/ production	Correct /k/ production
(c)ap	boo(k)
(k)eep	jo(ke)
de(ck)	(c)ool
ba(ck)	(c)ake
wa(ke)	so(ck)
bi(ke)	(c)aught

As both initial and final sounds are produced both correctly and incorrectly it seems clear that position is not the factor responsible for Child #008's errors. But as you will soon see, position is not the only factor that can create a limited (yet consistent) rule. In fact, there are at least 11 phonolinguistic factors that can help to obscure the consistency in speech which, upon first study, seems inconsistent. In the case of Child #008, for example, consider the vowels that are adjacent to the /k/ sounds in each of the words.

Adjacent vowels in correctly produced words: /ʊ/, /o/, /o/, / o/, / a/, /ɔ/

Adjacent vowels in incorrectly produced words: /æ/, /i/, /ɛ/, /æ/, /e/, /aɪ/

A pattern begins to emerge. Child #008 produces the /k/ correctly in words having a back vowel adjacent to the sound. However, if a front vowel is adjacent, Child #008 substitutes /t/ for /k/. Once again, we have a limited rule. Once again, misarticulations that seem to be inconsistent and randomly produced become consistent when studied in a systematic fashion.

Clinical Mastery Exercise—Ho Lee Moe Lee

Introduction

Ho (not his real name) was a very real 6-year-old boy who demonstrated several interesting behaviors. First of all, he was fully intelligible when tested on formal articulation tests. Yet he was mostly unintelligible during spontaneous conversation. Second, his speech seemed unyieldingly inconsistent. In fact, he even said the same word differently on a number of occasions. For example, if he was just saying the word *hot*, he would produce it correctly (i.e., /hat/). But in a two-word phrase like *hot foot*, he would leave off the final /t/ in *hot* (i.e., /hafʊt/). Yet in the two-word phrase *hot air*, the /t/ would again be produced correctly.

Refer to Ho's gloss on page 163. Because identification of the exact rule is not the goal here, we will skip the first two steps of the 6-step generic procedure and go right on to the Consistency Check. Study Ho's speech output for a few minutes and then place each phrase in either the *yes* (rule operating) or *no* (rule not operating) column of the abbreviated Consistency Checklist. (Notice that Ho's rule has arbitrarily been labeled "Strange Deletion Rule #1"). After all of Ho's phrases have been placed into either the *yes* or *no* columns, study the two lists and see if you can determine the consistent pattern underlying these seemingly inconsistent misarticulations. (Hint: Concentrate on the final consonants for each word. When does Ho delete the final consonants and when are the final consonants retained?)

(Solution on page 165)

PHONOLOGICAL RULE SUMMARY

Client: _Ho Lee Moe Lee_

Check	Target Word	Client Production	Rule(s) Operating
	hot foot	hafʊt	
	back up	bækʌp	
	big dog	bɪdɔg	
	big	bɪg	
	bag lady	bæwedi	
	big ape	bɪgep	
	big boy	bɪbɔɪ	
	that not	dænɔt	
	that over there	dætobʊdɛə	
	sick dog	tɪdɔg	

CONSISTENCY CHECKLIST

Initial Rule Description: _____

Rule Operating (Yes)	Rule Not Operating (No)

Solution

The abbreviated Consistency Checklist for Ho has been properly completed on page 166. For each phrase, the particular final consonant being studied has been circled. Upon close study, a pattern once again begins to emerge. Ho deletes final consonants in a word only when another consonant is adjacent, beginning the following word. So in *hot foot*, the /t/ in *hot* is deleted, because another consonant (/f/) begins the next word. But in *hot air*, the /t/ in *hot* is maintained because the following word begins with a vowel.

In short, the initial impression of inconsistent final consonant deletion has been shown to be inaccurate (or at least imprecise). What is really occurring: Ho consistently reduces clusters that arise across word boundaries. (As it turned out, he also reduced clusters within words. In other words, *stop* became /tap/. So his cluster reduction was actually consistent across all phonolinguistic contexts.)

CONSISTENCY CHECKLIST

Initial Rule Description: _Strange Deletion Rule #1_

Rule Operating (Yes)	Rule Not Operating (No)
ho(t)foot	hot foo(t) tha(t) over there
bi(g)dog	ba(ck)up sick do(g)
ba(g)lady	back u(p) b(g)
bi(g)boy	bigd(og)
tha(t)not	bi(g)ape
si(ck)dog	big (ape)
	thafn(ot)

Discussion

If one thing has been learned from the revolution in phonology, it is the fact that how something is observed often influences what is observed. Nowhere does this prove to be more true than in our search for consistency. As the previous examples have shown, speech that looks inconsistent often becomes consistent once we have organized our observations in a different way. Unsurpris-ingly, this is exactly what investigators have found as well. Camarata and Gandour (1984) reported on a child whose supposedly inconsistent speech became consistent after studying the vowel following the sound in question. Leonard and Leonard (1985) reported on another child whose supposedly inconsistent speech became consistent after considering the effect of the neighboring consonant. Other researchers have found additional factors that have served to mask consistent speech, such as linguistic task, listener status, part of speech, and others (Bowman, Parsons, & Morris, 1984; Leonard, 1985; Leonard & Brown, 1984; Schwartz, Messick & Pollock, 1983).

In all, there are at least 11 factors that can help create the look of inconsistency in what is, upon keener analysis, consistent speech. Let us consider each of these possible factors separately:

1. Phonetic context. The phonetic context of a target sound may determine how that sound is produced. For example, perhaps the vowel before or after the target sound is affecting the production of that sound. So maybe a child has labial assimilation only after or before vowels with lip rounding. Otherwise, no labial assimilation is seen. Alternatively, perhaps another consonant before or after the target sound is affecting the production of that sound. So maybe a child stops fricatives only in words that contain another stop. (For example, *sun* is produced correctly but *soup* becomes /tup/). Some other examples:

- Fronting of velars in words with /b/ or /p/.

- Deletion of final consonants in words with high vowels.

2. Position. This particular factor is one that historically has been considered by some speech pathologists performing traditional analyses, albeit perhaps not as systematically as possible. Actually, however, position-bound limited rules don't seem to occur all that often. It is just that, given our traditional familiarity with this form of limited rule, as analysts we tend to think of this factor first and most frequently; however, further analysis will usually confirm that a different factor is creating the seeming inconsistency. Nonetheless, position-bound limited rules do sometimes occur. Some examples:

- Fronting of initial velar sounds.
- Stopping of final fricatives.

3. Intra-class variability. Sometimes a rule will seem consistent except for one or two particular sounds. For example, sometimes children will delete most final consonants but maintain the final nasals correctly. So the child might say /ta/ for *top*, but then say the name *Tom* correctly. This is a sound-dependent limited rule in which the seeming inconsistency is caused by intra-class variability. Some additional examples:

- Stopping of fricatives except for /s/ and /z/ (i.e., stopping of nonalveolar fricatives).
- Labial assimilation except in words with /m/.

4. Syllable structure. Periodically a given rule will occur only in certain limited syllable structures. So a child might front velars only in words more complex than a CVC syllable structure. Again this is a rule that seems inconsistent until your systematic analysis uncovers the consistency. More examples:

- Deletion of final consonants only in words having CVC syllable structures.
- Stopping of fricatives in CV words only.

5. Word length. This factor is, of course, closely related to syllable structure. (Obviously, a longer word will have a more complex syllable structure, and vice versa.) A common limited rule bound by word length in unintelligible children is "Deletion of medial and final consonants in multisyllabic words" where the child might say *tell* correctly and might say *phone* with reasonable accuracy but *telephone* becomes /tɛʔʌʔo/ or *teh-uh-oh*.

6. Part of speech. Although this is most likely a rarely occurring factor, we have seen at least two children who have altered their articulation depending on the part of speech or word class of the target. For example, one child fronted velars in all parts of speech except verbs. A second child deleted final consonants except in verbs (this same child also deleted unstressed syllables except in verbs). In both children, the errors seemed inconsistent until the limitation by part of speech was discovered.

7. Morphological endings. A morphological ending communicates additional and different information to the listener than the body of a particular word. As such, it is unsurprising that some children would alter their basic articulation patterns in morphemes. For example, the child might normally stop fricatives, but produce the final /s/ or /z/ correctly when using the plural. In this case, inconsistent stopping of fricatives becomes stopping of fricatives except in morphemes. Another example: Deletion of unstressed morphemes, where the child includes all other unstressed syllables and all morphemes occurring in stressed syllables.

8. Syllable stress. A fairly common rule limitation relates to the stress of a given syllable. Unstressed syllables frequently tend to work differently than stressed syllables in the phonological systems of individuals with speech disorders. So one child might demonstrate fronting of velars only in unstressed syllables; in stressed syllables, on the other hand, velars are produced correctly. Inconsistent fronting of velars becomes consistent fronting of velars in unstressed syllables. Some other examples of limited rules mediated by syllable stress:

- Stopping of fricatives in unstressed syllables.
- Alveolar assimilation in unstressed syllables only.

9. Syllable boundary. Sometimes the positioning of the syllable boundary will have a systematic effect on the child's production of particular words. Indeed, limited rules related to syllable boundary are often the cause of unintelligible conversational speech in children who are mostly intelligible in single word articulation tests. So perhaps a child demonstrates cluster reduction only when a syllable boundary occurs between elements of the cluster. This child would say the word *star* correctly, but the word *mister* becomes /mɪtɚ/.

10. Elicitation mode. This is another primary factor creating the look of inconsistency in speech that is essentially consistent. Consider this scenario: A child is presented with a picture of a *cup* and is asked to label it. He says /tʌ/. However, you (the examiner) are not certain what he said so you ask him to say it again. This time he says /kʌ/. This time you decide to use imitation. "Say *cup*," you say. He says /kʌk/. Three attempts at the same word; three different productions. Is this child inconsistent? As indicated before, not necessarily. Attempt #1 occurred fairly spontaneously after being requested to name the picture. By the time attempt #2 occurred, the child most likely thought he was wrong the first time, so he probably tried to change something. Attempt #3 of course changed the conditions again. Thus, the child may consistently omit final consonants during spontaneous output. But he may also just as consistently include a final consonant appropriately after imitation. It is not that the child's output is inconsistent; it is instead the fact that the elicitation mode keeps changing.

Because many researchers have shown that the truest measure of a child's output occurs in spontaneous speech (e.g., see Dubois & Bernthal, 1978; Faircloth & Faircloth, 1970) it is important that, as much as possible, spontaneous speech or at least spontaneous picture naming be used to gather the data for performing a phonological analysis. Any deviation from this elicitation mode should be noted and if a child has a rule limitation that is mediated by the mode of elicitation (for example, deletion of final consonants except in imitation) that limitation should be noted.

11. Situational context. Some children demonstrate different speech patterns with different people. For example, we have seen several children who have "regressed" to more primitive speech patterns when playing with younger siblings. On a few other occasions, children have exhibited articulation errors *only* with their parents. The key is, the situational context of the interaction may indeed alter the client's phonological pattern—but this does not automatically indicate that the client is being inconsistent. Instead, he or she may be demonstrating a limited, but consistent rule.

A summary of the phonolinguistic factors just discussed appears on page 170. Any of these factors can lead the unwary examiner astray, creating the impression of inconsistency in speech output that is, in reality, consistent. In fact, after performing phonological analyses on hundreds of children and adults with speech disorders, we have recently arrived at a viewpoint that even we would have considered radical 5 years ago. Namely, that with only

three small exceptions, there is no such thing as inconsistent speech. Further, any inconsistency we think we see is due to our inability to decipher the consistent pattern. Now, this belief coincides with current phonological concepts of the child as a creator of an orderly rule-based system which has simplified the adult model. However, it threatens strongly our more traditional beliefs, where inconsistency was not only expected, but even thought to be positive by some. Nevertheless, as more clinicians analyze their clients' phonological systems more precisely, inconsistent errors are disappearing, to be replaced by consistent, yet limited rules. And as these same clinicians alter their therapy foci so that the clients' precise problems can now be targeted, improvement is enhanced and accelerated.

If one subscribes to the "no inconsistency" premise and one develops skill in discovering limited rules, does this mean that all inconsistency will disappear? Sadly no, not totally. Remember, there are three small exceptions to our "no inconsistency" premise; three conditions under which a small amount of inconsistent speech may still occur. Let us discuss those now:

1. Growth phases. When the child is in an active phonological growth phase, or when he or she is in the midst of effective therapy, you will undoubtedly see some inconsistency in his or her rule production.

2. Overlearned words. Both children (and adults) with phonological disorders periodically develop favored ways of articulating certain words. When this occurs, it becomes decidedly more difficult to change the errant pattern. Hence, many normal children continue saying "jammies" for *pajamas* right through their childhood years. For children with speech disorders, the overlearned words can be less socially acceptable, but just as resistant to change. So the child who has just eliminated fronting of velars from his or her error patterns may continue to say /ote/ for *okay*. For this child, a different therapy

Factors that can Create the Look of Inconsistency in Consistent Speech

1. **Position**
   Ex. Stopping of final fricatives
2. **Intra-Class Variability**
   Ex. Stopping of fricatives except for **s** and **z**
   or
   Stopping of non-alveolar fricatives
3. **Phonetic Context**
   Ex. Stopping of fricatives which follow high vowels
   or
   Stopping of fricatives in words with nasals
4. **Syllable Structure**
   Ex. Stopping of fricatives in CVC words
5. **Length of Word**
   Ex. Stopping of fricatives in multisyllabic words
6. **Part of Speech**
   Ex. Stopping of fricatives in non-nouns
7. **Morphological Endings**
   Ex. Deletion of unstressed morphemes
8. **Syllable Stress**
   Ex. Stopping of fricatives in unstressed syllables
9. **Syllable Boundary**
   Ex. Stopping of fricatives when the syllable boundary immediately precedes the fricative
10. **Elicitation Mode**
    Ex. Stopping of fricatives except in imitation
11. **Situational Context**
    Ex. Stopping of fricatives when playing with younger sister

approach would be needed to overcome this overlearned words phenomenon (see Chapter 14).

3. Transcription error. Probably the most frequently occurring residual inconsistency has nothing to do with the client. Unfortunately, human error is always a factor, even for phonetic transcribers who are well-practiced and, thus, highly skilled. Because most clinicians do not begin their sojourn into clinical phonology as expert phoneticists, the problem is compounded. However, the picture is not as bleak as it sounds. Because transcription errors tend to occur randomly, rarely if ever does it happen that identical transcription errors occur more than once or twice over several words. This makes these errors easy to detect and then discard upon inspection.

These three exceptions to our basic premise that all speech is consistent lead to two good rules of thumb. First, if during your analysis, you find a transcribed word or two that does not seem to fit in with the rest of your analysis, throw the word out. Ignore it; chances are that your transcription was inaccurate. On the other hand, if you find several instances in which your client produces a sound in one way, and several other instances in which she produces the sound in a different way, don't automatically assume that the client is being inconsistent. More likely, she is exhibiting a limited rule and you just have not yet been able to determine that limited rule.

Systematic Determination of Limited Rules

You will remember that in Chapter 6, we determined Farrell #2's limited rule just by placing the words in his sample into one of two columns (depending on whether or not the rule was exhibited) and then studying the data, looking for patterns. By looking at the two lists of words, we were able to discern a pattern whereby only final voiced consonants were devoiced; other voiced consonants maintained their voicing. Similarly, in the examples presented toward the beginning of this chapter, we were able to determine the limited rule just by looking at lists of *yes* words and *no* words, again grouped according to whether or not the rule was demonstrated.

Unfortunately, many clinicians, especially those with less practice in working with clinical phonology, are unable to discern limited rules just by studying the two lists of words. For this reason, the bottom two-thirds of the Consistency Checklist has been created. This bottom portion is essentially a worksheet that allows the clinician to systematically determine the consistency in lists of seemingly inconsistent words. But remember: If possible, the limited rule should be figured out just by studying the words in the *yes* and *no* columns and finding any patterns. If this search for patterns is unsuccessful, then the bottom worksheet portion can be utilized. In the remainder of this chapter, use of the worksheet portion of the Consistency Checklist will be explained and practice in figuring out some more subtle limited rules will be undertaken.

Understanding and Completing the Form: Child #007

In order to illustrate how the worksheet portion of the Consistency Checklist is meant to be used, we shall return for a bit to Child #007, J.B., who had the following speech sample:

Target	Child #007 Response
cup	/kʌp/
pick	/pɪt/
cat	/kæt/
car	/kaʊ/
rake	/wet/
sick	/tɪt/
cold	/kot/
cake	/ket/
book	/bʊt/
walk	/wɔt/
back	/bæt/

See the completed Consistency Checklist for Child #007 on page 173. As the procedure is presented and discussed, follow along with the completed form.

Step 1: *Visual inspection of* yes-no *columns*
  A. After listing each relevant word from the client's speech sample in either the *yes* column or the *no* column depending on whether or not the rule is in operation, study the two lists of words.
  B. Try to find a systematic difference between the words on the left (*yes* words) and the words on the right (*no* words). Make certain that any difference found is consistent for all the words on the list.
  C. If you determine the systematic difference by means of this visual inspection, skip down to the bottom of the checklist and fill in the newly discovered limited rule. (In the case of J.B., as discussed earlier in the chapter, it is easy to see, just through visual inspection, that the limited rule is Fronting of Final Velars. Normally we would fill in that newly determined rule on the bottom of our checklist and then continue with our generic analysis. However, in the interests of extra practice, let us assume that we could *not* determine the limitation by means of visual inspection and instead would have to use the worksheet to find the limited rule.)

Step 2: *Systematic Consistency Check*
  A. Evaluate phonetic context.
    1. Vowel preceding: For the yes words—/ɪ/, /e/, /ɪ/, /e/, /ʊ/, /ɔ/, and /æ/. For the *no* words—nothing; there are no vowels preceding the target /k/. As preceding vowels do not even exist for many of the words studied, this certainly cannot be

CONSISTENCY CHECKLIST

Initial Rule Description: _Fronting of Velars_

Rule Operating **(Yes)**	Rule Not Operating **(No)**
pi(ck) c(up)	
ra(ke) (cat)	
si(ck) (jar)	
ca(ke) (cold)	
boo(k) (cake)	
wa(lk)	
b(ack)	

Check for Consistency	Yes Words	No Words	Sig. Diff.
1. Phonetic Context	/ɪ/,/e/,/ɪ/,/e/,/ʊ/,/ɔ/,/æ/	Not Applicable	NO
— List vowel preceding	Not Applicable	/ʌ/,/æ/,/a/,/o/,/e/	NO
— List vowel following	/p/,/r/,/s/,/k/,/b/,/w/,/b/	Not Applicable	NO
— List consonant preceding	Not Applicable	/p/,/t/,/d/,/k/	NO
— List consonant following			
— List other sig. non-adjacent sounds	Visual Check ——————————————→		No
2. Position	F,F,F,F,F,F,F	I,I,I,I,I	Yes!
— List I, M, F for initial medial, final			
3. Intra-class Variability			
— List correct/incorrect sounds, search for intra-class patterns			
4. Syllable Structure/ Word Length			
— List syllable structures			
5. Part of Speech/Morphological Endings			
— List grammatical categories			
6. Syllable Stress			
— List U, S for unstressed, stressed			
7. Syllable Boundary			
— List words/Draw line between syllable boundaries; Note differences			

Note other factors: Elicitation mode, situational context, overlearned words, etc.

Final Rule Description: _Fronting of Final Velars_

173

the factor creating the significant difference between the two lists of words and causing the look of inconsistency.

2. Vowel following: For *yes* words—nothing. No vowels follow the target in the *yes* words. For *no* words—/ʌ/, /æ/, /a/, /o/, and /e/. Once again, as half of the words don't even have a "following vowel," this factor is eliminated in our search for the cause of the seeming inconsistency.

3. Consonant preceding: For *yes* words—/p/, /r/, /s/, /k/, /b/, /w/, and /b/. For *no* words—no preceding consonants. This again cannot be the factor we are seeking.

4. Consonant following: For *yes* words—no following consonants. For *no* words—/p/, / t/, /d/, and /k/. Again, with several words having no following consonant, this factor cannot be creating the limitation.

5. Other significant nonadjacent sounds: A visual check of the two word lists yields no other sounds that seem to be occurring more often in one list than the other. This is most likely not the factor.

B. Evaluate position.

1. List position of the target sounds: For the *yes* words—F, F, F, F, F, F, F. For the *no* words—I, I, I, I, I.

2. A significant difference exists between the *yes* words and the *no* words. The rule is operating when the target sound is in the final position. When the target sound is in the initial position, however, the rule is not in operation. We have found our limitation.

3. Because the limitation has been found, there is no need to continue further with the systematic consistency check. Only one more step remains.

Step 3: *Describe the final rule.*

A. Based on the analysis completed in Step 2, create a new rule that accounts for the limitation that was observed (in this case, Fronting of Final Velars).

B. Record that new rule on the appropriate line at the bottom of the worksheet.

Discussion

Several elements of the analytic process involved in the systematic consistency check might profitably be highlighted here.

1. Because the purpose of the systematic consistency check is to determine which of the factors listed earlier in this chapter is responsible for the seeming inconsistency between the two word lists, once that factor is found, there is no need or reason to continue the analysis. Thus, in most cases, you will not have to go through the test for each of the factors. This will shorten the time needed considerably.

2. In several instances, you will be able to discount a factor just by making a visual check, rather than having to go through each of the words in each list. For example, when we were looking at the phonetic context of words, a visual check quickly told us that several of the words had no preceding vowel. Others had no following vowel. Thus, just by looking at the words, we could tell that the preceding or following vowel *could not* possibly be the factor that we were looking for.

3. If words in the *no* column and words in the *yes* column contain the same identical elements, we also know that the factor is not the one we are seeking. For example,

suppose that for J.B., we did not get such a neat division between the *yes* words and *no* words when analyzing position. Suppose that for some *yes* words the target sound occurred in the initial position and for others, it occurred in the final position. If this were the case, the position section of the worksheet would have looked something like this:

---

2. Position
   - List I, M, F for ⎢I,F F,I,F,I⎢ F,F,I,I,I,F,I ⎢
     initial, medial, final

Since both *yes* and *no* words would be sharing identical elements of the factor being studied, we would not be able to say that that factor is the cause of the difference between the lists of words.

4. As you achieve more practice in performing systematic consistency checks, you will find that the process of determining the factor responsible for the rule limitation will speed up greatly. Eventually, you will need the worksheet only for the most subtle limited rules; in most cases, you will find that you can recognize the limitation just by studying the two lists of words.

Clinical Mastery Exercise—Tip A. Canout

Introduction

Tip was a 7-year-old boy who also demonstrated seemingly inconsistent Fronting of Velars. See his gloss on the opposite page. Once again, because you have been given the name of the rule, we will skip the first 2 steps of the 6-step generic procedure and proceed to the Consistency Check. A blank Consistency Checklist is provided on page 178. First place Tip's words into either the *yes* or *no* column, depending on whether or not the rule is exhibited. Then, study the two lists of words to see whether you can decipher the limitation just through visual analysis. Finally, whether or not you have determined the limitation, perform the systematic consistency check in the worksheet portion of the Consistency Checklist. Try to go through the process yourself prior to reading the solution.

(Solution on page 179)

PHONOLOGICAL RULE SUMMARY

Client: _Tip A. Canoût_

Check	Target Word	Client Production	Rule(s) Operating
	gun	gʌn	correct
	cap	kæp	correct
	skate	stet	
	queen	twin	
	quick	twɪt	
	kate	ket	correct
	back	bæk	correct
	basket	bæstət	
	box	bats	
	dog	dɔg	correct
	tiger	taɪdɚ	
	sick	sɪk	correct
	goose	gus	correct
	ghost	dost	

177

CONSISTENCY CHECKLIST

Initial Rule Description: _____

Rule Operating **(Yes)**	Rule Not Operating **(No)**

Check for Consistency	**Yes** Words	**No** Words	Sig. Diff.
1. **Phonetic Context**			
— List vowel preceding			
— List vowel following			
— List consonant preceding			
— List consonant following			
— List other sig. non-adjacent sounds			
2. **Position**			
— List I, M, F for initial medial, final			
3. **Intra-class Variability**			
— List correct/incorrect sounds, search for intra-class patterns			
4. **Syllable Structure/ Word Length**			
— List syllable structures			
5. **Part of Speech/Morphological Endings**			
— List grammatical categories			
6. **Syllable Stress**			
— List U, S for unstressed, stressed			
7. **Syllable Boundary**			
— List words/Draw line between syllable boundaries; Note differences			

Note other factors: Elicitation mode, situational context, overlearned words, etc.

Final Rule Description: _____

178

Solution

In order to discover the consistent limitation to the Fronting of Velars rule, we will first place each word from Tip's speech sample into either the *yes* (rule operating) or *no* (rule not operating) columns of the Consistency Checklist as appropriate. Then, we will try to discover the limitation by visually inspecting the two lists of words and attempting to decipher the systematic difference between the lists. Finally, if visual inspection is insufficient, we will progress through the worksheet until the limitation is discovered.

I. *Place words from speech sample into* yes *and* no *columns, as appropriate.*
   A. The words *skate, queen, quick, basket, box, tiger,* and *ghost* should be placed in the *yes* column, indicating that the Fronting of Velars rule is working for those words.
   B. The words *gun, cap, kate, back, dog, sick,* and *goose* should be placed in the *no* column, signaling that they do not exhibit Fronting of Velars.
II. *Visual inspection of word lists.*
   A. Study the two lists of words. Try to find a systematic difference between the words exhibiting Fronting of Velars and those that do not. Make certain that any difference found is consistent for all the words on the list.
   B. If you determine the systematic difference by means of this visual inspection, go to the bottom of the checklist and label the newly discovered limited rule. (In this case, although it certainly is possible that you may have discovered the limitation by means of visual inspection, we will proceed as if we haven't; just for the extra practice, you may also want to continue with the systematic consistency check, regardless of whether or not you have found the limitation yet.)
III. *Systematic consistency check*
   A. Evaluate phonetic context.
      1. Vowel preceding the target error: For the *yes* words—none, none, none, /ɪ/, /æ/, /a/, /aɪ/, none. For the *no* words—none, none, none, /æ/, /ɔ/, /ɪ/, none. *Conclusion:* Not only do several words in both lists have no preceding vowel, automatically eliminating this factor, but of the vowels that do precede the target, several are the same for both the *yes* and the *no* words. This is not the factor.
      2. Vowel following the target error: For the *yes* words—/e/, /i/, /i/, none, /ə/, none, /ɚ/, /o/. For the *no* words—/ʌ/, /æ/, /e/, none, none, none, /μ/. *Conclusion:* Again, several words in both lists have no following vowel. Also, the *yes* and *no* words again share at least one of the vowels. Thus, with respect to the "following vowel," there is essentially no difference between the *yes* and *no* words. Once again, this cannot be the factor.
      3. Consonant preceding: *Yes* words—/s/, none, none, /k/, /s/, /b/, /t/, none. *No* words—none, none, none, / b/, /d/, /s/, none.

Conclusion: The two word lists have similar preceding consonants. Also, several words in both lists do not even have a preceding consonant. This is not the factor.

4. Consonant following: *Yes* words—/t/, /n/, /k/, none, /t/, /s/, none, /s/. *No* words—/n/, /p/, /t/, none, none, none, /s/. *Conclusion:* Same story; the following consonants are similar in both lists and several words have no following consonant. This cannot be the factor.

5. Other significant nonadjacent sounds: A visual check indicates that there are no other sounds that systematically occur in the *yes* words yet do not occur in the *no* words. *Conclusion:* This cannot be the factor creating the limited rule.

B. Evaluate position.

1. Position of target sounds for *yes* words—M, I, I, F. M, M, M, I. Position of target sounds for *no* words—I, I, I, F. F. F. I.

2. *Conclusion:* Actually, we can tell that position is not the factor creating the limitation just by looking at the *yes* words, in which the target sounds occur in all three possible positions. The position seems to be irrelevant to whether the error occurs or not.

C. Evaluate the intraclass variability.

1. In this case, we are interested in whether some systematic difference between the members of the class of sounds being studied (velars) is responsible for the limitation. In essence, we want to find out whether the client treats the /k/ sound differently than he or she does the /g/ sound.

2. Class members appearing in *yes* words: /k/, /k/, /k/, / k/, /k/, /k/, /g/, /g/. Class members appearing in *no* words: /g/, /k/, /k/, /k/, /g/, /k/, /g/.

3. *Conclusion:* This cannot be a factor because all members of the class of sounds being studied occur in both lists of words.

D. Evaluate syllable structure/word length.

1. Syllable structure for *yes* words: CCVC, CCVC, CCVC, CVCCVC, CVCC, CVCV, CVCC. Syllable structure for *no* words: CVC, CVC, CVC, CVC, CVC, CVC, CVC.

2. *Conclusion:* There is most definitely a significant difference between the two lists of words. All of the words with Fronting of Velars have a syllable structure that is more complex than CVC. On the other hand, all of the words without the rule have only a CVC syllable structure.

3. A new, limited rule can be formulated: Fronting of Velars in words having syllable structures more complex than CVC. This rule should be noted on the bottom of the Consistency Checklist. The systematic consistency check is now finished and if a full 6-step generic analysis were being undertaken, the clinician would now return to Step 4 of that analysis. (See completed Consistency Checklist on page 181.)

CONSISTENCY CHECKLIST

Initial Rule Description: _Fronting of Velars_

Rule Operating (Yes)	Rule Not Operating (No)
skate, queen, quick, qui(ck), basket, box, tiger, ghost	gun, cap, skate, back, dog, sick, goose

Check for Consistency	Yes Words	No Words	Sig. Diff.
1. Phonetic Context — List vowel preceding	none, none, none, /ɪ/, /æ/, /ə/, /aɪ/, none	none, none, none, /æ/, /ɔ/, /ɪ/, none	No
— List vowel following	/e/, /i/, none, /ə/, /ər/, /o/	/ʌ/, /æ/, /e/, none, /u/	No
— List consonant preceding	/s/, none, /k/, /b/, /t/	none, /b/, /d/, /s/	No
— List consonant following	/t/, /n/, /k/, none, /t/, /s/	/n/, /p/, /t/, none, /s/	No
— List other sig. non-adjacent sounds	Visual check ————————→		No
2. Position — List I, M, F for initial medial, final	M, I, I, F, M, M, I	I, I, I, F, F, F, I	No
3. Intra-class Variability — List correct/incorrect sounds, search for intra-class patterns	/k/, /k/, /k/, /k/, /k/, /k/, /g/, /g/	/g/, /k/, /k/, /k/, /g/, /k/, /g/	No
4. Syllable Structure/ Word Length — List syllable structures	CCVC, CCVC, CCVC, CVCCVC, CVCC, CVCV, CVCC	CVC, CVC, CVC, CVC, CVC, CVC	Yes!
5. Part of Speech/Morphological Endings — List grammatical categories			
6. Syllable Stress — List U, S for unstressed, stressed			
7. Syllable Boundary — List words/Draw line between syllable boundaries; Note differences			

Note other factors: Elicitation mode, situational context, overlearned words, etc.

Final Rule Description: _Fronting of Velars in words with syllable structures more complex than CVC._

181

Discussion

Tip's output is another example of speech that seems inconsistent until a consistency check is undertaken. With closer analysis, inconsistent Fronting of Velars becomes consistent Velar Fronting in more complex syllable structures. Why is this subtle difference important? If you were to work on the originally formulated inconsistent rule, chances are that several of your therapeutic materials and stimuli would be inappropriate for the child's real problem. Now that we know the precise rule, only stimuli having syllable structures more complex than CVC will be used in therapy. Undoubtedly, this use of appropriate stimuli will accelerate Tip's improvement.

Clinical Mastery Exercise—Clara Bell

Introduction

When first seen, Clara was a 6-year-old girl who exhibited some very strange speech. She had only one error: She omitted medial position alveolars. Unfortunately, this one error rendered her extremely difficult to understand in conversational speech. What made the problem worse was that she seemed to be almost totally and stubbornly inconsistent in her errors. Her clinicians could never predict when she was going to say a word correctly as opposed to when she was going to omit an alveolar in the middle of a word or phrase. The height of frustration was reached with Clara after one and one-half years of therapy, when a third or fourth reevaluation yielded the fact that virtually no change had occurred in her overall conversation. She was still leaving out alveolars, and she was still seemingly inconsistent. It was just about at that time when we began questioning our own earlier thoughts about inconsistency. Although the worksheets in this book were not yet developed, we became convinced that we were missing something in our analysis. We decided to look at that inconsistency more closely.

Part of Clara's speech sample, obtained at the age 7 years 6 months, appears on page 184. Perform a consistency check and see if you can come up with the limitation it took us more than a year and a half to discover. A blank Consistency Checklist appears on page 185.

(Solution on page 186)

PHONOLOGICAL RULE SUMMARY

Client: _Clara Bell_

Check	Target Word	Client Production	Rule(s) Operating
	boy dog	bɔɪdɔg	correct
	bottle	baʔəl	
	on top of	antapʌv	correct
	baton	bətan	correct
	caterpillar	kæʔɚpɪʔɚ	
	butterfly	bʌʔɚflaɪ	
	necktie	nɛktaɪ	correct
	turtle	tɝʔəl	
	balloon	bəlun	correct
	poison	pɔɪʔən	
	sweater	swɛʔɚ	
	bazaar	bəzar	correct
	bicycle	baɪʔɪkəl	
	relay race	rileres	correct
	return	ritɝn	correct

CONSISTENCY CHECKLIST

Initial Rule Description: _Strange Deletion Rule #2_

Rule Operating (Yes)	Rule Not Operating (No)

Check for Consistency	Yes Words	No Words	Sig. Diff.
1. Phonetic Context			
— List vowel preceding			
— List vowel following			
— List consonant preceding			
— List consonant following			
— List other sig. non-adjacent sounds			
2. Position			
— List I, M, F for initial medial, final			
3. Intra-class Variability			
— List correct/incorrect sounds, search for intra-class patterns			
4. Syllable Structure/ Word Length			
— List syllable structures			
5. Part of Speech/Morphological Endings			
— List grammatical categories			
6. Syllable Stress			
— List U, S for unstressed, stressed			
7. Syllable Boundary			
— List words/Draw line between syllable boundaries; Note differences			

Note other factors: Elicitation mode, situational context, overlearned words, etc.

Final Rule Description: _____

Solution

I. *Place words/phrases from speech sample into* yes/no *columns, as appropriate.*

   A. The following words/phrases go into the *yes* column: *battle, caterpillar, butterfly, turtle, poison, sweater, bicycle.* Medial alveolars are being deleted in these words.

   B. The following words/phrases should be placed in the *no* column: *boy dog, on top of, baton, blue tie, balloon, bazaar, relay race, return.* In these words, the medial alveolars are maintained.

II. *Visual inspection of the word lists.*

   A. Study the columns of *yes* and *no* words. Try to find a systematic difference between the words exhibiting Medial Alveolar Deletion and those that do not. Make certain that any difference found is consistent for all of the words on the checklist.

   B. If you are able to determine the systematic difference by means of this visual inspection, go to the bottom of the checklist and label the newly discovered limited rule. (In this case, although you may have already discovered the limitation, we will once again proceed with the worksheet as if we haven't; hopefully you will, too.)

III. *Systematic consistency check.*

   A. Evaluate phonetic context.

     1. Vowel preceding the target error: For the *yes* words—/a/, /æ/, /ɪ/, /ʌ/, /ɜ/, /ɔɪ/, /ɛ/, /aɪ/. For the *no* words—/ɔɪ/, /a/, /ə/, /ɛ/, /ə/, /ə/, /i/, /ɪ/. *Conclusion:* Because the *yes* words and the *no* words share some of the same preceding vowels, this cannot be the factor separating the two groups of words.

     2. Vowel following the target: For the *yes* words—/ɚ/, /ɚ/, /ɚ/, /ɚ/, /ə/, /ɪ/, /ɚ/, /ɪ/. For the *no* words—/ɔ/, /a/, /a/, /aɪ/, /ar/, /µ/, /e/, /ɜ/. *Conclusion:* Something very interesting is happening here. There indeed seems to be at least some difference between the two groups. In all the *yes* words, the following vowel is unstressed. On the other hand, in the *no* words, the target is always followed by a stressed vowel. Although we probably could terminate the systematic consistency check here and call our limited rule Deletion of Medial Alveolars that Precede Unstressed Vowels, we will avoid this for the time being and continue with the worksheet. As you will see, there is a more precise way of describing this limited rule. However, if you came up with a limited rule based on unstressed vowels, you are most certainly on the right track.

     3. Consonant preceding: *Yes* words—/b/, /k/, /p/, /b/, /t/, /p/, /w/, /b/. *No* words—/b/, /n/, /b/, /k/, /b/, /b/, /r/, /r/. *Conclusion:* Although there are a few differences between the two lists of words, several of the consonants overlap both groups. This is not the factor.

     4. Consonant following: *Yes* words—none, /p/, none, /f/, none, /n/, none, /k/. *No* words—/g/, /p/, /n/, none, /n/, none, /r/. *Conclusion:* This is certainly not the factor. Not only do some sounds overlap both word groups, but several words do not even have a following consonant.

5. Other significant nonadjacent sounds: A visual check of the *yes* and *no* word lists indicates that there are no other sounds that systematically occur in one list yet do not occur in the other. *Conclusion:* This cannot be the factor creating the limited rule.

B. Evaluate position.

1. A quick visual check indicates that this is not the factor creating the seeming inconsistency. All of the alveolars being studied, in both the *yes* and *no* lists, occur in the medial position of the utterance. (Although it is possible to analyze position by words rather than overall utterance, as we have just done, the conclusion would remain the same: the position of the sound is irrelevant to the presence or absence of alveolars in the word.)

C. Evaluate intraclass variability.

1. Class members appearing in *yes* words—/d/, /d/, /l/, /d/, /d/, /z/, /d/, /s/. Class members appearing in *no* words—/d/, /t/, /t/, /t/, /l/, /z/, /l/.

2. *Conclusion:* This cannot be a factor because words having the error contain the same alveolars as do words not having the errors.

D. Evaluate syllable structure/word length.

1. A visual check indicates that the word length of the two groups of words seems fairly equivalent. This seems not to be the factor. However, we will check out the syllable structure in a more systematic fashion.

2. Syllable structure for *yes* words: CVCVC, CVCVCVCV, CVCVCCV, CVCVC, CVCVC, CCVCV, CVCVCVC. Syllable structure for *no* words: CVCVC, VCCVCVC, CVCVC, CCVCV, CVCVC, CVCV, CVCVCVC.

3. *Conclusion:* Although there is some variability in syllable structure between the *yes* and *no* words, there is much more similarity between the two lists of words. This is not the factor.

E. Evaluate part of speech/morphological endings.

1. This is an easy category to eliminate as a factor just by means of a visual check. Words in which the rule is operating are all nouns. Words in which the rule is not operating are more varied; however, nouns still abound. This is not the factor.

F. Evaluate syllable stress.

1. Stress of target syllable in *yes* words: U, U, U, U, U, U, U, U. Stress of target syllable in *no* words: S, S, S, S, S, S, S.

2. There is clearly a significant difference between the two lists of words. In all of the words having Deletion of Medial Alveolars, the rule occurs when the alveolar begins an unstressed syllable. However, when the alveolar begins a stressed syllable (as in the *no* words), there is no deletion.

3. A new limited rule can be formulated: Deletion of Medial Alveolars that Begin Unstressed Syllables. This rule should be noted on the bottom of the Consistency Checklist. The systematic consistency check is now completed. (See the completed form on the next page.)

CONSISTENCY CHECKLIS.

Initial Rule Description: _Strange Deletion Rule #2_

Rule Operating (Yes)	Rule Not Operating (No)
battle caterpillar caterpillar butterfly turtle poison sweater bicycle	boy dog on top of baton **necktie** balloon bazaar relay race return

Check for Consistency	Yes Words	No Words	Sig. Diff.
1. Phonetic Context	/a/,/æ/,/ɪ/,/ʌ/,/ɜ/,/ɔɪ/, /ɛ/,/aɪ/	/ɔɪ/,/a/,/ɔ/,/ɛ/,/ɔ/,/ə/, /i/,/ɪ/	No
— List vowel preceding	/ɚ/,/ə/,/ɪ/	/ɔ/,/a/,/aɪ/,/ʌ/,/arl/,/el/,/ɜ/	?
— List vowel following	/b/,/k/,/p/,/t/,/w/	/b/,/n/,/k/,/r/	No
— List consonant preceding	none,/p/,/f/,/n/,/k/	/g/,/p/,/n/,none,/r/	No
— List consonant following			
— List other sig. non-adjacent sounds	Visual Check ———————→		No
2. Position	Visual Check ———————→		No
— List I, M, F for initial medial, final			
3. Intra-class Variability	/d/,/l/,/z/,/s/	/d/,/t/,/l/,/z/	No
— List correct/incorrect sounds, search for intra-class patterns			
4. Syllable Structure/ Word Length	CVCVC, CVCVCV, CVCVCV, CCVCV	CVCVC, VCCVCVC, CCVCV, CVCV, CVCVCVC	No
— List syllable structures			
5. Part of Speech/Morphological Endings	Visual Check ———————→		No
— List grammatical categories			
6. Syllable Stress	U,U,U,U,U,U,U,U	S,S,S,S,S,S,S,S	Yes⬇
— List U, S for unstressed, stressed			
7. Syllable Boundary			
— List words/Draw line between syllable boundaries; Note differences			

Note other factors: Elicitation mode, situational context, overlearned words, etc.

Final Rule Description: _Deletion of Medial Alveolars which begin unstressed syllables._

Why is Deletion of Medial Alveolars that Begin Unstressed Syllables a better limited rule than the one we proposed earlier, based on vowels (Deletion of Medial Alveolars that Precede Unstressed Vowels)? At the least, we would have saved a lot of work.

There are two answers to this question. First, the rule referring to unstressed syllables is not "better." It is, however, more precise. Unstressed vowels only occur in unstressed syllables. Thus, the syllable is the controlling element here. So it is not the phonetic context but the syllabification that is the linguistic element responsible for the error occurring. In practical terms, it may not make a difference, but if the goal is precision, the latter rule comes closest. Besides, if we had accepted the earlier rule, you would not have had near the same amount of practice in performing the systematic consistency check.

Discussion

At this point, you may be wondering how a rule that is so obvious after the analysis could have been missed by a competent clinician for more than one and one-half years. The answer lies in the mindset of this traditionally trained clinician. For him, inconsistency was expected; it was not a phenomenon which required particular study. So no systematic attempt had ever been made to study it. In other words, this clinician, like most of us, saw what he expected to see. And if it was frustrating, so be it. Articulation training, especially at the conversational speech levels, often was frustrating. It was not until the mindset changed that the clinician began to question his original diagnosis and look more closely at the supposed inconsistency. Of course, once the additional analysis was undertaken, the limitation to the rule was found, inconsistent became consistent, and appropriate therapeutic stimuli and procedures could be utilized.

This issue has been raised once more to underline the importance of mindset. Currently, the mindset of most clinicians and investigators in the area of phonology is that inconsistency is accepted and expected. Unfortunately, unless this thinking changes, and is replaced with a "no inconsistency" framework, the unnecessary and unsuccessful time and energy spent in trying to help Clara will continue to be a model for our profession.

By the way, there are two postscripts to Clara's story. First, after the correct limited rule was identified and appropriate stimuli and procedures were introduced, it took less than 3 months for Clara to learn the contrast, generalize it to her conversational speech, and be dismissed. Second, the clinician in this true story was your author.

Clinical Mastery Exercise—Irwin Erwin

Introduction

Irwin, like Clara, was an older child (close to 8 at the time of the speech sample you are about to see). Like Clara, he was periodically unintelligible in conversational speech. Like Clara, he had speech that seemed inconsistent if not totally random, and like Clara, he had been receiving speech therapy for a while before the true nature of his errors was discovered.

The gloss contains a relevant sample of Irwin's speech. You will notice some strange errors: /sp/ → /t/ sometimes, but not always (sometimes it remains /sp/); /sk/ → /ks/ again sometimes, although at times it also remains unchanged; /st/ → /s/ at times, but on other occasions it remains /st/. These errors have all been grouped together and labeled the Strange Cluster Rule. Try to find the limited rule, doing your work on the blank Consistency Checklist.

(Solution on page 193)

PHONOLOGICAL RULE SUMMARY

Client: _Irwin Erwin_

Check	Target Word	Client Production	Rule(s) Operating
	I spy	aɪfaɪ	
	I scream	aɪksrim	
	space	fes	
	he stopped	hisapt	
	teaspoon	tifun	
	bedspread	bɛdfrɛd	
	outerspace	aʊdɚfes	
	boyscout	bɔɪksaʊt	
	hospital	haspɪtl̩	correct
	aspirin	æsprɪn	correct
	eskimo	ɛskɪmo	correct
	suspicion	səfɪʃən	
	basket	bæskət	correct
	ice cream	aɪskrim	correct
	presto	prɛsto	correct
	lipstick	lɪpsɪk	
	bluesky	bluksaɪ	
	housetool	haʊstul	correct

CONSISTENCY CHECKLIST

Initial Rule Description: _Strange Cluster Rule #3_

Rule Operating (Yes)	Rule Not Operating (No)

Check for Consistency	Yes Words	No Words	Sig. Diff.
1. Phonetic Context			
— List vowel preceding			
— List vowel following			
— List consonant preceding			
— List consonant following			
— List other sig. non-adjacent sounds			
2. Position			
— List I, M, F for initial medial, final			
3. Intra-class Variability			
— List correct/incorrect sounds, search for intra-class patterns			
4. Syllable Structure/ Word Length			
— List syllable structures			
5. Part of Speech/Morphological Endings			
— List grammatical categories			
6. Syllable Stress			
— List U, S for unstressed, stressed			
7. Syllable Boundary			
— List words/Draw line between syllable boundaries; Note differences			

Note other factors: Elicitation mode, situational context, overlearned words, etc.

Final Rule Description: _____

Solution

I. *Place words from speech sample into* yes/no *columns, as appropriate.*
   A. The following words/phrases should be placed in the *yes* column, indicating that the Strange Cluster Rule is operating for this output: *I spy, I scream, space, He stopped, teaspoon, bedspread, outerspace, boyscout, suspicion, lipstick, blue sky.*
   B. The following words/phrases should be placed in the *no* column, indicating that the Strange Cluster Rule is not working for this output: *hospital, aspirin, eskimo, basket, ice cream, presto, house tool.*
II. *Visual inspection of word lists.*
   A. Study the two lists of words. Try to find a systematic difference between the words exhibiting the Strange Cluster Rule and those not demonstrating the rule. Make certain that any difference found is consistent for all the words on the list.
   B. If you decipher the systematic difference by means of this visual inspection, go to the bottom of the checklist and label the newly discovered limited rule. Otherwise, perform the systematic consistency check.
III. *Systematic consistency check.*
   A. Evaluate phonetic context.
      1. Vowel preceding: *Yes* words—/aɪ/, none, /aɪ/, /i/, /i/, /ɛ/, /ɚ/, /ɔɪ/, /ə/, /ɪ/, /µ/. *No* words—/a/, /æ/, /ɛ/, /æ/, /aɪ/, /ɛ/, /aʊ/. *Conclusion*: Some of the same vowels are in *yes* words as are in *no* words. Thus, the two lists of words are not significantly different and this is not the factor.
      2. Vowel following: *Yes* words — /aɪ/, /e/, /i/, /a/, /µ/, /ɛ/, /aʊ/, /ɪ/. *No* words — /ɪ/, /ə/, /ɪ/, /ə/, /i/, /o/, /u/. *Conclusion*: Again, some vowels appear in both word lists. Thus, the following vowel cannot be the significantly different factor creating the limitation.
      3. Consonant preceding: A quick visual check will indicate that this is not a relevant factor. For example, several words in both lists have no preceding consonant. How can this be the factor causing the problem if the factor doesn't exist in many of the words? It cannot.
      4. Consonant following: Once again, a quick visual check indicates that this is an irrelevant dimension. Several words have no following consonant and the following consonants that do exist are pretty much equivalent across the two lists.
      5. Other significant nonadjacent sounds: Yet again, a visual check reveals no sounds that systematically occur in the *yes* words yet do not occur in the *no* words. Conclusion: This is not the factor.
   B. Evaluate position.
      1. This factor also can be dismissed easily after very short study. However, for the sake of practice, we will fill out the worksheet.
      2. Position of target: *Yes* words—M, I, M, M, M, M, M, M, M, M. Position of target: *No* words—M, M, M, M, M, M, M.
      3. *Conclusion*: Nothing could be clearer; position is certainly not the factor separating the two groups of words.

   C. Evaluate intraclass variability.
1. In this case, we are interested in whether there is a particular subclass of clusters in which the rule operates as opposed to another subclass in which the rule is absent.
2. Class members appearing in *yes* words: /sp/, /sp/, /sk/, /st/, /sp/, /sp/, /sp/, /sk/, /sp/, /st/, /sk/. Class members appearing in *no* words: /sp/, /sp/, /sk/, /sk/, /sk/, /st/, /st/.
3. *Conclusion*: All class members that appear in the *yes* words also appear in the *no* words. This cannot be the factor creating the seeming inconsistency.
   D. Evaluate syllable structure/word length.
1. A quick visual check indicates that words in the *yes* column and those in the *no* column are essentially equivalent with respect to syllable structure or word length. This is not the factor.
   E. Evaluate part of speech/morphological endings.
1. Again, this factor is easily eliminated after a visual check. No significant difference exists between the words that have the rule operating and those that do not.
   F. Evaluate syllable stress.
1. Stress of target syllable in *yes* words: S, S, S, S, U, U, S, U, S, U, S. As the rule operates in both stressed and unstressed syllables, we can already reason that syllable stress is not the factor. However, something very interesting occurs when attempting to determine the stress of the target syllable in *no* words, so we will continue.
2. Stress of target syllable in *no* words: This cannot be determined. For example, take the first word *hospital*—half of the cluster (i.e., /s/) occurs in the stressed syllable; the other half (i.e., /p/) is part of the unstressed syllable. The same thing occurs in all the other words.
3. *Conclusion:* Although we know that syllable stress is not the factor we are looking for, we *have* seen some evidence that something systematic is occurring, that it has something to do with the syllable, and that it reflects differently on the *yes* words than it does on the *no* words.
   G. Evaluate syllable boundary.
1. To assess this factor, list the words/phrases on the worksheet; draw a line between the syllable boundaries bordering our target cluster; then look for systematic differences.
2. Location of syllable boundary in *yes* words: before cluster, before, before, before, before, before, before, before, before, before, before. Location of syllable boundary in *no* words: between the elements of the cluster, between, between, between, between, between, between.
3. *Conclusion*: An extremely clear differentiation between the two word lists has emerged. Irwin misarticulates his clusters when the syllable boundary occurs before the cluster. However, his "cluster" is maintained when the syllable boundary appears between the two elements of the "cluster."
4. A new limited rule can be formulated: Strange Cluster Rules in Words in Which the Syllable Boundary Precedes the Cluster. The systematic consistency check is now completed. (See the completed checklist on the next page.)

CONSISTENCY CHECKLIST

Initial Rule Description: _Strange Cluster Rule #3_

Rule Operating (Yes)	Rule Not Operating (No)
lipstick I spy hospital	
blue sky space aspirin	
I scream eskimo	
he stopped basket	
teaspoon ice cream	
bedspread presto	
outerspace house tool	
boyscout	
suspicioun	

Check for Consistency	Yes Words	No Words	Sig. Diff.
1. Phonetic Context	/aɪ/, –, /aɪ/, /i/, /i/, /ɛ/, /ɚ/, /ɔɪ/, /ə/, /ɪ/	/ə/, /æ/, /ɛ/, /aɪ/, /ɛ/, /aʊ/	No
— List vowel preceding			
— List vowel following	/aɪ/, /e/, /i/, /b/, /u/, /ɛ/, /ɪ/	/ɛ/, /ə/, /i/, /o/, /u/	No
— List consonant preceding	Not Applicable (NA)	NA	No
— List consonant following	NA	NA	No
— List other sig. non-adjacent sounds	NA	NA	No
2. Position	Visual Check →		No
— List I, M, F for initial medial, final			
3. Intra-class Variability	sp → F st → s	sp → sp st → st	No
— List correct/incorrect sounds, search for intra-class patterns			
4. Syllable Structure/ Word Length	Visual Check →		No
— List syllable structures			
5. Part of Speech/Morphological Endings	Visual Check →		No
— List grammatical categories			
6. Syllable Stress	S, S, S, S, U, U, S, U, S, U	Syllable boundary on both sides	?
— List U, S for unstressed, stressed			
7. Syllable Boundary	I/spy tea/spoon	hospital ice/cream	Yes!
— List words/Draw line between syllable boundaries; Note differences	I/space bed/spread I/scream outer/space he/stopped boy/scout	as/pirin pres/to es/kimo house/tool bas/ket	

Note other factors: Elicitation mode, situational context, overlearned words, etc.

Final Rule Description: _Cluster Reduction when syllable Boundary precedes cluster_

Discussion

Try this little exercise: Say the phrases *I scream* and *Ice cream* aloud to yourself at a normal conversational speed. Do you hear any difference between the two? Probably not. Yet Irwin said these two seemingly "identical" words differently. But now say these words again to yourself and prolong both the vowels and the fricative /s/. You will notice something interesting begin to occur. In *ice cream*, the /s/ will seem connected to the vowel before it; in *I scream*, the vowel /aɪ/ will seem to stand alone. In reality, although the speed of normal conversation makes it difficult to hear, there is a subtle difference between the way at least many of us produce the two phrases. Irwin incorporated this subtle difference into his rule system. For him, when a syllable boundary occurred between the two elements of a consonant cluster, he produced both elements; perhaps they no longer even functioned as a true cluster for him. When the syllable boundary occurred before the cluster, he exhibited his strange cluster rule. In short, as you will find is frequently the case, there was some bizarre logic in Irwin's limited rule. It not only was consistent, but it was logical in its own way.

A short postscript on Irwin: Once again, when the correct limited rule was determined, appropriate therapy materials could be prepared. Following more than a year of virtually no improvement, with continued frequent unintelligibility, Irwin was dismissed after 4 months, with no remaining speech errors.

The Paperwork Burden

If a clinician were forced to go through an entire Consistency Checklist for every rule their clients exhibited, the time and paperwork needed would be unbearable. Luckily, there are two factors that help in this regard. First, with increased experience, most clinicians come to the point where they no longer need to use the worksheet portion of the Consistency Checklist.

Instead, after some practice, they can usually determine the limitation just by visually analyzing the lists of *yes* and *no* words. Second, after a while, certain limitations become more predictable, and thus require only verification rather than true analysis. Although Final Consonant Devoicing is perhaps the most obvious example of a predictable limited rule, you will find that with more phonolinguistic experience, you will start formulating possible limitations immediately. So for a child who has seemingly inconsistent labial assimilation, you may start looking initially at the nearby vowels to see if the presence of lip rounded vowels is contributing to the limited rule.

Once again, we see the importance of internalized place, manner and voicing knowledge for speeding up the analytic process. And although the learning process is not necessarily pleasurable, the payoff can be immense, as was the case with Clara and Irwin.

Conclusion

Throughout this chapter, much as been made of the importance of clinical "mindset"; how this mental inclination or predisposition on our parts will often affect what we see. Nowhere has this been more true than in our concepts regarding inconsistency. We have been taught that inconsistency is the norm, so we are unsurprised if our clients seem inconsistent and our analysis ends. Unfortunately, this not only gives the wrong idea regarding our clients' problems, but it leads us astray in our therapy.

Perhaps you are not yet at the point where you believe that most if not all speech is consistent (aside from the three exceptions noted earlier). This belief will come with time and practice. After all, it takes time to overcome the clinical mindsets we have all been taught. For now, just realize that what we think we see is not necessarily what exists. Look a little more closely . . . and your clients will benefit.

CHAPTER ◆ 8

Description of Commonly Seen Phonological Rules

In all fairness, this chapter should be preceded with a warning. Perhaps the following will suffice:

> WARNING: This chapter may be harmful to your phonological health. Use the material presented herein with caution.

Why the disclaimer? Remember, the entire focus thus far has been to determine the rule *after* systematically examining each of the parameters of articulatory constraint. It has been stated more than once that the exact name of a rule is less important than is a clear reliable description of what is taking place. It has been cautioned that if one begins with a corpus of rules and then compares the client's output to those rules (as formal, or macroanalytic, tests of phonology), then much information might be missed.

So why have a chapter delineating the commonly seen phonological rules? For the same reason that we have used the accepted terminology in our examples (e.g., Fronting of Velars) rather than an equally descriptive alternative (e.g., Alveolarization of Velars). In other words, it will help your understanding of phonology if your know that these rules are frequently seen and it will help your communication with other professionals if you have learned the conventional labels. However, creating a checklist of the rules and using this list to evaluate your client will leave you with the same problems and limitations of current formal macroanalytic tests of phonology. So read with caution.

Placement Rules

This category includes rules that are caused by inappropriate location of articulatory valving within the vocal tract, in the absence of contextual considerations. The following placement rules are commonly seen:

1. *Fronting of Velars*—Velars become alveolars, so /k/, /g/ becomes /t/, /d/. Example: *cup* → /tʌp/.
2. *Fronting of all sounds*—In the past, the attempt has been made to create a more generalized fronting rule, which could account for more sound errors at once. (Thesis: If you could work on this generalized fronting rule, not only did /k/ and /g/ become /t/ and /d/, but /ʃ/ and /ʒ/ became /s/ and /z/ and other selected fronting errors would periodically be seen as well (for example, /t/ going to /p/). Examples: *cup* → /tʌp/ and *shoe* → /su/ and, perhaps, sun → /fʌn/.

3. *Fronting of Palatals*—Palatals become alveolars, so /ʃ/, /ʒ/, /t/, and /d/ become /s/, /z/, /ts/, and /dz/ respectively. Examples: *shoe* → /su/; *church* → /tsɜ̍ts/.

4. *Backing of Alveolars*—Alveolars become velars. Examples: *two* → /kµ/; *sun* → /kʌn/ (here embedded with Stopping of Fricatives); *door* → /gɔr/ (here embedded with Vocalization).

5. *Labialization*—A very primitive rule whereby many sounds move to the labial position. Somewhat equivalent to Tetism or a Systematic Sound Preference but concentrated in the labial position. Examples: *cow* → /pa/ (here embedded with Vowel Neutralization); *ten* → /pɛm/; *dog* → /ba/ (here embedded with Final Consonant Deletion).

6. *Tetism* (sometimes referred to as Consonant Neutralization)—Another primitive rule whereby many sounds move to the alveolar position. It is important that this not be mixed up with Alveolar Assimilation, which looks identical if there is a culprit in the word. Examples: bee → /di/; cow →/tau/; four → /sɔr/.

7. *Alveolarization of Fricatives*—A not quite as primitive relation of Tetism, whereby all fricatives move to the alveolar position. Examples: *four* → /sɔr/; *thick* → /sɪk/; *shoe* → /sµ/.

8. *Glottal Replacement*—Although investigators have typically designated this a substitution rule (e.g., see Weiner, 1979), it is probably more accurately described as a syllable structure rule. Thus, it will be discussed later.

Manner Rules

Rules in this category are caused by inappropriate degree or type of articulatory constriction during the sound production. The following manner rules are the most commonly seen:

1. *Stopping of Fricatives*—Fricatives become stops. Examples: *zoo* → /dµ/; *fish* → /pɪt/; *five* → /paɪb/.

2. *Gliding of Fricatives*—Very primitive rule not generally seen in normal phonological development; usually indicative of a need for intervention regardless of child's age. Fricatives become glides. Usually occurs in limited form, only in the initial position, with final fricatives being deleted or stopped. Examples: *fish* → /wɪt/ (here limited to initial position only); *sun* → /jʌn/; *shoe* → /ju/; *frog* → /wag/ (here embedded with Cluster Reduction); *soap* → /jop/.

3. *H'ing of Stops*— Stops are replaced with the glottal fricative (i.e., /h/). This is a primitive rule that has sometimes been referred to as a Systematic Sound Preference. In most cases, this rule occurs in limited form, usually only referring to initial sounds and often only initial, voiceless stops. Examples: *cow* → /haʊ/; *big* → /hɪ/ (here embedded with Final Consonant Deletion); *tie* → /haɪ/.

4. *Deaffriction*—An affricate loses either its stopping aspect or its fricative aspect. (The latter is most common). So /tʃ/ becomes either /ʃ/ or /t/, depending on which element is omitted. Likewise, /dʒ/ becomes either /ʒ/ or /d/. Notice that if the fricative element is lost, the sound also changes placement, to the alveolar position. This is an artifact created by the fact that there is no natural palatal stop and the error should not be regarded as "Fronting," despite the position change. Examples: *chew* → /ʃµ/ or /tµ/; *Jack* → /ʒæk/ or /dæk/.

5. *Affrication*—An uncommon rule that usually represents a halfway step in a child's elimination of Stopping of Fricatives. Where the child used to produce a stop for a fricative, he or she now produces an affricate instead of the fricative. This rule is often a by-

product of traditional intervention strategies. Examples: *sun* → /tsʌn/; *zoo* → /dzu/; *four* → /pfɔ/.

6. *Denasalization*—Nasals become denasal. Not very common, except if the client has a cold. Examples: *mom* →/bab/; *neck* → /dɛk/.

7. *Gliding of Liquids*—A very common rule in both children who are normally developing and those who are phonologically disordered. Liquids becomes glides so /r/ becomes /w/ and /l/ becomes /j/ or /w/. Examples: *red* → /wɛd/; *light* → /waɪt/ or /jaɪt/.

8. *Vocalization*—In this rule, final position vocalic /l/ and /r/ sounds becomes the rounded vowel /µ/ or /o/. Examples: *table* → /tebo/; *butter* → /bʌto/; *bottle* → /bato/.

9. *Lateralization of Fricatives*—A rule that causes many speech pathologists to shudder involuntarily. Interestingly, this error does not seem to occur as frequently to children with severely disordered phonology as it does to children with mild disorders. Clients demonstrating this rule lower the sides of their tongue during production of /s/, /z/, /ʃ/, and/or /ʒ/ causing lateral emission of air and a characteristic acoustic quality.

Voicing Rules

In that there are so few alternatives in the voicing parameter, it is unsurprising that only a restricted number of voicing rules have been observed. The two most frequently occurring voicing rules are both limited and a discussion of these rules follows:

1. *Prevocalic Voicing*—A rule in which voiceless sounds occurring before vowels or other voiced sounds become voiced. (Because this is a contributing factor here, some investigators consider this an assimilation problem rather than

a problem of voicing, per se. In the end, as we will see when we get to the section on therapy, it probably doesn't make much of a difference.) Examples: *top* → /dap/; *cookie* → /gʊgi/; *pie* → /baɪ/.

2. *Devoicing of Final Consonants* (also called Final Consonant Devoicing)—Final voiced consonants become voiceless. (Again, some investigators consider this an assimilation error, claiming that the silence after the word is assimilating to the final voiced consonant, causing it to become voiceless. Again, it probably doesn't matter.) Examples: *red* → /rɛt/; *bug* → /bʌk/.

Context Rules

Rules in this category are caused when the target sound is produced incorrectly because of the influence of another sound in the word. Remember, it is always important to determine whether a particular error is caused by assimilation or one of the other parameters. This can only be done by means of a Parameter Confusion Test or a Consistency Check. The following context rules are the most commonly seen:

1. *Labial Assimilation*—When there is a labial culprit in the word, other sounds go to the labial position. Examples: *cup* → /pʌp/; *thumb* → /fʌm/; *birthday* → /bɪrfde/.

2. *Alveolar Assimilation*—When there is an alveolar culprit in the word, other sounds go to the alveolar position. Examples: *cat* → /tæt/; *dog* → /dɔd/; *bottle* → /dato/ (here embedded with vocalization).

3. *Velar Assimilation*—When there is a velar culprit in the word, other sounds go to the velar position. Examples: *kitty* → /kɪki/; *dog* → /gɔg/; *back* → /gæk/.

4. *Nasal Assimilation*—When there is a nasal culprit in the word, other sounds become nasal. If this rule exists, it will be discovered during the consistency

check, not as a result of the Parameter Confusion Test. Examples: *lunch* → /nʌnʃ/; *Emily* → /ɛməni/.

Structure Rules

Rules in this category are caused when some difficulty with phonemic structure of the intended word has caused the client to alter the phonemic structure. Structure rules occur frequently in unintelligible children and adults (the latter usually due to influences of foreign dialect). Several structure rules are commonly seen:

1. *Deletion of Final Consonants* (alternately called Final Consonant Deletion) — Extremely common rule in children who have reduced intelligibility. Final consonants are omitted. Examples: *cup* → /kʌ/; *walk* → /wa/; *bread* → /bɛ/ (here embedded with Cluster Reduction).

2. *Deletion of Initial Consonant*—An uncommon rule that is usually indicative of an unusually primitive phonological system. In this case, initial consonants are omitted, often along with Final Consonant Deletion. Examples: *cup* → /ʌ/ (here embedded with Deletion of Final Consonants); *sun* →/ʌn/; *bread* → /ɛd/.

3. *Deletion of Unstressed Syllables*—In this rule, unstressed syllables are deleted from multisyllabic words and/or unstressed single syllable words are deleted from phrases. Although this rule will contribute substantially to unintelligibility, it does not occur as frequently as you might guess, because the language level of many children with speech disorders is not complex enough to include sufficient multisyllabic words and multiword phrases. Nevertheless, in children who are difficult to understand but have fairly constant verbal output, Deletion of Unstressed Syllables is often a primary culprit. Examples: *telephone* → /tɛfo/ (here embedded with Final Consonant Deletion); *pajamas* → /dæməz/; *I want to go* → /aɪ wa go/. (In this case, notice that what might be misconstrued as a language problem—deletion of the infinitive *to*—can be explained as a phonological problem—Deletion of Unstressed Syllables.)

4. *Cluster Reduction* (within words) — This is another rule that is seen frequently both in children developing normally and in children with phonological disorders. Thus, the decision about therapy usually revolves around the age of the child exhibiting this rule, rather than the rule itself. In Cluster Reduction, the child omits one of the members of a consonant cluster or blend. Examples: *stop* → /dap/; *black* → /bæk/; *bread* → /bɛd/; *nest* → /nɛt/.

5. *Cluster Reduction Across Words*—By its nature, this rule can only exist in phrases. In two-word phrases in which the first word ends with a consonant and the second begins with a consonant, the client omits one of those consonants. This rule is often mistaken for inconsistent Final Consonant Deletion. Examples: *wish to* → /wɪ tµ/: *big boy* →/bɪ bɔɪ/; *is happy* → /ɪ hæpi/.

6. *Epenthesis*—A rule that often occurs as a result of regional or foreign dialect rather than disorder or deviance. In this rule, a schwa is inserted between the two elements of a cluster, creating an additional syllable. Examples: *bread* → /bərɛd/; *elm* → /ɛləm/.

7. *Migration*—This refers to the movement of a sound to another position in the word. This change will often (though not always) change the syllable structure of the word. Examples: *blue* → /bala/; *cry* → /kawə/ (here embedded with Gliding of Liquids); *phone* → /nop/ (here embedded with Stopping of Fricatives).

8. *Metathesis*—A special form of migration, popularly referred to as a spoonerism.

In this case, the position of two sounds is reversed, although both sounds are produced correctly. Examples: *ask* → /æks/; *animals* → /æmɪnəlz/; *spaghetti* → /pɪsgɛti/.

9. *Reduplication*—One of the most primitive rules that a child can exhibit. Children demonstrating reduplication convert most multisyllabic utterances to two syllables, where the second syllable mirrors the first. Normal children in early babbling go through a stage of reduplication; however, this generally disappears with the onset of true speech. Children with phonological disorders can maintain this behavior for a long time prior to intervention. These children are often those inaccurately referred to as apraxic. Examples: *rabbit* → /wawa/ (here embedded with Gliding of Liquids); *wagon* → /wawa/; *bottle* → /baba/.

10. *Glottal Replacement*—In this rule, a consonant is replaced by a glottal stop. The fact that a glottal stop is supposedly being substituted for a consonant is probably one reason that investigators have typically considered this a substitution rule. However, a glottal "stop" is not really a stop at all, in the typical sense, but is probably no more than a byproduct of the fact that a sound has been omitted. In other words, the "stop-like" physiological action of vocal cord closure, air buildup, and explosion is really little more than an artifact caused by the fact that an omission requires a stoppage and the following vowel requires a re-initiation of phonation. Unsurprisingly, our experience with therapy has verified the structural nature of the glottal replacement rule. Children improve much more quickly when a structural concept is taught then they do when a substitution concept is introduced. Examples: *butter* → /bʌʔɚ/; *telephone* → /tɛʔəʔon/; *Santa Claus* → /tæʔʌʔɔd/ (here embedded with Stopping of Fricatives).

Semantic and Syntactic Rules

Most of the rules occurring in this category are limited and sometimes they have their basis in linguistic rather than phonological problems. However, all clinicians have at one time or another seen a child who knows *in* and *on* receptively 100% of the time, who can imitate a phrase or short sentence with those prepositions, but includes them erratically or not at all during conversation. Very possibly this child has a limited phonologically based problem that manifests itself in unstressed functor words (like *in* or *on*) only. While phonologically based semantic and syntactic rules seem to occur only rarely, the following rules have been observed in the past and the discovery of a phonological basis on the part of clinicians has enhanced therapy immensely:

1. *Deletion of Unstressed Functor Words*—A limited form of Deletion of Unstressed Syllables whereby only the functor words (prepositions, articles, infinitives, etc.) are involved. Example: *I wanna go to the store* becomes *I wan go store*.

2. *Deletion of Unstressed Bound Morphemes*—This is another limited version of Unstressed Syllable Deletion that may occur more frequently than we think. When we have a client who omits bound morphemes (e.g., *ing, es* [plural], *ed* [past]) our initial reaction is usually to treat it as a language problem. However, we have recently found that clients seem to be responding more positively in therapy if we treat the errors as a structurally based phonological problem. We have also found that we could work on several bound morphemes at once and achieve improvement across the entire class—something we have not found possible when treating the morpheme deletion as a language problem. Of course, this is not at all meant to imply that all mor-

pheme deletions are phonologically rather than linguistically based. They are not. But it certainly stands to reason that some limited phonological rules might revolve around particular linguistic structures, and that is precisely what we are seeing.

3. *Stopping of Fricatives Except in Verbs*— Strange, but it has been reported— more than once.

4. *Glottal Replacement in the Copula and Auxiliary "is"*—Actually, this is a fairly frequently occurring rule, especially when a child with both speech *and* language delay is first learning the verb *is*. Two observations concerning this rule are noteworthy: First, it is frequently mistaken for a language problem, although it is clearly a phonological structure difficulty. This distinction becomes very important during therapy. Second, as long as the marker (i.e., /I/) is present, you may not want to make the inclusion of the missing sound a top priority in therapy. (We have observed that frequently a child will after a while include the missing sound on his or her own, without direct intervention.) Example: *The boy is eating* → /bɔɪ ɪ itɪŋ/ (here embedded with deletion of the missing article).

Other Rules

Although the rules listed previously represent a state of the art compendium of those that are most accepted and used by investigators and clinicians, several other rules have been described by one or another investigator. With only one possible exception, these rules can exist (though the terminology is used infrequently) so they are presented and described below, along with the investigator responsible for the label.

1. *Lisping* (Ingram, 1976)— Substitution of *th* for other sounds. A *th* for *s* substitu-

tion is the traditional lisp all clinicians are aware of, but Ingram describes some others (for example, *th* for *t*).

2. *Stopping of Liquids* (Ingram, 1976)— Liquids become stops. Examples: *yellow* → /jɛdo/; *light* → /daɛt/; *red* → /dɛd/.

3. *Systematic Sound Preference* (Weiner, 1981b)—Some children have a particular favored sound which comprises the bulk of their speech errors. For example, H'ing of stops, described previously, would be one example of a Systematic Sound Preference. However, the sound preference can be any sound for a particular child.

4. *Coalescence* (Hodson, 1986)—Replacement of two sounds by a new one that combines features of both original sounds. For example, if *thread* becomes /fɛd/, the /r/ cluster becomes /f/, a sound that combines the fricative feature of /θ/ and the labial feature of /r/ after it has glided to /w/. Examples: *spoon* → /fμn/; *three* → /fi/ (here embedded with Gliding of Liquids).

5. *Stridency Deletion* (Hodson & Paden, 1983; Khan & Lewis, 1986)—The term strident is a holdover from the Chomsky and Halle (1968) distinctive feature system and refers to fricatives and affricates produced with much noise. Sounds included in the strident classification are /s/, /z/, /ʃ/, /ʒ/, /tʃ/, and /dʒ/. On the other hand, /θ/ and /ð/ are not considered strident, because they are supposedly less noisy sounds.

Although the term Stridency Deletion is used by several phonologists, we must admit to some skepticism concerning either the validity or the value of its usage. For example, the term was developed by Chomsky and Halle (1968) in order to be able to distinguish /θ/ and /ð/ from the other fricatives and affricates. According to this system, a child who had a frontal lisp (e.g., *thick/sick*) would be deleting stridency in the word. Yet as most clinicians know, children with frontal lisps generally produce the lisp with more stridency that a normal /ɵ/. So at least for the speech-disordered population, the term seems to be unproductive. Further, Hodson and Paden's (1983) use of the term is inconsistent with every other pattern described in their system. For example, they say that one manifestation of Stridency Deletion occurs when one of the strident sounds is omitted. In other words, if a strident sound is omitted, the feature is absent. This is a throwback to the McReynolds and Engmann (1975) approach to feature analysis where an omitted sound indicated several absent features. It is also inconsistent with Hodson and Paden's own seemingly more logical approach to analysis of all other patterns where a deletion is a syllable structure problem, unrelated to other errors (e.g., Stopping of Fricatives) demonstrated by the client.

In summary, there seems to be little value in creating a separate phonological category of strident. Division into fricatives and affricates seems to be sufficient for describing the errors that we see in our clients, and since children with frontal lisps tend to produce these /ɵ/ sounds with stridency anyway, it seems better to focus on the true error dimension in these particular cases— placement.

6. *Palatization* (Hodson & Paden, 1983)— Alveolar fricatives become palatals. Example: *sun* → /ʃʌn/.

7. *Fricative Enhancement* (Klein)—Strengthening of the fricative quality in voiceless stop-liquid clusters, usually accompanied by some Coalescence. For example, in the word *tree*, the /tr/ cluster is actually an affricate (try it aloud to yourself and listen for the affricate quality). So if a child says /fi/ for *tree*, the child is enhancing the fricative nature of the /tr/ cluster. The labial fricative is produced because of the /r/ which glides to /w/, thus establishing the labial position. Examples of Fricative Enhancement combined with Coalescence: *drum* → /vʌm/; *try* → /faɪ/; *truck* → /fʌk/ (sorry . . . but this is a common childhood misarticulation that has a logical explanation, but drives parents crazy).

8. *Dissimilation* (Grunwell, 1987)—A rule in which the child avoids the production of two like consonants in the same word. Examples: *cake* → /kep/; *pipe* → /paɪk/.

9. *Manner Assimilation* (Harmony) (Grunwell, 1987)—When there is a culprit having a particular manner in a word (i.e., stop, fricative, affricate, lateral, etc.), other sounds in the word take on the same manner. Examples: *shoot* → /ʃʉs/; *kiss* → /kɪt/ (this must be distinguished from Stopping of Fricatives); *best* → /vɛst/.

Conclusion

Undoubtedly, as the field of clinical phonology grows, more rules will be added to these lists. Better terms will be developed for some of the common rules, and some rules will be considered obsolete or unproductive. The important things to remember are first, these are only the most commonly occurring rules. They are certainly not an exhaustive listing of all possible patterns. Second, and for the last time, there is nothing magical about the labels. If you find that one is unproductive for you, change it, just remembering to explain your new terminology to your readers and/or listeners.

CHAPTER ◆ 9

Microanalysis of Phonology, Part 3: Advanced Generative Analysis

Up until this point, in order to teach you the basics of generative phonological analysis, we have concentrated on methodology and details. Now it is time to shift the focus to "The Big Picture," so that you can begin reaping the benefits of generative phonology with your clients. No new material will be presented in this chapter. Instead, the attempt will be made to help you internalize the learning you have already acquired. All clinical mastery exercises will provide examples of real children. Although the analyses may be somewhat more complex, you will see that the process remains the same, regardless of the number of rules exhibited by a given client. Finally, you will be provided with ways to speed up the analytical process, so that the time factor required for analysis becomes reasonable within a clinical caseload.

The mountain has just about been climbed. Although you might not see it just yet, the end of the trail is just around the next bend, a few hours down the road. So stick with it for just a while longer, as the attempt is made to bridge that often difficult gap between theory and practice.

Clinical Mastery Exercise — Cora A. Appel

Introduction

Cora's speech sample provides you with the opportunity for refamiliarizing yourself with the 6-step generic process. Immediately following Cora's analysis several alternatives for speeding up the analysis will be presented. However, in Cora's case, we will stick to the entire procedure; the review will be valuable after the "interruption" of the last two chapters.

Cora has four phonological rules operating in her speech. Some of these rules are embedded with other rules in given words, and at least one of these rules is limited. As usual, begin the analysis with the first word and continue in an orderly manner until all four rules have been figured out.

Worksheets required for Cora Appel (in correct order of use)
- Phonological rule summary
- Generic 6-step procedure
- Parameter Confusion Test
- Consistency Check Form
- Generic 6-step procedure
- Consistency Check Form
- Generic 6-step procedure
- Consistency Check Form
- Generic 6-step procedure
- Consistency Check Form

(Solution on page 217)

PHONOLOGICAL RULE SUMMARY

Client: *Cora Appel*

Check	Target Word	Client Production	Rule(s) Operating
	pot	pɑp	
	cat	kæt	
	shoot	tut	
	dog	dɔ	
	pig	pɪ	
	soup	pʌp	
	sock	tɑ	
	kiss	kɪt	
	shake	te	
	ship	pɪp	
	nose	non	
	bed	bɛb	
	duck	dʌ	
	meat	mim	
	neat	nin	
	feet	pip	
	neck	nɛ	
	might	mɑɪm	
	come	mʌm	
	tame	mem	

PROCEDURE FOR PHONOLOGICAL ANALYSIS — GENERIC WORKSHEET

I. <u>Take one error and choose possible parameters</u>

        ERROR:
        ANALYSIS: **Manner?**   ⟶

                    Voicing?   ⟶

                    Placement? ⟶

                    Context?   ⟶

                    Structure? ⟶

                    Linguistic? ⟶

                    Semantic? ⟶

> If unclear as to whether placement or context, perform Parameter Confusion Test (See Form). Otherwise go to Step II.

II. <u>Make initial conclusion re: rule by describing the difference between target and client production.</u>

      _____ PARAMETER

          Description: _____

          Rule: _____

III. <u>Perform Consistency Check (See Consistency Check Form)</u>

IV. <u>Describe rule in Final Form</u>

          Rule: _____

V. <u>Go to phonological rule summary, find all words for which rule is operating, and note.</u>

VI. <u>Perform final check</u>

        — Make sure all changes in target word can be explained by rule. If so, check the word off. If not, leave until next analysis.

PLACEMENT CONTEXT. PARAMETER CONFUSION CHECK

<u>Target Word:</u>   _____

<u>Client Production:</u>   _____

<u>Choose Test Word:</u>   _____
     (Word in which there's no culprit; i.e no
       chance for assimilation to occur).

<u>Error Still Occur?</u> _____Yes

                 _____No

    <u>Yes</u> = Placement error; even though chance for assimilation has been
           removed, error still occurs.

    <u>No</u> = Assimilation error; error disappears when culprit is removed.

<u>Return to Step 1 – Generic Worksheet</u>

CONSISTENCY CHECKLIST

Initial Rule Description: _____

Rule Operating (Yes)	Rule Not Operating (No)

Check for Consistency	Yes Words	No Words	Sig. Diff.
1. Phonetic Context			
— List vowel preceding			
— List vowel following			
— List consonant preceding			
— List consonant following			
— List other sig. non-adjacent sounds			
2. Position			
— List I, M, F for initial medial, final			
3. Intra-class Variability			
— List correct/incorrect sounds, search for intra-class patterns			
4. Syllable Structure/ Word Length			
— List syllable structures			
5. Part of Speech/Morphological Endings			
— List grammatical categories			
6. Syllable Stress			
— List U, S for unstressed, stressed			
7. Syllable Boundary — List words/Draw line between syllable boundaries; Note differences			

Note other factors: Elicitation mode, situational context, overlearned words, etc.

Final Rule Description: _____

PROCEDURE FOR PHONOLOGICAL ANALYSIS — GENERIC WORKSHEET

I. Take one error and choose possible parameters

ERROR:

ANALYSIS: Manner? ⟶

Voicing? ⟶

Placement? ⟶

Context? ⟶

Structure? ⟶

Linguistic? ⟶

Semantic? ⟶

> If unclear as to whether placement or context, perform Parameter Confusion Test (See Form). Otherwise go to Step II.

II. Make initial conclusion re: rule by describing the difference between target and client production.

_____ PARAMETER

Description:_____

Rule:_____

III. Perform Consistency Check (See Consistency Check Form)

IV. Describe rule in Final Form

Rule:_____

V. Go to phonological rule summary, find all words for which rule is operating, and note.

VI. Perform final check

— Make sure all changes in target word can be explained by rule. If so, check the word off. If not, leave until next analysis.

CONSISTENCY CHECKLIST

Initial Rule Description: _____

Rule Operating (Yes)	Rule Not Operating (No)

Check for Consistency	Yes Words	No Words	Sig. Diff.
1. Phonetic Context			
— List vowel preceding			
— List vowel following			
— List consonant preceding			
— List consonant following			
— List other sig. non-adjacent sounds			
2. Position			
— List I, M, F for initial medial, final			
3. Intra-class Variability			
— List correct/incorrect sounds, search for intra-class patterns			
4. Syllable Structure/ Word Length			
— List syllable structures			
5. Part of Speech/Morphological Endings			
— List grammatical categories			
6. Syllable Stress			
— List U, S for unstressed, stressed			
7. Syllable Boundary — List words/Draw line between syllable boundaries; Note differences			

Note other factors: Elicitation mode, situational context, overlearned words, etc.

Final Rule Description: _____

PROCEDURE FOR PHONOLOGICAL ANALYSIS — GENERIC WORKSHEET

I. **Take one error and choose possible parameters**

ERROR:
ANALYSIS: Manner? ————▶

Voicing? ————▶

Placement? ————▶

Context? ————▶

Structure? ————▶

Linguistic? ————▶

Semantic? ————▶

> If unclear as to whether placement or context, perform Parameter Confusion Test (See Form). Otherwise go to Step II.

II. **Make initial conclusion re: rule by describing the difference between target and client production.**

_____ PARAMETER

Description:_____

Rule:_____

III. **Perform Consistency Check (See Consistency Check Form)**

IV. **Describe rule in Final Form**

Rule:_____

V. **Go to phonological rule summary, find all words for which rule is operating, and note.**

VI. **Perform final check**

— Make sure all changes in target word can be explained by rule. If so, check the word off. If not, leave until next analysis.

CONSISTENCY CHECKLIST

Initial Rule Description: _____

Rule Operating **(Yes)**	Rule Not Operating **(No)**

Check for Consistency	Yes Words	No Words	Sig. Diff.
1. Phonetic Context			
— List vowel preceding			
— List vowel following			
— List consonant preceding			
— List consonant following			
— List other sig. non-adjacent sounds			
2. Position			
— List I, M, F for initial medial, final			
3. Intra-class Variability			
— List correct/incorrect sounds, search for intra-class patterns			
4. Syllable Structure/ Word Length			
— List syllable structures			
5. Part of Speech/Morphological Endings			
— List grammatical categories			
6. Syllable Stress			
— List U, S for unstressed, stressed			
7. Syllable Boundary			
— List words/Draw line between syllable boundaries; Note differences			

Note other factors: Elicitation mode, situational context, overlearned words, etc.

Final Rule Description: _____

PROCEDURE FOR PHONOLOGICAL ANALYSIS — GENERIC WORKSHEET

I. Take one error and choose possible parameters

       ERROR:
      ANALYSIS: **Manner?** ——————▶

                 Voicing? ——————▶

                 Placement? ————▶

                 Context? ——————▶

                 Structure? —————▶

                 Linguistic? ————▶

                 Semantic? —————▶

> If unclear as to whether placement or context, perform Parameter Confusion Test (See Form). Otherwise go to Step II.

II. Make initial conclusion re: rule by describing the difference between target and client production.

       _____ PARAMETER

         Description:_____

         Rule:_____

III. Perform Consistency Check (See Consistency Check Form)

IV. Describe rule in Final Form

         Rule:_____

V. Go to phonological rule summary, find all words for which rule is operating, and note.

VI. Perform final check

         — Make sure all changes in target word can be explained by rule. If so, check the word off. If not, leave until next analysis.

CONSISTENCY CHECKLIST

Initial Rule Description: _____

Rule Operating (Yes)	Rule Not Operating (No)

Check for Consistency	Yes Words	No Words	Sig. Diff.
1. Phonetic Context			
— List vowel preceding			
— List vowel following			
— List consonant preceding			
— List consonant following			
— List other sig. non-adjacent sounds			
2. Position			
— List I, M, F for initial medial, final			
3. Intra-class Variability			
— List correct/incorrect sounds, search for intra-class patterns			
4. Syllable Structure/ Word Length			
— List syllable structures			
5. Part of Speech/Morphological Endings			
— List grammatical categories			
6. Syllable Stress			
— List U, S for unstressed, stressed			
7. Syllable Boundary			
— List words/Draw line between syllable boundaries; Note differences			

Note other factors: Elicitation mode, situational context, overlearned words, etc.

Final Rule Description: _____

Solution

I. *Take one error and choose possible parameters.*
   A. Fill in the error being analyzed (*pot* → /pap/).
   B. Ask question: Manner? (Answer: *No*. Both the /t/ in *pot* and the final /p/ in /pap/ have the same manner.)
   C. Voicing? (Answer: *No*.)
   D. Placement? (Answer: *Maybe*. It is possible that Cora has a speech problem whereby she does not produce alveolars, shifting them to the labial position instead.)
   E. Context? (Answer: *Maybe*. The other possible explanation is that the /t/ is changing to /p/ because there is a labial culprit in the word. Maybe Cora has difficulty with production of /t/ only when it is in the context of a labial.)
   F. Structure? (Answer: *No*. Both *pot* and /pap/ have the same syllable structures.)
   G. Linguistic? (Answer: *Unlikely*.)
   H. Semantic? (Answer: *Unlikely*.)
   I. Because there exists confusion regarding whether placement or context is the parameter responsible for the error, we must perform a Parameter Confusion Test.

I-a. *Parameter Confusion Test*
   A. On the appropriate form, note the target word on the correct line (i.e., *pot*).
   B. Indicate the client's production on the next line (i.e., /pap/).
   C. Choose test word. An appropriate test word will contain an alveolar, but will not have a labial culprit. (The very next word in the list, *cat*, meets our needs.)
   D. Does the error still occur? (Answer: *No*. When the labial culprit is removed from the word, assimilation no longer occurs and the alveolar is produced correctly.)
   E. Return to Step 1 of the 6-step procedure. Cross out the *maybe* after placement and write *no*. Then cross out the *maybe* after context and indicate *yes*. We can now proceed with Step 2. (See Appendix A for correctly completed Parameter Confusion Test worksheet.)

II. *Make initial conclusion re: rule by describing the difference between target and client production.*
   A. Fill in the violated parameter, as per Step 1 (i.e., context).
   B. Describe what the client is doing: When there is a labial in a word, other sounds assimilate to the labial position.
   C. Label the rule: Labial Assimilation.

III. *Perform Consistency Check.*
   A. Go to Consistency Checklist and place the word analyzed in Steps 1 and 2 (*pot*) into the *yes* column.
   B. Systematically go to each word in the sample having the possibility for labial assimilation (*pig, soup, ship, bed, meat, feet, might, come, tame*). Does

labial assimilation occur in these words? If so, put the word in the *yes* column; if not, put it in the *no* column. (Answer: *Yes* for *soup, ship, bed, meat, feet, might, come, tame.* How about *pig*? Well, we cannot say *yes*, because the final g does not change to a labial. But we cannot say *no* either. Because of the final sound omission we are in a position of not knowing for certain whether labial assimilation would have occurred in the word had the final consonant been retained. So we skip the word in our consistency analysis, reasoning that there is no chance for labial assimilation to occur given the structural error. The word *pig* is put into neither the *yes* nor the *no* columns.)

   C. Since all words having a chance for labial assimilation do indeed exhibit that rule, we know that the rule is consistent. Fill in the final rule description (i.e., Labial Assimilation) on the bottom line of the Consistency Checklist. (See Appendix A for completed checklist.)

IV. *Describe rule in final form.*

   A. Transfer the final rule description from the bottom of the Consistency Checklist to the appropriate space on the generic worksheet.

V. *Go to phonological rule summary. Find all words for which rule is operating and note.*

   A. On the rule summary sheet, go to each word having Labial Assimilation and record that rule in the appropriate column.

VI. *Perform final check.*

   A. Return to the first error listed on the phonological rule summary (i.e., *pot*)—Ask question: Is the error now totally explained by the rule listed? (Answer: *Yes.* Check off the word.)

   B. Ask the same question with the other words. (The only other word that can be checked off is *bed*. The other words [i.e., *soup, ship, meat, feet, might, come,* and *tame*] have at least one more rule operating in them and cannot as yet be checked off.)

Having determined the first of Cora's rules, our next step is to proceed to the next error in the speech sample (i.e., the *sh* in *shoot*) and repeat the process.

  I. *Take one error and choose possible parameters.*

   A. Fill in the error being analyzed (*shoot* → /tμt/).

   B. Manner: (Answer: *Yes.* The *sh* sound is a fricative whereas the /t/ sound is a stop.)

   C. Voicing? (Answer: *No.*)

   D. Placement? (Answer: *No.* The /t/ position is the natural stopping place for *sh*.)

   E. Context? (Answer: *No.*)

   F. Structure? (Answer: *No.*)

   G. Linguistic? (Answer: *Unlikely.*)

   H. Semantic? (Answer: *Unlikely.*)

   I. Because we have one *yes* and no confusion, we can go on to Step 2.

 II. *Make initial conclusion re: rule by describing the difference between target and client production.*

   A. Fill in the violated parameter, as per Step 1 (in this case, manner).

    B. Describe what the client is doing: A fricative is becoming a stop.

    C. Label the rule: Stopping of Fricatives.

III. *Perform Consistency Check.*

    A. Go to Consistency Checklist and put the word analyzed in Steps 1 and 2 into the *yes* column.

    B. One by one, evaluate the other words in the speech sample that have a possibility for Stopping of Fricatives (*soup, sock, kiss, shake, ship, nose, feet*). Does Stopping of Fricatives occur? If so, put the given word in the *yes* column; otherwise, put it in the *no* column. (Answers: *Yes* for all words.)

    C. Fill in the final rule description (i.e., Stopping of Fricatives) on the bottom line of the Consistency Checklist. (See Appendix 1 for completed checklist.)

IV. *Describe rule in final form.*

    A. Transfer the final rule description from the bottom of the Consistency Checklist to the appropriate space on the generic worksheet.

V. *Go to phonological rule summary. Find all words for which rule is operating, and note.*

    A. On the rule summary sheet, go to the eight words that have Stopping of Fricatives and record that rule in the appropriate column.

VI. *Perform final check.*

    A. Return to the first occurrence of Stopping of Fricatives on the phonological rule summary (i.e., *shoot*). Ask question: Is the error now totally explained by the rule listed? (Answer: *Yes*. Check off the word.)

    B. Ask the same question with *soup*. (Answer: *Yes*. *Soup* → /tup/ after Stopping of Fricatives and /tup/ → /pup/ as a result of the Labial Assimilation. Check off the word.)

    C. Ask same question with *sock*. (Answer: *No*. *Sock* goes to /tak/ as a result of the rule, but that is not what Cora is saying.)

    D. Ask same question with *kiss*. (Answer: *Yes*. *Kiss* is a golden word for Stopping of Fricatives.)

    E. Ask same question with *shake*. (Answer: *No*, for the same reason as *sock*.)

    F. Ask same question with *ship*. (Answer: *Yes*. *Ship* becomes /fɪp/ due to Labial Assimilation and /fɪp/ → /pɪp/ after Stopping of Fricatives. Check off the word.)

    G. Ask same question with *nose*. (Answer: *No*. *Nose* becomes /nod/ due to Stopping of Fricatives, but we haven't yet explained the /d/ → /n/ when Cora says /non/.)

    H. Ask same question with *feet*. (Answer: *Yes*. *Feet* → /pit/ [Stopping of Fricatives] and /pit/ → /pip/ [Labial Assimilation]. Check off the word.)

We have now deciphered two of Cora's rules. However, we still have two more to go. Once again, we go to the next error in the sample and repeat the process.

    I. *Take one error and choose possible parameters.*

        A. Fill in the error being analyzed (*dog* → /dɔ/).

        B. Manner? (Answer: *No*.)

        C. Voicing? (Answer: *No*.)

        D. Placement? (Answer: *No*.)

E. Context? (Answer: *No*.)

F. Structure? (Answer: *Yes*. A CVC syllable structure has become CV.)

G. Linguistic? (Answer: *Unlikely*.)

H. Semantic? (Answer: *Unlikely*.)

I. We have one *yes* and no confusion, so we proceed with Step 2.

II. *Make initial conclusion re: rule by describing the difference between target and client production.*

A. Fill in the violated parameter, as per Step 1 (in this case, structure).

B. Describe what the client is doing: A final consonant is being omitted from the word.

C. Label the rule: Deletion of Final Consonants.

III. *Perform Consistency Check.*

A. Go to Consistency Checklist and put the word analyzed in Steps 1 and 2 into the *yes* column.

B. One by one, evaluate each of the other words with final consonants. Does the rule occur? If so, put the given word in the yes column; otherwise, put it in the *no* column. (Answers: *Yes* for *dog, pig, sock, shake, duck,* and *neck. No* for all other words.)

C. Visual inspection of word lists.

1. Study the two lists of words. Try to find a systematic difference between the words exhibiting the deletion rule and those not demonstrating the rule.

2. If you figure out the systematic difference by means of this visual inspection, go to the bottom of the checklist and label the newly discovered rule. Otherwise, perform the systematic consistency check. (In this case, it will be assumed that the limitation could not be deciphered upon visual inspection alone; as such, we shall undertake a systematic consistency check.)

D. Systematic consistency check.

1. Evaluate phonetic context.

a. Vowel preceding: *Yes* words—/ɔ/, /ɪ/, /a/, /e/, /ʌ/, /ɛ/. *No* words—/a/, /æ/, /µ/, /ɪ/, /o/, /ɛ/, /i/, /aɪ/, /ʌ/, /e/. *Conclusion*: As we have more *no* words, more vowels appear for that group. But overall, there are no significant differences between the preceding vowels of the *yes* words and those of the *no* words.

b. Vowel following: *Conclusion*: Not applicable as we are studying final consonants only.

c. Consonant preceding: *Yes* words—/d/, /p/, /s/, /ʃ/, /d/, /n/. *No* words—/p/, /k/, /ʃ/, etc. *Conclusion*: Already there are overlaps between *yes* and *no* words. No significant difference exists in the preceding consonants.

d. Consonant following: *Conclusion*: Again, not applicable as only final consonants are being evaluated.

e. Other significant nonadjacent sounds: A visual check reveals no sounds that systematically occur in the *yes* words yet do not occur in the *no* words. *Conclusion*: This is not a factor.

2. Evaluate position.
   a. This factor need not even be evaluated here, as we are interested in final consonants only.
3. Evaluate intraclass variability.
   a. In this case, we are interested in whether there is a particular subclass of final sounds in which the rule operates as opposed to another subclass in which the rule is absent.
   b. Class members appearing in *yes* words: /g/, /g/, /k/, /k/, /k/, /k/. Class members appearing in *no* words: /t/, /t/, /t/, /p/, /s/, /p/, /z/, /d/, /t/, /t/, /t/, /t/, /m/, /m/.
   c. *Conclusion:* This is the factor we have been looking for. All *yes* words contain velars in the final position; all *no* words contain nonvelars, or other sounds.
   d. A new, limited rule can be formulated: Deletion of Final Velars. This rule should be noted on the bottom of the Consistency Checklist. The systematic consistency check is now complete and we can return to our generic analysis. (See Appendix A for completed Consistency Checklist.)

IV. *Describe rule in final form.*
   A. Transfer the final rule description (in this case, Deletion of Final Velars) from the bottom of the Consistency Checklist to the appropriate space on the generic worksheet.

V. *Go to phonological rule summary. Find all words for which rule is operating, and note.*
   A. On the rule summary sheet, go to the six words that have Deletion of Final Velars and record that rule in the appropriate column.

VI. *Perform final check.*
   A. Return to the first occurrence of Deletion of Final Velars on the phonological rule summary (i.e., *dog*). Ask question: Is the error now totally explained by the rule listed? (Answer: *Yes.* Check off the word.)
   B. Ask the same question with *pig.* (Answer: *Yes.* Check off the word.)
   C. Ask the same question with *sock.* (Answer: *Yes. Sock* becomes /tak/ due to Stopping of Fricatives, which then becomes /ta/ after Deletion of Final Velars. Check off the word.)
   D. Ask the same question with *shake.* (Answer: *Yes. Shake* → /ʃe/ [Deletion of Final Velars] and /ʃe/ → /te/ [Stopping of Fricatives]. Check off the word.)
   E. Ask the same question with *duck.* (Answer: *Yes.* Check off the word.)

This completes our analysis of the third rule. Only one to go. Let us proceed to the next error on the list.

I. *Take one error and choose possible parameters.*
   A. Fill in the error being analyzed (*nose* → /non/).
   B. Manner? (Answer: *Yes.* A nonnasal sound is becoming nasalized.)

C. Voicing? (Answer: *No.*)

D. Placement? (Answer: *No.* Both the /z/ in *nose* and the /n/ in /non/ are alveolars.)

E. Context? (Answer: *No.* However, if this answer bothers you, see the footnote[6] below.)

F. Structure? (Answer: *No.*)

G. Linguistic? (Answer: *Unlikely.*)

H. Semantic? (Answer: *Unlikely.*)

I. Because we have one *yes* and no confusion, we can proceed with Step 2.

II. *Make initial conclusion re: rule by describing the difference between target and client production.*

A. Fill in the violated parameter, as per Step 1 (in this case, manner).

B. Describe what the client is doing: A nonnasal sound is becoming nasalized.

C. Label the rule: Nasalization.

III. *Perform Consistency Check.*

A. Go to Consistency Checklist and put the word analyzed in Steps 1 and 2 into the *yes* column.

B. One by one, evaluate each of the other words with nonnasal sounds (which, of course, includes all of the other words). Does the rule occur in those words? If so, put the given word in the *yes* column: otherwise, put it in the *no* column. (Answers: *nose, meat, neat, might, come,* and *tame* go into the *yes* column. All other words belong in the *no* column.)

C. Visual inspection of the word lists.

1. Study the two lists of words. Try to find a systematic difference between the words exhibiting the nasalization rule and those that do not.

2. If you figure out the systematic difference by means of this visual inspection, go to the bottom of the checklist and label the newly discovered limited rule. Otherwise, perform the systematic consistency check.

3. After studying the two lists, it is quite easy to see that the error is occurring only when there is another nasal sound in the word. When the other sound in the word is not nasal, no "nasalization" occurs. So a nasal sound anywhere in the word acts as a culprit to change the other

---

[6]If your initial answer was *maybe* rather than *no,* you are not incorrect. One might very well say that the initial /n/ in *nose* could be a nasal culprit, causing the final sound to become nasalized. However, remember that in Chapters 5 and 6, we decided by convention to analyze confusions between placement and context only. We further claimed that any rare manner-context confusions (e.g., stop assimilation, or, in this case, nasal assimilation) would be resolved during the consistency check. As you will see, this will be the case with Cora. Although this decision risks an accusation of some arbitrariness in the development of the analytic process, the major purpose throughout has been ease of learning rather than procedural parsimony. It is all probably moot anyway, because in the next section, methods of speeding up the analytical process and eliminating the entire first step of the 6-step procedure will be presented.

consonant in the word to a nasal. Nasal Assimilation seems to be occurring after all. This new, limited rule should be noted on the bottom of the Consistency Checklist. (See Appendix A for completed checklist.)

IV. *Describe rule in final form.*

    A. Transfer the final rule description (in this case, Nasal Assimilation) from the bottom of the Consistency Checklist to the appropriate space on the generic worksheet.

V. *Go to phonological rule summary, find all words for which rule is operating, and note.*

    A. On the rule summary sheet, go to the six words having Nasal Assimilation and record that rule in the appropriate column.

VI. *Perform final check.*

    A. Return to the first occurrence of Nasal Assimilation. Ask question: Is the error now totally explained by the rule listed? (Answer: *Yes. Nose* → /nod/ [Stopping of Fricatives] and /nod/ → /non/ [Nasal Assimilation]. Check off the word.)

    B. Ask the same question with *meat*. (Answer: *Yes. Meat* becomes /min/ as a result of Nasal Assimilation and / min/ → /mim/ after Labial Assimilation. Check off the word.)

    C. Ask the same question with *neat*. (Answer: *Yes.* Check off the word.)

    D. Ask the same question with *might*. (Answer: *Yes. Might* becomes /maɪp/ [Labial Assimilation] and /maɪp/ → /maɪm/ [Nasal Assimilation]. Check off the word.)

    E. Ask the same question with *come*. (Answer: *Yes. Come* → /pʌm/ [Labial Assimilation] and /pʌm/ → /mʌm/ [Nasal Assimilation]. Check off the word.)

    F. Ask the same question with *tame*. (Answer: *Yes. Tame* becomes /nem/ after Nasal Assimilation and /nem/ becomes /mem/ as a result of Labial Assimilation.)

    G. As all misarticulated words have now been checked off, Cora's analysis is now complete. (See the completed phonological rule summary for Cora.)

PHONOLOGICAL RULE SUMMARY

Client: _Cora Appel_

Check	Target Word	Client Production	Rule(s) Operating
✓	pot	pap	LA
✓	cat	kæt	Correct
✓	shoot	tut	SF
✓	dog	dɔ	DFV
✓	pig	pI	DFV
✓	soup	pup	SF; LA
✓	sock	tɑ	SF; DFV
✓	kiss	kIt	SF
✓	shake	te	SF; DFV
✓	ship	pIp	LA
✓	nose	non	SF; NA
✓	bed	bɛb	LA
✓	duck	bʌ	DFV
✓	meat	mim	LA; NA
✓	neat	nin	NA
✓	feet	pip	LA; SF
✓	neck	nɛ	DFV
✓	might	maIm	LA; NA
✓	come	mʌm	LA; NA
✓	tame	mem	LA; NA

Discussion

Something was probably occurring to many of you while proceeding through Cora's analysis. Although Cora exhibited only 4 phonological rules, already the time and paperwork required for the procedure was becoming burdensome and unwieldy. Imagine a client with 8 rules. Or 10. If you had to complete a full 6-step generic procedure for each of those rules, along with any associated Parameter Confusion Tests and Consistency Checks, you would probably opt for retirement instead. Happily, the burden of excessive time and paperwork can be eased considerably, with the use of a few shortcuts.

Speeding Up the Analytical Process

Let us return for a moment to the unanalyzed phonological rule summary for Cora (see page 226). Rather than taking the first error and subjecting it to the first two steps of the generic procedure, as we did earlier, this time just glance casually through the speech sample. Look for a golden word that immediately signals a familiar rule. For example, just glancing at Cora's substitution of /kɪt/ for *kiss* probably brings to mind Stopping of Fricatives almost immediately.

Now that you have a tentative rule, quickly scan the other words in the speech sample, focusing on the fricatives. See if you can find any examples of a fricative which is *not* stopped. In other words, you are looking for any examples that might invalidate your rule. Not finding any in this case, you would then note the rule in the appropriate column on the summary sheet and check off any words for which the rule listed has totally explained the error.

Next, return to the speech sample and look for another golden word that might cue a familiar rule. The error in /pap/ for *pot* looks very familiar. In fact, without even going through the first step of the generic procedure, we have seen this error

frequently enough to know that one of two things is happening: Either the rule is Labial Assimilation or the client has a fronting rule whereby the alveolar /t/ is being fronted to the labial position. To find out which, let us try a *mental* Parameter Confusion Test. We will find a word without a labial culprit and see if the /t/ sound still changes position. Of course (as is seen in the word *cat*), the error disappears when the culprit is removed, so we know that the rule is Labial Assimilation.

Once again, now that a tentative rule has been determined, quickly scan the other words in the speech sample, focusing on words with labials. See if you can find any words with labials in which Labial Assimilation does *not* occur. Because there are no discrepancies with Cora, the final step is to note the rule as appropriate on the summary sheet and check off any additional words in which the error has been explained.

If you timed the described activities, you would find that the entire procedure for a given rule need take no longer than 1–2 minutes, even with the extra step of the mental Parameter Confusion Test. That means that for Cora, half of her analysis would be completed in 2–4 minutes.

When is more than 1–2 minutes needed? Sometimes you will be faced with a sound error that does not immediately suggest to you a familiar rule. On these occasions, you may have to return to Step 1 of the 6-step generic process and systematically go through each of the parameters of articulatory constraint, until you arrive at the correct rule. You will find, however, that this will occur less and less frequently as you become more familiar with the most common rules. In fact, at some point in the future, you will undoubtedly be able to discard the first two steps of the process totally. So much the better! In reality you will not really be abandoning those first two steps so much as performing them mentally.

The other time when more than 1–2 minutes is needed will occur when you

PHONOLOGICAL RULE SUMMARY

Client: _Cora Appel_

Check	Target Word	Client Production	Rule(s) Operating
	pot	pap	
	cat	kæt	
	shoot	tut	
	dog	dɔ	
	pig	pɪ	
	soup	pʌp	
	sock	ta	
	kiss	kɪt	
	shake	te	
	ship	pɪp	
	nose	non	
	bed	bɛb	
	duck	dʌ	
	meat	mim	
	neat	nin	
	feet	pip	
	neck	nɛ	
	might	maɪm	
	come	mʌm	
	tame	mem	

find words in which your originally hypothesized rule does not occur. On these occasions, unfortunately, the only answer is to go back to the *yes* (rule occurring) and *no* (rule not occurring) columns of the Consistency Checklist, and try to determine the limitation. Although this procedure will definitely take some time, as we have seen, it is time well worth spending. Further, you will find that with more experience, your ability to begin sensing the limitations that do occur will improve. This will translate into less need for the systematic consistency check, the part of the procedure that is the most time intensive. Finally, keep in mind that for most rules there will be no limitation. Because our "new streamlined procedure" now only requires a consistency check when some limitation is found, you will only be engaging in this time intensive procedure for a small percentage of your clients' rules.

In summary, three suggestions have been made for speeding up what could be a time-consuming process of phonological analysis. These suggestions are summarized below:

1. Search for Golden Words—Scan the client's speech sample for a golden word that immediately suggests a familiar rule. If this can be done for several of the rules exhibited by a given client, much time will be saved.

2. Perform a Mental Parameter Confusion Test—The more familiar you become with the possible effects of assimilation, the easier it will be for you to do the Parameter Confusion Test in your head, rather than on paper. Remember, you will always be testing for the same thing: Whether a particular sound is produced incorrectly because of a culprit or because of a problem the client has with the sound itself. As long as you locate a word, then, which eliminates the culprit, the test is easy.

3. Perform a Visual Consistency Check First—After determining a probable rule, scan the speech sample and determine whether the rule is consistent. If so, no further paperwork related to this step is necessary. If not, place the relevant words from the speech sample into the *yes* and *no* columns as you would have done originally. Then determine the limitation. You will find that the visual consistency check will save a tremendous amount of time and paperwork.

Finally, in your attempt to save time, there are a few shortcuts that might tempt you, but should be avoided nevertheless. For example:

1. If, after you have determined a rule, your visual check reveals some inconsistency, *resist the temptation to skip the full consistency check*. Success with your client is going to depend heavily on determining the precise rule that the client uses. Without having identified the precise limited rule, you may very well target the wrong goal in therapy.

2. Avoid terminating your analysis until you have checked off all of the words on the client's speech sample—Unless all words have been checked off, something has been missed—perhaps an embedded rule; perhaps a limitation—but something. The only way that you can assure yourself of a correct, completed, and precise analysis is to see check marks beside each of the words in the speech sample.

Additional Practice

The remainder of this chapter will provide you with practice in performing an accelerated phonological analysis. Whenever possible, try to use the previous suggestions for speeding up the analysis. Only go through the entire 6-step procedure when you feel you have to, but try to avoid any sacrifice of precision in your work.

Clinical Mastery Exercise—Leonardo Smackmustard

Introduction

Leonardo was a 4-year-old with greatly reduced intelligibility when first seen for evaluation. If you glance quickly through his speech sample, you will see why. Everything is reduced to a basic CVC syllable structure and there seems to be an overabundance of labials and stops.

You will find that Leonardo's speech has 7 rules. However, you will be provided with fewer worksheets than would be required if you were to complete every step of the 6-step procedure for every rule. If you need additional worksheets, feel free to copy some additional forms from Appendix B. Fill out the Phonological Rule Summary in its entirety, until all words in the sample are checked off. On the other hand, try to use the previous suggestions to minimize your worksheet work and maximize your mental analysis.

One hint (to be read only after you have almost completed the analysis, but find yourself stuck on one element): Your initial hypothesis about one of the more unusual rules is most likely going to be inaccurate and you will end up with some words that you will not be able to check off (e.g., *rock* or *Rick*). To find a solution for this dilemma, you will have to find an explanation for those words that addresses the question of how they got to the labial position. Without answering that question for these words, you will not be able to complete the analysis.

Worksheets provided for Leonardo Smackmustard
- Phonological rule summary
- Two generic 6-step procedures
- Two Parameter Confusion Tests
- Four Consistency Check Forms

(Solution on page 238)

PHONOLOGICAL RULE SUMMARY

Client: *Leonardo Smackmustard*

Check	Target Word	Client Production	Rule(s) Operating
	keep	pip	(correct)
	cot	kɑt	
	many	bɛbt	
	light	dɑɪt	
	yes	dɛt	
	hello	ʔɛdo	
	soup	pʌp	
	sheep	pip	
	shoe	tu	
	fake	pep	
	sky	kɑɪ	
	dog	dɔk	
	big	bɪp	
	you	du	
	red	bɛp	
	cold	kot	
	neck	dɛk	
	meat	bip	
	need	dit	
	rob	bɑp	
	rock	bɑp	
	leg	dɛk	
	one	bʌp	
	wet	bɛp	
	glass	gæt	
	bee	bi	(correct)
	Rick	bɪp	
	stop	pap	

PROCEDURE FOR PHONOLOGICAL ANALYSIS — GENERIC WORKSHEET

I. <u>Take one error and choose possible parameters</u>

        ERROR:

        ANALYSIS: **Manner?** ————➤

                  Voicing? ————➤

                  Placement? ———➤

                  Context? ————➤

                  Structure? ———➤

                  Linguistic? ———➤

                  Semantic? ————➤

> If unclear as to whether placement or context, perform Parameter Confusion Test (See Form). Otherwise go to Step II.

II. <u>Make initial conclusion re: rule by describing the difference between target and client production.</u>

           _____ PARAMETER

               Description:_____

               Rule:_____

III. <u>Perform Consistency Check (See Consistency Check Form)</u>

IV. <u>Describe rule in Final Form</u>

               Rule:_____

V. <u>Go to phonological rule summary, find all words for which rule is operating, and note.</u>

VI. <u>Perform final check</u>

        — Make sure all changes in target word can be explained by rule. If so, check the word off. If not, leave until next analysis.

PROCEDURE FOR PHONOLOGICAL ANALYSIS — GENERIC WORKSHEET

I. **Take one error and choose possible parameters**

    ERROR:
    ANALYSIS: **Manner?** ⎯⎯⎯►

                  Voicing? ⎯⎯⎯►

                  Placement? ⎯⎯►

                  Context? ⎯⎯⎯►

                  Structure? ⎯⎯►

                  Linguistic? ⎯⎯►

                  Semantic? ⎯⎯⎯►

> If unclear as to whether placement or context, perform Parameter Confusion Test (See Form). Otherwise go to Step II.

II. **Make initial conclusion re: rule by describing the difference between target and client production.**

        _____ **PARAMETER**

            Description: _____

            Rule: _____

III. **Perform Consistency Check (See Consistency Check Form)**

IV. **Describe rule in Final Form**

            Rule: _____

V. **Go to phonological rule summary, find all words for which rule is operating, and note.**

VI. **Perform final check**

         — Make sure all changes in target word can be explained by rule. If so, check the word off. If not, leave until next analysis.

PLACEMENT CONTEXT. PARAMETER CONFUSION CHECK

Target Word: _____

Client Production: _____

Choose Test Word: _____
    (Word in which there's no culprit; i.e no
      chance for assimilation to occur).

Error Still Occur? _____Yes

            _____No

    Yes = Placement error; even though chance for assimilation has been
           removed, error still occurs.

    No = Assimilation error; error disappears when culprit is removed.

Return to Step 1 — Generic Worksheet

PLACEMENT CONTEXT. PARAMETER CONFUSION CHECK

Target Word: _____

Client Production: _____

Choose Test Word: _____
   (Word in which there's no culprit; i.e no
     chance for assimilation to occur).

Error Still Occur? _____Yes

                   _____No

   Yes = Placement error; even though chance for assimilation has been
          removed, error still occurs.

   No = Assimilation error; error disappears when culprit is removed.

Return to Step 1 - Generic Worksheet

CONSISTENCY CHECKLIST

Initial Rule Description: _____

Rule Operating (Yes)	Rule Not Operating (No)

Check for Consistency	Yes Words	No Words	Sig. Diff.
1. Phonetic Context			
— List vowel preceding			
— List vowel following			
— List consonant preceding			
— List consonant following			
— List other sig. non-adjacent sounds			
2. Position			
— List I, M, F for initial medial, final			
3. Intra-class Variability			
— List correct/incorrect sounds, search for intra-class patterns			
4. Syllable Structure/ Word Length			
— List syllable structures			
5. Part of Speech/Morphological Endings			
— List grammatical categories			
6. Syllable Stress			
— List U, S for unstressed, stressed			
7. Syllable Boundary — List words/Draw line between syllable boundaries; Note differences			

Note other factors: Elicitation mode, situational context, overlearned words, etc.

Final Rule Description: _____

CONSISTENCY CHECKLIST

Initial Rule Description: _____

Rule Operating (Yes)	Rule Not Operating (No)

Check for Consistency	Yes Words	No Words	Sig. Diff.
1. **Phonetic Context**			
— List vowel preceding			
— List vowel following			
— List consonant preceding			
— List consonant following			
— List other sig. non-adjacent sounds			
2. **Position**			
— List I, M, F for initial medial, final			
3. **Intra-class Variability**			
— List correct/incorrect sounds, search for intra-class patterns			
4. **Syllable Structure/ Word Length**			
— List syllable structures			
5. **Part of Speech/Morphological Endings**			
— List grammatical categories			
6. **Syllable Stress**			
— List U, S for unstressed, stressed			
7. **Syllable Boundary**			
— List words/Draw line between syllable boundaries; Note differences			

Note other factors: Elicitation mode, situational context, overlearned words, etc.

Final Rule Description: _____

CONSISTENCY CHECKLIST

Initial Rule Description: _____

Rule Operating (Yes)	Rule Not Operating (No)

Check for Consistency	Yes Words	No Words	Sig. Diff.
1. Phonetic Context			
— List vowel preceding			
— List vowel following			
— List consonant preceding			
— List consonant following			
— List other sig. non-adjacent sounds			
2. Position			
— List I, M, F for initial medial, final			
3. Intra-class Variability			
— List correct/incorrect sounds, search for intra-class patterns			
4. Syllable Structure/ Word Length			
— List syllable structures			
5. Part of Speech/Morphological Endings			
— List grammatical categories			
6. Syllable Stress			
— List U, S for unstressed, stressed			
7. Syllable Boundary — List words/Draw line between syllable boundaries; Note differences			

Note other factors: Elicitation mode, situational context, overlearned words, etc.

Final Rule Description: _____

CONSISTENCY CHECKLIST

Initial Rule Description: _____

Rule Operating (Yes)	Rule Not Operating (No)

Check for Consistency	Yes Words	No Words	Sig. Diff.
1. **Phonetic Context**			
— List vowel preceding			
— List vowel following			
— List consonant preceding			
— List consonant following			
— List other sig. non-adjacent sounds			
2. **Position**			
— List I, M, F for initial medial, final			
3. **Intra-class Variability**			
— List correct/incorrect sounds, search for intra-class patterns			
4. **Syllable Structure/ Word Length**			
— List syllable structures			
5. **Part of Speech/Morphological Endings**			
— List grammatical categories			
6. **Syllable Stress**			
— List U, S for unstressed, stressed			
7. **Syllable Boundary**			
— List words/Draw line between syllable boundaries; Note differences			

Note other factors: Elicitation mode, situational context, overlearned words, etc.

Final Rule Description: _____

Solution

The format for presenting the solution to this analysis will be changed, in order to correspond to the accelerated analytical procedure introduced in the last section.

Rule One

I. *Scan the speech sample for a golden word that will immediately cue one of the client's rules.*
   A. *Shoe* is a golden word when it becomes /tµ/. This error is very familiar, cuing the rule Stopping of Fricatives.
II. *Perform a visual check for consistency.*
   A. Visually evaluate each fricative, to see if the rule is consistent.
   B. If you find any answers of *no*, perform a full Consistency Check using the appropriate worksheet. (In this case, all fricatives in the words *yes, hello, soup, sheep, fake, glass,* and *stop* are stopped. The rule is consistent.)

What about sky? *You didn't label this word a* yes, *yet you are not calling it a* no. *Since the /s/ is omitted in the word, why isn't it called a* no?

Sky to /kaɪ/ cannot be called a *yes* for Stopping of Fricatives because the sound in question is omitted. However, it cannot be deemed a *no* either, because the deletion has made it impossible for stopping to occur. In this case, the deletion is what is known as an *overriding* or *dominant* rule. Whenever you have a dominant rule embedded with a subservient rule (in this case, stopping) you cannot say that the subservient rule is not occurring. Instead, one has to say that there has been no chance for occurrence due to the overriding nature of the dominant rule. So in terms of the consistency check, one skips the word, designating it *No Chance*.

III. *Note the rule for each involved word on the summary sheet and check off the word if it has been explained.*
   A. The rule is noted after the words *yes, hello, soup, sheep, shoe, fake, glass, stop.*
   B. The word *shoe* is checked off; the remaining words have additional rules working.

One of the 7 rules has now been easily and quickly determined. We shall now go on to the second rule in operation.

Rule Two

I. *Scan the speech sample for a golden word that will immediately cue one of the client's rules.*
   A. The rule operating in the first word, *keep,* looks like one we have seen many times before. We know that the /k/ → /p/ either due to Labial Assimilation or some type of fronting rule. We have to get rid of the culprit and perform a mental Parameter Confusion Test to be sure.

I-a. *Perform mental Parameter Confusion Test.*
   A. Find a word that has a /k/ sound but no labial culprit. (The word *cot* is attractively available.)
   B. The error no longer occurs once the culprit is eliminated, thus Labial Assimilation is the cause of *keep* → /pip/.

II. *Perform a visual check for consistency.*
   A. Visually evaluate each word having a labial and another consonant to see if Labial Assimilation is consistently occurring in the relevant words.
   B. If you find any answers of *no*, perform a full Consistency Check using the appropriate worksheet. (In this case, all words with labials and other sounds demonstrate Labial Assimilation. The rule is consistent.)

III. *Note the rule for each involved word on the summary sheet and check off the word if it has been explained.*
   A. The rule is noted after the words *keep, many, soup, sheep, fake, big, meat, rob, one, wet,* and *stop.*

Why isn't the rule noted for rock, *for which Leonardo says* /bap/, *or* red, *for which he says* /bɛp/?

Because neither of these words has a labial in the target, we cannot yet attribute any of the errors to Labial Assimilation. This does not mean that Labial Assimilation is *not* occurring as part of the client's error. It's just that we cannot yet claim this rule because there is not yet a labial culprit.

   B. The words *keep, soup, sheep,* and *fake* are checked off. The remaining words have additional rules working.

Rule Three

I. *Scan the speech sample for a golden word that will immediately cue one of the client's rules.*
   A. There are several golden words for this next rule; we will choose *dog* (for which Leonardo says /dɔk/).
   B. Although the first reaction might be Devoicing of Consonants, we can already tell from *dog* that that rule would be limited. After scanning the speech sample once more to verify our hypothesis, we decide to label the rule Devoicing of Final Consonants.

II. *Perform a visual check for consistency.*
   A. Visually evaluate each word with a voiced final consonant to see if it becomes unvoiced, as per our rule.
   B. If any answers of *no* are found, perform a full Consistency Check using the appropriate worksheet. (In this case, all final voiced consonants become voiceless, so the rule is consistent.)

III. *Note the rule for each involved word on the summary sheet and check off the word if it has been explained.*
   A. Devoicing of Final Consonants is noted after the words *dog, big, red, cold, need, rob, leg,* and *one.*

B. The word *dog* is checked off. All other words continue to have additional rules at work.

Rule Four

I. *Scan the speech sample for a golden word that will immediately cue one of the client's rules.*

   A. The next rule, Denasalization, is identifiable in many golden words (for example, the /m/ in *many* makes that word golden, as does the /n/ in *neck* or *need* or the /m/ in *meat*).

II. *Perform a visual check for consistency.*

   A. Visually evaluate each word with a nasal sound to see if it becomes denasal.

   B. If any answers of *no* are found, perform a full consistency check using the appropriate worksheet. (In this case, all nasal sounds become denasal; thus the rule is consistent.

III. *Note the rule for each involved word on the summary sheet and check off the word if it has been explained.*

   A. Denasalization is noted twice for the word *many* and once for *neck, meat, need*, and *one*.

   B. A few more words can now be checked off. *Many* becomes /mɛmi/ (Labial Assimilation) which then becomes /bɛbi/ (Denasalization). Since this is Leonardo's output, the word is checked off. Likewise, *neck, meat*, and *need* can be checked off.

Rule Five

I. *Scan the speech sample for a golden word which will immediately cue one of the client's rules.*

   A. We next notice *sky* → /kaɪ/. Although we have not had much formal experience with this rule in earlier examples, the rule itself is easily identifiable: Cluster Reduction.

II. *Perform a visual check for consistency.*

   A. Visually evaluate each word having a consonant cluster to see if one element in the cluster is omitted.

   B. If any answers of *no* are found, perform a full Consistency Check using the appropriate worksheet. (In this case, all clusters are reduced to a single consonant. The rule is consistent.)

III. *Note the rule for each involved word on the summary sheet and check off the word if it has been explained.*

   A. The rule is noted after the words *sky, cold, glass*, and *stop*.

   B. All words with clusters—*sky, cold, glass*, and *stop*—can be checked off.

We have now completed our analysis of Leonardo's less difficult rules. Unfortunately, the remainder of the analysis will be more problematic. In anticipating some of these problems, we will now revert back to the longer 6-step procedure. Nonetheless, we will continue to take some shortcuts if we believe that the quality of the analysis can be maintained.

Rule Six

I. *Take one error and choose possible parameters.*
   A. Fill in the errors being analyzed (*light* → /daɪt/; *you* → /dʌ/)

Why have you picked two errors to analyze?

A quick scan of the speech sample indicates that the same thing seems to be happening to both liquids and glides. Because those two sound categories are closely related to one another, it is possible that Leonardo has one rule that encompasses both groups. Further, considering the two groups together will inevitably speed up the analysis. So it makes sense to do so here.

   B. Manner? (Answer: *Yes.* In one instance a liquid is becoming a stop; in the other, a glide is turning into a stop.)
   C. Voicing? (Answer: *No.*)
   D. Placement? (Answer: *No.* All liquids and glides remain in their original positions with the exception of /j/, which goes to its natural stopping place.)
   E. Context? (Answer: *No.*)
   F. Structure? (Answer: *No.*)
   G. Linguistic? (Answer: *Unlikely.*)
   H. Semantic? (Answer: *Unlikely.*)
   I. Because there is no confusion as to which parameter has been violated, we can proceed to Step 2.
II. *Make initial conclusion re: rule by describing the difference between target and client production.*
   A. Fill in the violated parameter, as per Step 1 (i.e., manner).
   B. Describe what the client is doing: Liquids and glides are becoming stops.
   C. Label the rule: Stopping of Liquids and Glides.
III. *Perform Consistency Check.*
   A. To speed up the procedure, we will attempt a visual check for consistency first, visually evaluating each word having a liquid or a glide, to see if it becomes stopped.
   B. If any answers of *no* are found, perform a full consistency check using the appropriate worksheet. (In this case, all liquids and glides are stopped. Thus, no limitation exists.)
IV. *Describe rule in final form.*
   A. Final rule description: Stopping of Liquids and Glides.
V. *Go to phonological rule summary, find all words for which rule is operating, and note.*
   A. On the rule summary sheet, go to each word having Stopping of Liquids and Glides and record that rule in the appropriate column.

VI. *Perform final check.*

A. Return to the first word on the rule summary sheet that has the rule being analyzed (i.e., *light*). Ask question: Is the error now totally explained by the rule or rules listed? (Answer: *Yes.* Check off the word.)

B. Ask the same question with the other words. (*Yes, hello, you, rob, leg, one,* and *wet* can be checked off. However, *red, rock,* and *Rick* cannot be checked off. For example, *red* → /dɛd/ [Stopping of Liquids and Glides] which then becomes /dɛt/ [Devoicing of Final Consonants] but the child says /bɛp/. How has that word terminated in the labial position? We have no rule to explain this. Similarly *rock* → /dak/ [Stopping of Liquids and Glides] but we have no rule to get it to /bap/, Leonardo's utterance.)

In fact, we have a problem at this point. Our speech sample is now explained with the exception of three words. (See the "almost-finished" analysis.) In each of those three words, the consonants terminate in the labial position. Yet no rule has been discovered that might explain this phenomenon.

In order to solve this problem, some way must be found to move words like *rock* from the middle to the front of the mouth. Can you think of a solution to the problem? (Hint: This "position change" has to occur only in words having /r/. There is a very common rule that regularly moves /r/ to the labial position.)

Of course! Gliding of Liquids will move /r/ to /w/ (a labial). In reality, our earlier rule—Stopping of Liquids and Glides—was incorrect. Instead, Leonardo has two rules—Gliding of Liquids and Stopping of Glides. Unfortunately, the Gliding of Liquids rule is totally hidden in most words, because the Stopping of Glides rule masks our ability to study the two sound classes separately—*except in words with /r/!* Because words with /r/ glide to the labial /w/, the stopping will now occur in the labial position; if the gliding was not occurring, on the other hand, the /r/ would have been stopped in the /d/ position.

Now we have to redo the final two steps of the analysis, correcting our incorrect rule. In the case of *light,* Stopping of Liquids and Glides is crossed out, to be replaced with Gliding of Liquids (light → /jaɪt/) and Stopping of Glides (/jaɪt/ → /daɪt/). The following changes are also made:

1. For *yes,* rule is now Stopping of Glides.
2. For *hello,* Stopping of Liquids and Glides is replaced with Gliding of Liquids (*hello* → /hɛjo/) and Stopping of Glides (/hɛjo/ → /hɛdo/) to go with Stopping of Fricatives (/hɛdo/ → /ʔɛdo/). The word can again be checked off.
3. For *you,* change rule to Stopping of Glides.
4. For *red,* these rules are now working:

Devoicing of Final Consonants	(*red* → /rɛt/)
Gliding of Liquids	(/rɛt/ → /wɛt/)
Labial Assimilation	(/wɛt/ → /wɛp/)
Stopping of Glides	(/wɛp/ → /bɛp/)

PHONOLOGICAL RULE SUMMARY

Client: *Leonardo Smackmustard*

Check	Target Word	Client Production	Rule(s) Operating
✓	keep	pip	LA
✓	cot	kat	(correct)
✓	many	bɛbɨ	LA; DEN; DEN
✓	light	daɪt	SLG
✓	yes	dɛt	SF; SLG
✓	hello	ʔɛdo	SF; SLG
✓	soup	pup	SF; LA
✓	sheep	pip	SF; LA
✓	shoe	tu	SF
✓	fake	pep	SF; LA
✓	sky	kaɪ	CR
✓	dog	dɔk	DFC
✓	big	bɪp	LA; DFC
✓	you	du	SLG
?	red	bɛp	DFC; SLG
✓	cold	kot	DFC; CR
✓	neck	dɛk	DEN
✓	meat	bip	LA; DEN
✓	need	dit	DFC; DEN
✓	rob	bap	LA; SLG; DFC
✓	rock	bap	SLG
?	leg	dɛk	DFC; SLG
✓	one	bʌp	LA; DFC; DEN; SLG
✓	wet	bɛp	LA; SLG
✓	glass	gæt	SF; CR
✓	bee	bi	(correct)
?	Rick	bɪp	SLG
✓	stop	pap	SF; LA; CR

243

5. For *rob*, these rules are working:

Gliding of Liquids	(*rob* → /wab/)
Stopping of Glides	(/wab/ → /bab/)
Devoicing of Final Consonants	(/bab/ → /bap/)

6. For *rock*:

Gliding of Liquids	(*rock* → /wak/)
Labial Assimilation	(/wak/ → /wap/)
Stopping of Glides	(/wap/ → /bap/)

7. For *leg*:

Gliding of Liquids	(*leg* → /jɛg/)
Stopping of Glides	(/jɛg/ → /dɛg/)
Devoicing of Final Consonants	(/dɛg/ → /dɛk/)

8. For *one*:

Denasalization	(*one* → /wʌd/)
Labial Assimilation	(/wʌd/ → /wʌb/)
Stopping of Glides	(/wʌb/ → /bʌb/)
Devoicing of Final Consonants	(/bʌb/ → /bʌp/)

9. For *wet*:

Stopping of Glides	(*wet* → /bɛt/)
Labial Assimilation	(/bɛt/ → /bɛp/)

10. For *Rick*:

Gliding of Liquids	(*Rick* → /wɪk/)
Labial Assimilation	(/wɪk/ → /wɪp/)
Stopping of Glides	(/wɪp/ → /bɪp/)

All of these words can now be checked off and Leonardo's analysis is complete. (See the corrected finished analysis on the opposite page.)

PHONOLOGICAL RULE SUMMARY

Client: _Leonardo Smackmustard_

Check	Target Word	Client Production	Rule(s) Operating
✓	keep	pip	LA
✓	cot	kat	
✓	many	bɛbɨ	LA; DEN'; DE
✓	light	daɪt	GL; SG
✓	yes	dɛt	SF; SG
✓	hello	ʔɛdo	SF; GL; SG
✓	soup	pup	SF; LA
✓	sheep	pip	SF; LA
✓	shoe	tu	SF
✓	fake	pep	SF; LA
✓	sky	kaɪ	CR
✓	dog	dɔk	DFC
✓	big	bɪp	LA; DFC
✓	you	du	SG
✓	red	bɛp	DFC; GL; SG; LA
✓	cold	kot	DFC; CR
✓	neck	dɛk	DEN
✓	meat	bip	LA; DEN
✓	need	dit	DFC; DEN
✓	rob	bap	GL; SG; DFC
✓	rock	bap	GL; SG; LA
✓	leg	dɛk	GL; SG; DFC
✓	one	bɪp	LA; DFC; DEN; SG
✓	wet	bɛp	LA; SG
✓	glass	gæt	SF; CR
✓	bee	bi	(correct)
✓	Rick	bɪp	GL; SG; LA
✓	stop	pap	SF; LA; CR

Now that Leonardo's 7 rules have been determined, it is possible to predict what he will say for practically any word. Prediction becomes very important when it comes to choosing stimuli for therapy. For example, consider the word *lamb*. The following changes would occur in Leonardo's use of that word:

lamb → /jæm/	(Gliding of Liquids)
/jæm/ → /wæm/	(Labial Assimilation)
/wæm/ → /wæb/	(Denasalization)
/wæb/ → /wæp/	(Devoicing of Final Consonants)
/wæp/ → /bæp/	(Stopping of Glides)

With 5 rules working, *lamb* becomes a very poor stimulus word to use during therapy. Obviously, prediction is more difficult in a child like Leonardo (with 7 rules) than it was for Sissy or Parsippany in Chapter 6, both of whom had 2 rules working. The following list of words represents your final practice exercise for prediction. Try to predict how Leonardo would produce the following words (answers in Appendix A):

1. *rug* →
2. *sand* →
3. *pig* →
4. *feed* →
5. *know* →
6. *zoo* →
7. *spin* →
8. *frog* →
9. *thin* →
10. *tomato* → (be careful!)

Discussion

In Leonardo's speech sample, we see our first example of two totally embedded rules. Gliding of Liquids is never observed directly because as soon as the liquids become glides, the glides are then stopped, as a result of Stopping of Glides. In fact, our only evidence of Gliding of Liquids at all is inferential—because the /r/ in *rock* shifts to the labial position, we infer that Gliding of Liquids is occurring.

Why is this important? Imagine that you have engaged in therapy with Leonardo and have now eliminated his Stopping of Glides. How will he now produce *rock*? Right— /wap/. *Leg*, which was originally produced as /dɛk/ will now become /jɛk/. In both instances, it will seem as if as a result of your therapy Leonardo has developed a new error: Gliding of Liquids. In reality, Leonardo has had the gliding rule all along; it was just hidden by the stopping rule. So your therapy has not worsened Leonardo's speech; it has just allowed a previously embedded rule to surface.

Clinical Mastery Exercise—Theodora Haversingersmith

Introduction

Theodora's speech is the type that encourages gray hair in parents and clinicians alike. As you can see from her speech sample, her speech is easily the most primitive output we have observed thus far in our examples. Although two of Theodora's rules should be fairly easy to discover, the precise identification of at least two others will be difficult and extremely challenging. (The syllable structure rule[s] especially may be a "tough nut to crack.")

Some hints: Try to determine the two "easier" rules first; this will leave you with a better feel for Theodora's speech system by the time you get to the more difficult rules. Additionally, don't let the primitiveness of the output "throw" you; follow the same systematic procedures for determining the rules that you have used in earlier exercises. Finally, several of the rules you discover will be limited. Don't forget to return to the full Consistency Checklist if necessary. One more thing: Beginning with this exercise, blank worksheets for the 6-step generic procedure and the Parameter Confusion Test will no longer be provided along with the speech sample. It is hoped that this will encourage less reliance on those worksheets during our attempts to speed up the analytical process. (Additional blank worksheets, if needed, can be copied from the forms that appear in Appendix B.)

Worksheets provided for Theodora
- Phonological rule summary
- Three Consistency Check Forms

(Solution on page 253)

PHONOLOGICAL RULE SUMMARY

Client: _Theodora Haversingersmith_

Check	Target Word	Client Production	Rule(s) Operating
	top	at	
	shoe	ku	
	soup	ut	
	up	ʌt	
	key	ki	(correct)
	neck	ɛk	
	light	aɪk	
	dog	ɔk	
	cat	æk	
	tooth	ut	
	stop	ka	
	one	ʌn	
	him	ɪm	
	say	ke	
	big	ɪk	
	bread	tɛ	
	bed	ɛk	
	stone	ko	
	now	naʊ	
	ten	ɛn	
	eat	ɪk	
	see	ki	
	like	aɪk	(correct)
	me	mi	
	step	kɛ	
	pie	taɪ	
	juice	uk	
	zoo	ku	
	bye	taɪ	
	sheep	it	
	mouse	aʊk	
	Scott	ka	
	lime	aɪm	
	sad	æk	
	space	te	
	cub	ʌt	
	hive	aɪt	

CONSISTENCY CHECKLIST

Initial Rule Description: _____

Rule Operating (Yes)	Rule Not Operating (No)

Check for Consistency	Yes Words	No Words	Sig. Diff.
1. **Phonetic Context**			
— List vowel preceding			
— List vowel following			
— List consonant preceding			
— List consonant following			
— List other sig. non-adjacent sounds			
2. **Position**			
— List I, M, F for initial medial, final			
3. **Intra-class Variability**			
— List correct/incorrect sounds, search for intra-class patterns			
4. **Syllable Structure/ Word Length**			
— List syllable structures			
5. **Part of Speech/Morphological Endings**			
— List grammatical categories			
6. **Syllable Stress**			
— List U, S for unstressed, stressed			
7. **Syllable Boundary**			
— List words/Draw line between syllable boundaries; Note differences			

Note other factors: Elicitation mode, situational context, overlearned words, etc.

Final Rule Description: _____

CONSISTENCY CHECKLIST

Initial Rule Description: _____

Rule Operating (Yes)	Rule Not Operating (No)

Check for Consistency	Yes Words	No Words	Sig. Diff.
1. **Phonetic Context**			
— List vowel preceding			
— List vowel following			
— List consonant preceding			
— List consonant following			
— List other sig. non-adjacent sounds			
2. **Position**			
— List I, M, F for initial medial, final			
3. **Intra-class Variability**			
— List correct/incorrect sounds, search for intra-class patterns			
4. **Syllable Structure/ Word Length**			
— List syllable structures			
5. **Part of Speech/Morphological Endings**			
— List grammatical categories			
6. **Syllable Stress**			
— List U, S for unstressed, stressed			
7. **Syllable Boundary** — List words/Draw line between syllable boundaries; Note differences			

Note other factors: Elicitation mode, situational context, overlearned words, etc.

Final Rule Description: _____

CONSISTENCY CHECKLIST

Initial Rule Description: _____

Rule Operating (Yes)	Rule Not Operating (No)

Check for Consistency	Yes Words	No Words	Sig. Diff.
1. Phonetic Context			
— List vowel preceding			
— List vowel following			
— List consonant preceding			
— List consonant following			
— List other sig. non-adjacent sounds			
2. Position			
— List I, M, F for initial medial, final			
3. Intra-class Variability			
— List correct/incorrect sounds, search for intra-class patterns			
4. Syllable Structure/ Word Length			
— List syllable structures			
5. Part of Speech/Morphological Endings			
— List grammatical categories			
6. Syllable Stress			
— List U, S for unstressed, stressed			
7. Syllable Boundary			
— List words/Draw line between syllable boundaries; Note differences			

Note other factors: Elicitation mode, situational context, overlearned words, etc.

Final Rule Description: _____

Solution

It is probably a good idea just to study the speech sample for a few moments initially. This will give you a better feel for Theodora's phonological system and will underline the primitive nature of her output. It will also indicate clearly that her crude syllable structure will be a major element of her rule system.

Rule One
I. *Scan the speech sample for a golden word that will immediately cue one of the client's rules.*
   A. The change from /θ/ to /t/ in *tooth* makes that word a golden word for Stopping of Fricatives.[7]
II. *Perform a visual check for consistency.*
   A. Visually evaluate each fricative, to see if the rule is consistent.
   B. If you find any answers of *no*, perform a full Consistency Check using the appropriate worksheet. (In this case, all fricatives in the words *shoe, tooth, say, see, juice, zoo, mouse,* and *hive* are stopped. [Because of the deletion rule, other fricatives are ignored in that there is No Chance for stopping to be evaluated.] The rule is consistent.)
III. *Note the rule for each involved word on the summary sheet and check off the word if it has been explained.*
   A. The rule is noted after the words *shoe, tooth, say, see, juice, zoo, mouse,* and *hive*.
   B. No words are checked off; additional rules are operating in each of the words.

Rule Two
I. *Scan the speech sample for a golden word that will immediately cue one of the client's rules.*
   A. Another very familiar rule is exhibited when *dog* becomes /ɔk/. Devoicing of Consonants is our hypothesized rule.
II. *Perform a visual check for consistency.*
   A. Visually evaluate each voiced consonant to see if it becomes unvoiced.
   B. If you find any answers of *no*, perform a full Consistency Check using the appropriate worksheet. (In this case, the word *one*, only four words after *dog*, has a final /n/ that is not devoiced. A full Consistency Check must be undertaken.)
II-a. *Place words from speech sample into* yes/no *columns, as appropriate.*
   A. The following words demonstrate Devoicing of Consonants and go into the *yes* column: *dog* (with the focus on the final /g/), *big* (focus

---

[7]Interestingly, *tooth* is the only golden word for Stopping of Fricatives in the entire sample. However, by now, you are probably becoming adept enough at rule identification that you can recognize many rules even when they are embedded together in the same word. So much the better! For example, in *shoe* → /kμ/, Stopping of Fricatives is embedded with another rule. Yet this does not prevent us from recognizing the fact that the fricative /ʃ/ has been stopped. The point to be gained from this is that, although it is valuable to have many golden words in a speech sample, rules can sometimes be deciphered in nongolden words also.

on final /g/), *bread* (focus on initial cluster), *bed* (focus on final /d/), *zoo, bye, sad, cub,* and *hive*.

B. The following words should be placed in the *no* column: *one* (focus on the final /n/), *him, now, ten, me* and *lime* (focus on the final /m/). In these words the voiced consonant remains voiced.

II-b. *Visual inspection of the word lists.*

A. Study the columns of *yes* and *no* words. Try to find a systematic difference between the words that exhibit Devoicing of Consonants and those that do not.

B. If you are able to determine the systematic difference by means of this visual inspection, label the newly discovered limited rule and continue with the analysis. (In this case, it is easy to see that there is a different class of voiced consonants in the *yes* column than there is in the *no* column. Essentially, voiced consonants are devoiced except in the case of nasals, which maintain their voicing. The newly formulated limited rule: Devoicing of Nonnasal Consonants.)

III. *Note the rule for each involved word on the summary sheet and check off the word if it has been explained.*

A. The rule, Devoicing of Nonnasal Consonants, is noted after the words *dog, big, bread, bed, zoo, bye, sad, cub,* and *hive*.

B. Once again, no words can be checked off. All words are subject to additional rules.

Rule Three

I. *Scan the speech sample for a golden word that will immediately cue one of the client's rules.*

A. The first word (i.e., *top* → /at/) cues this first more difficult rule. The natural first tendency of clinicians at this point in the learning process is to call this rule "Backing of Labials." However, by attaching "of Labials" to the label, a limitation is added that may not, indeed, be occurring. This leads to a good rule-of-thumb: Always make your original statement of a given rule *as general as possible*; if a limitation exists, you will discover it later, as part of the consistency check. Back to Theodora, even a quick glance at other words will indicate that backing is occurring to a wider array of sounds than just labials. A more general, better initial statement of this rule, then, is Backing of Consonants.

II. *Perform a visual check for consistency.*

A. Visually evaluate each consonant to see if it shifts its placement backward in the mouth.

B. If you find any answers of *no*, perform a full Consistency Check using the appropriate worksheet. (In this case, it does not take long to find a *no*—the word *key*, for example, which stays in the velar position rather than shifting to the glottal. A full Consistency Check is needed.)

II-a. *Place words from speech sample in* yes/no *columns as appropriate.*

A. The following words demonstrate Backing of Consonants and should be placed in the *yes* column: *top* (focus on /p/), *shoe, soup* (focus on

/p/), *up*, *light* (focus on /t/), *eat*, *tooth* (focus on /θ/), *stop* (focus on /st/), *say*, *bread* (focus on /br/), *bed* (focus on /d/), *stone* (focus on /st/), *eat*, *see*, *step* (focus on /st/), *pie*, *juice* (focus on /s/), *zoo*, *bye*, *sheep* (focus on /p/), *mouse* (focus on /s/), *sad* (focus on /d/), *space* (focus on /sp/), *cub* (focus on /b/), and *hive* (focus on /v/).

B. These words belong in the *no* column: *key*, *neck* (focus on /k/), *dog* (focus on /g/), *one* (focus on /n/), *him* (focus on /m/), *big* (focus on /g/), *now*, *ten* (focus on /n/), *like* (focus on /k/), *me*, and *lime* (focus on /m/).

II-b. *Visual inspection of word lists.*

A. Study the columns of *yes* and *no* words. Try to find a systematic difference between the words that exhibit Backing of Consonants and those that do not.

B. If you are able to determine the systematic difference by means of this visual inspection, label the newly discovered limited rule and continue with the analysis. (In this case, it is fairly easy to see that words in the *yes* list are indeed significantly different from those in the *no* list. Backing of Consonants affects all sound classes except for nasals and velars. Thus, the newly formulated limited rule is Backing of Nonnasal, Nonvelar Consonants.)

III. *Note the rule for each involved word on the summary sheet and check off the word if it has been explained.*

A. The rule, Backing of Nonnasal, Nonvelar Consonants, is noted after the words *top*, *shoe*, *soup*, *up*, *light*, *cat*, *tooth*, *stop*, *say*, *bread*, *bed*, *stone*, *eat*, *see*, *step*, *pie*, *juice*, *zoo*, *bye*, *sheep*, *mouse*, *sad*, *space*, *cub*, and *hive*.

B. The following words can be checked off: *shoe*, *up*, *say*, *eat*, *see*, *pie*, *zoo*, and *bye*.

Well, we cannot avoid it any longer. We must tackle the syllable structure rule that pervades Theodora's output so completely.

Rule Four

I. *Scan the speech sample for a golden word that will immediately cue one of the client's rules.*

A. The first word, *top*, immediately suggests the rule Deletion of Initial Consonants. Although we can already tell from the second word (i.e., *shoe*) that the rule will be a limited one, we will accept Deletion of Initial Consonants as our preliminary description.

II. *Perform a visual check for consistency.*

A. As just stated, we do not have to go far to find a seeming inconsistency; the initial consonant in *shoe* is not deleted. A full Consistency Check will be needed.

II-a. *Place words from speech sample into* yes/no *columns, as appropriate.*

A. The following words exhibit Deletion of Initial Consonants and should be placed in the *yes* column: *top*, *soup*, *neck*, *light*, *dog*, *cat*, *tooth*, *one*, *him*, *big*, *bed*, *ten*, *like*, *juice*, *sheep*, *mouse*, *lime*, *sad*, *cub*, and *hive*.

B. The following words go into the *no* column because they do not exhibit the deletion rule: *shoe, key, stop, bread, stone, now, me, step, zoo, bye,* and *space.*

II-b. *Visual inspection of word lists.*

A. Study the columns of *yes* and *no* words. Try to find a systematic difference between the words that exhibit Deletion of Initial Consonants and those that do not.

B. If you are able to discover the systematic difference by means of this visual inspection, label the newly discovered limited rule and continue with the analysis. (In this case, the difference can be most clearly seen if you divide the *no* words into two groups: *shoe, key, now, me, zoo,* and *bye* belong in one group and *stop, bread, stone, step,* and *space* go into the other. What can now be easily seen is a systematic difference in the syllable structures of the *yes* words and the *no* words. The initial sound is deleted in CVC words only. In CV words, the syllable structure remains unchanged. In CCVC words, the syllable structure is reduced to CV. The new limited rule can now be formulated: Deletion of Initial Consonants, except CV → CV and CCVC → CV.)

III. *Note the rule for each involved word on the summary sheet and check off the word if it has been explained.*

A. The rule, Deletion of Initial Consonants, except CV → CV and CCVC → CV, is noted after the words *top, soup, neck, light, dog, cat, tooth, stop, one, him, big, bread, bed, stone, ten, like, step, juice, sheep, mouse, Scott, lime, sad, space, cub,* and *hive.*

B. All the remaining words can now be checked off. Theodora's analysis is complete. (See the completed phonological rule summary for Theodora on the opposite page.)

PHONOLOGICAL RULE SUMMARY

Client: _Theodora Haversingersmith_

Check	Target Word	Client Production	Rule(s) Operating
	top	æt	BNNNVC; DICX
	shoe	ku	SF; BNNNVC
	soup	ut	BNNNVC; DICX
	up	ʌt	BNNNVC
	key	ki	(correct)
	neck	ɛk	DICX
	light	aɪk	BNNNVC; DICX
	dog	ɔk	DNNC; DICX
	cat	æk	BNNNVC; DICX
	tooth	ut	SF; BNNNVC; DICX
	stop	ka	BNNNVC; DICX
	one	ʌn	DICX
	him	Im	DICX
	say	ke	SF; BNNNVC
	big	ɪk	DNNC; DICX
	bread	tɛ	DNNC; BNNNVC; DICX
	bed	ɛk	DNNC; BNNNVC; DICX
	stone	ko	BNNNVC; DICX
	now	naʊ	(correct)
	ten	ɛn	DICX
	eat	Ik	BNNNVC
	see	ki	SF; BNNNVC
	like	aɪk	DICX
	me	mi	(correct)
	step	kɛ	BNNNVC; DICX
	pie	taɪ	BNNNVC
	juice	uk	SF; BNNNVC; DICX
	200	ku	SF; DNNC; BNNNVC
	bye	taɪ	DNNC; BNNNVC
	sheep	it	BNNNVC; DICX
	mouse	aʊk	SF; BNNNVC; DICX
	Scott	ka	DICX
	lime	aɪm	DICX
	sad	æk	DNNC; BNNNVC; DICX
	space	te	BNNNVC; DICX
	cub	ʌt	DNNC; BNNNVC; DICX
	hive	aɪt	SF; DNNC; BNNNVC; DICX

Discussion

It is highly likely that your own analysis of Theodora's speech resulted in more than the four errors presented here. You were not incorrect. In fact, a valid argument can be made that the advantage of parsimony that might accrue from describing the syllable structure rule using only a single sentence with two exceptions in no way offsets the possible lack of clarity and imprecision that the shortened description creates. After all, three seemingly separate errors are occurring: Initial consonants are omitted in CVC words, clusters are reduced, and final consonants are deleted in words with initial clusters. Why not just describe three separate rules? We could have, and it would not have changed anything much except to make this chapter longer. (And truthfully, the errors *were* described separately during Theodora's initial evaluation.) However, an interesting thing occurred secondary to intervention which convinced us that the original hypothesis of three separate rules may have been inaccurate after all.

After several weeks of teaching Theodora the concept of initial consonants in CVC syllable structures, we began to notice more improvement than we had bargained for. In her conversational speech, Theodora was not only beginning to include some initial consonants in CVC words, but she was also beginning to include some final consonants in CCVC structures. Sure enough, by the time Theodora had stabilized her use of initial consonants, all final consonants were also being included, although no attempt had been made to teach that concept. (Importantly, she continued to reduce clusters at this point.) What we belatedly hypothesized was that Theodora had in reality had two rules operating: Cluster Reduction and an Absent CVC Syllable Structure Concept. While we were attempting to teach Theodora initial consonants in CVC words, what she really was learning was the concept of the CVC syllable structure. Once this learning had taken place, transfer occurred easily and she readily began to include final consonants in CCVC words.

What is to be learned from this exercise? Most of the time it is best to describe a rule in as general and holistic a manner as is possible. If you have overgeneralized your rule description (a situation which can, indeed, occur), you will become very aware of this during intervention, when one sound or class of sounds will not respond as readily. Then another rule can be generated. The good news is, as you develop more experience with phonological analysis, you will also develop a better feel for rule description, often knowing intuitively when speech errors are working separately, or together as a class.

Clinical Mastery Exercise—Carmine Crayola

For this final exercise, you are mostly on your own. In order to save space, no detailed solution will be presented. Instead, you are directed to Appendix A, where a list of the rules appears. Copy forms from Appendix B as needed; however, try to do as much of the analysis as possible without the use of forms other than the phonological rule summary. (Some use of the Consistency Checklist will of course be needed to determine limited rules.)

The phonological rule summary for Carmine follows.

PHONOLOGICAL RULE SUMMARY

Client: _Carmine Crayola_

Check	Target Word	Client Production	Rule(s) Operating
	turn	hɜn	
	comb	hom	
	chair	hɛr	
	lime	waɪm	
	pear	hɛr	
	juice	dʒus	
	jello	dʒɛwo	
	coat	hot	
	goat	dot	
	shoes	suz	
	pig	hɪ	
	mouse	maʊs	(correct)
	duck	dʌ	
	dog	da	
	deer	dir	(correct)
	red	wɛd	
	cat	hæ	
	sheep	si	
	chick	hɪ	
	brown	baʊn	
	shot	sat	
	vet	vɛ	
	gun	dʌn	
	lid	wɪd	
	get	dɛ	
	boat	bot	(correct)
	hat	hæ	
	Stacey	fesi	
	sponge	fʌnz	
	little	wɪdl	
	tic-tac-toe	hɪhæho	
	shoot	sut	
	ball	bɔl	
	roll	wol	
	glass	gæs	
	sky	faɪ	

Returning to the Semantic and Linguistic Parameters of Constraint

Very little space has been devoted thus far to the Semantic and Linguistic parameters of articulatory constraint. In fact, aside from a few examples of some linguistically based limited rules, the term we have used most often when considering these constraint categories has been "unlikely." This has not been meant to imply that semantically or linguistically based phonological errors do not occur. They do, and more frequently than many clinicians realize. The problem is, a full mastery of the basic concepts of clinical phonology is an important prerequisite to accurate recognition and differential diagnosis of these language based phonological errors. Yet, as you will see, at this point in the learning process, the discussion becomes rather elementary.

From a diagnostic perspective, phonology and the other components of language (morphology, syntax, semantics) have several points of intersection. Five possible sources of diagnostic confusion result from this interaction:

1. Phonological error masquerading as a morphological error. This is a fairly common occurrence which creates much ambiguity during the evaluation process. For example, if a client omits a substantial number of morphological endings (plurals, past tense -ed, etc.), the common initial reaction is that this client has a language problem. Intervention may very well (and often does) proceed on this basis. Yet the fact is that many plurals, most past tense markers, and several other morphological markers are part of consonant clusters or unstressed syllables within words. So the client may not have a language problem after all; instead he or she may have a phonological problem which just looks like a problem with morphology. Obviously, if therapy is to be effective, the appropriate linguistic element must be targeted.

2. Phonological error masquerading as a syntactic error. If a client has a shortened length of utterance and leaves out several words (e.g., articles, adjectives, prepositions), again the usual first reaction is that this client has a problem with syntax. Yet, the common phonological rule, Deletion of Unstressed Syllables, will present the same behaviors. Once again, an accurate differential diagnosis is essential if intervention is to be effective.

3. Phonological error masquerading as a semantic error. This type of confusion occurs less frequently but can be just as important. If a young child has a very primitive phonological system, his or her output will often be limited to very few utterances that can be differentiated from one another. This will give many listeners the initial impression of a restricted lexicon. Yet this impression may very well be false, created only because of the primitive phonology. Historically, clinicians have been puzzled by children demonstrating receptive vocabulary much superior to the vocabulary seen expressively. Perhaps many of these children have not had expressive vocabulary problems after all; instead the primitive phonological system has falsely given the impression of a semantic disorder.

4. Errors of phonolinguistic interaction. Sometimes errors will occur not due solely to phonological problems, nor due solely to linguistic factors, but instead due to the interaction of those factors. For example, the word *unsqueezed* presents difficult tasks both phonologically and morphologically. Perhaps the overall phonolinguistic "load" is so heavy that the child will have problems producing the word. So an individual might not normally have problems with clusters and might not normally have problems with morphemes. But when a word contains a cluster that also includes a morpheme, then the client has difficulty; thus the limited rule Cluster Reduction in Morphemes.

5. Language error masquerading as a phonological error. To gain a balanced perspective, it is important to realize that a confusion can occur in either direction. In other words, what looks like a speech problem may indeed be caused because of an inadequate or deviant linguistic system.

What can be done about these possible sources of diagnostic confusion? Most importantly, be aware of the possibility of their occurrence. When you see a child who says /pʌp/ for *cup* from now on, you will probably automatically reason "This is either labial assimilation or fronting; I have to test to see which is accurate. Just by being aware of the possible confusion between placement and context, you can avoid a misdiagnosis. Likewise, by being aware of the possible confusion between structure and morphology, for example, you can also perform a test that will indicate the violated parameter. So once again, the more you are aware of all the constraint parameters and the alternatives available under each parameter, the more accurate an analysis you can do.

Procedure for a Phonological Analysis

Our discussion thus far has been limited to the analytical components of performing a phonological analysis. At this point, if you are presented with a list of words, you will probably be able to perform some level of phonological analysis on that list. What we have not discussed yet is how you go about compiling that list of words, or gloss, from the client.

Theoretically, we are most interested in the client's spontaneous speech abilities. If we could easily do so, we would regularly transcribe 50 to 100 spontaneous utterances produced by the client and analyze those utterances. The problem is, we have neither the time nor the transcription ability to transcribe 100 utterances from a

client who is very difficult to understand. Luckily, we probably don't have to.

Standardized articulation tests serve the function of presenting a vast array of words that contain all relevant speech sounds and numerous opportunities for evaluating a client's rule system. The only problem presented by some standardized tests is that there is less opportunity to evaluate the client's syllable structure system, because only single words are utilized. For these reasons, we typically recommend an evaluation procedure that combines administration of a standard single word articulation test with transcription of 20–25 two to three word phrases uttered by the client. We find that this combination is both time effective and flexible enough to allow us to continue our transcriptions until we feel we've gathered a complete picture of the client's phonological systems.

Specifically, we recommend the following procedures:

1. Administration of a standardized articulation test, such as the *Goldman-Fristoe Test of Articulation*. Note: It is important that you transcribe each of the words; do not limit your attention only to the sounds highlighted by the test device.
2. Transcribe 20–25 two to three word phrases during the client's conversation. Even if the client's utterance length is greater than two to three words, limit your transcription attempts to no more than three words from those longer phrases. (If you try to transcribe output more than two to three words at a time, your accuracy will decrease substantially.)
3. Make certain that your final sample of transcribed words is varied enough to allow full evaluation of all the parameters of articulatory constraint.

The Next Step

Do you now feel fully comfortable in your ability to perform a complex phonological analysis? Probably not. Nor should you at this point. Starting tomorrow, or next week, or the next time you evaluate a child or adult with phonological disorders, the real learning will begin. Try to give yourself enough time and opportunity for practice, reread if necessary, use the forms you like—discard the others, but most importantly, keep working at it. Within 6 months' time, not only will you find that your comfort level has improved, but you will notice that your way of looking at clients with speech disorders has changed forever. So at the risk of sounding like an old cliche, the rest is up to you. Best wishes.

CHAPTER ◆ 10

Macroanalysis of Phonology: Formal and Informal Procedures

Michael J. Moran, Ph.D.
Auburn University

The underlying thesis of a phonological approach to studying deviant articulation is that the client has developed a set of phonological rules that simplifies his or her speech and sets it apart from community norms. The purpose of phonological assessment is to ascertain those rules in as comprehensive a fashion as possible. Several formal tests have been developed which attempt to allow the clinician to accomplish this goal. All of these tests evaluate a predetermined list of rules. The examiner's role is to determine the presence or absence of these predefined rules in the client's speech. Some of the tests use specific stimuli in order to obtain a speech sample; others require that the examiner elicit a spontaneous speech sample from the client. All of these tests, however, have the same problem that any macroanalytic test would have. If the client's phonological rule system does not match the predefined framework of the given test, assessment results will be incomplete and inconsistent.

A question that may occur to you at this point is if macroanalytic tests of phonology are flawed, why even discuss them in this text? There are two reasons: First, although

generative, or microanalytic, procedures represent the cutting edge in phonological assessment, more traditional formal tests are still used widely and will probably continue to be used by many clinicians. The popularity of such tests among clinicians is most likely rooted in tradition and in the perceived practicality of such instruments. Many formal tests of phonology are relatively quick and quite easy to administer. Some of these tests provide normative data, severity ratings, and suggestions regarding where and how to begin treatment. Most have a carefully selected list of words to ensure that all phonemes are examined and that the selected processes have ample opportunity to occur, thus saving the clinician from having to devise her own list or combing the literature to find an appropriate speech sample. Most of the tests provide specific stimulus items to aid the elicitation of the desired speech sample. All of these features may be quite appealing to clinicians who have a large caseload and little time.

A reason for the popularity of formal tests of phonology among school-based clinicians relates to regulations governing assessment in the schools. Most school districts require some form of standardized testing in order to qualify a student for services and to justify dismissal from treatment. Also, most of us feel comfortable using those methods in which we were trained and with which we have experience.

Finally, we believe that formal tests are used frequently because the procedures and objectives are clear and easily explained in a few pages in the test manual. On the other hand, the discussion regarding clinical application of microanalytic procedures or generative phonology has all too often been presented in a theoretical abstract context. Such descriptions of clinical application have sometimes served more as a barrier than an encouragement to the conversion of clinical practitioners.

The likelihood then, that formal tests of phonology will fall into disuse in the immediate future is slim. Therefore it seems appropriate and valuable to survey the current state of the art regarding these formal tests and to investigate how closely the various tests come to meeting our clinical needs for accurate and precise phonological description.

The second reason we feel that it is appropriate to discuss macroanalytic procedures is that despite their shortcomings, these procedures are not completely without merit. Most tests of phonology provide more clinically relevant data than do the traditional speech sound inventories. The specific processes assessed in the various tests are included because they are generally the most commonly occurring patterns demonstrated by children with phonological disorders. The tests aid in identifying patterns of errors and assist the clinician in targeting those patterns in treatment. For some children the proper administration and scoring of a commercially available test of phonology might completely define the child's phonological system and suggest to the clinician an appropriate place to begin intervention.

With the previous discussion as justification, we will now review several of the commonly used phonological tests.

Formal Assessments

Test: *Compton-Hutton Phonological Assessment*

Authors: Arthur J. Compton and J. Stanley Hutton

Date of Publication: 1978

Sample and Method of Elicitation: A total of 50 black and white pictures are named twice by the subject. According to the authors, the pictures represent "A phonetically balanced sampling of each initial consonant, final consonant, and consonant blend which occurs in English" (p. 2). Some frequently misarticulated consonants are sampled more than once, and all vowels are represented in the stimulus items. As the child names each item, the examiner phonetically transcribes the child's productions of the target consonants in the initial and final position in spaces provided on a response sheet.

Scoring: The child's productions of each target consonant on the response sheet are transferred to a "Pattern Analysis" sheet. On this sheet, correct productions are recorded in black and incorrect productions in red. Color-coded tally marks are placed after each phonetic representation to indicate the number of times it occurred. The pattern analysis sheet organizes the target phonemes according to 40 phonological rules that could potentially affect the production of those sounds. The examiner then identifies which of the phonological rules provided on the "Phonological Rule Analysis" sheet are present in the child's speech sample.

Time Required: The manual states that the entire analysis can be performed in 45 to

60 minutes: 20 to 25 minutes for the sample, 15 to 20 minutes for the pattern analysis and 10 to 15 minutes for the phonological rule analysis.

Comment: Unlike the other instruments discussed in this chapter, the *Compton-Hutton Phonological Assessment* yields linguistically written rather than descriptive phonological rules. The rules are written in the manner associated with linguistic rules, for example [s] → [t] or [s] → [ʃ]. Most of these phonological rules, however, represent the same sound changes as the more commonly used descriptive rules. For example, the rule stated as [b, d, g] → [p, t, k] in the final position would be called final consonant devoicing in a process oriented analysis. Finally, the authors indicate that their phonological rules are based on principles of generative phonology. This use of generative phonological theory is not, however, the same kind of generative approach discussed in the present text.

Test: *Phonological Process Analysis (PPA)*

Author: Frederick F. Weiner

Date of Publication: 1979

Sample and Method of Elicitation: A total of 136 black and white drawings, each featuring a character named "Uncle Fred," are used to elicit responses from the subject. Each response is designed to provide an opportunity for 1 of 16 phonological pro-cesses to occur. Each response is elicited twice, once as a single word through "de-layed imitation" and once in the context of a sentence through "sentence recall." (Actually the sentence recall response is usually a phrase rather than a sentence.) For example, one picture depicts Uncle Fred holding a bug. To elicit the delayed imitation response, the examiner says, "Here is a bug. Uncle Fred is holding a _____." To which the child responds, "bug." To elicit the sentence recall response the examiner says, "What is Uncle Fred doing?" to which the child responds, "Holding a bug."

Scoring: A chart is provided on which the examiner records the number of times each process was elicited when it was being tested and the number of times each process was elicited when another process was being tested. The examiner then makes a decision as to whether the process should be considered part of the child's phonological pattern. No criteria are provided for this decision. Space is provided for the examiner to describe other processes. There is also space provided to record the child's phonetic inventory.

Time Required: The instruction section of the *PPA* indicates that "A skilled examiner should be able to complete the PPA in 45 minutes with a cooperative subject" (p. 1).

Processes Examined: Sixteen processes are examined:

Deletion of final consonants
Weak syllable deletion
Cluster reduction
Glottal replacement
Labial assimilation
Alveolar assimilation
Prevocalic voicing
Final consonant devoicing
Stopping
Gliding of fricatives
Affrication
Fronting
Denasalization
Velar assimilation
Gliding of liquids
Vocalization

Comment: The *PPA* was the first commercially available instrument specifically designed to assess phonological processes. As such it has some historical significance. The lack of criteria for determining the presence of a process as well as the length of time to administer the test have made it a less useful instrument than some more recent tests. Bankson and Bernthal (1982) reported that using either of the response modes of the *PPA* (delayed imitation or sentence recall) yielded results that were essentially equivalent to those obtained by administering the entire test.

Test: *Natural Process Analysis (NPA)*

Authors: Lawrence D. Shriberg and Joan Kwiatkowski

Date of Publication: 1980

Sample and Method of Elicitation: A spontaneous speech sample of approximately 200 to 250 words is elicited using one or more of several techniques suggested by the authors. The sample is tape recorded and then transcribed orthographically (glossed) utterance by utterance on transcription sheets. Each utterance is then transcribed phonetically. The analysis is based largely on 80 to 100 different words selected from the sample.

Scoring: The first occurrences of the 80 to 100 words to be used are entered on one of three coding sheets. The child's productions are then coded to indicate the presence of one of the test processes. Finally, the information from the coding sheets is transferred to a summary sheet which indicates the frequency of occurrence of each process on a continuum of always occurs, sometimes occurs, or never occurs. All sound changes must be accounted for by only a single process. The summary sheet also allows for a phonetic inventory. Instructions are provided for an analysis of context/function variables associated with inconsistent process use.

Time Required: According to the authors, clinicians experienced with the procedure can complete the analysis in about 90 minutes in addition to the time needed to elicit the sample. Less-experienced clinicians require considerably more time.

Processes Examined: Only eight processes are directly tested in this procedure.

Final consonant deletion
Velar fronting
Stopping
Palatal fronting
Liquid simplification
Assimilation
Cluster reduction
Unstressed syllable deletion

Comment: Rather than a specific test instrument like the other procedures discussed here, the NPA is probably better considered an instruction manual for conducting a phonological process analysis from a spontaneous speech sample. The authors provide forms to aid in organizing the sample but no specific stimuli are provided. The authors also go a step beyond the other procedures in their attempt to distinguish *phonological rules*, which they describe as "descriptive," from true *phonological processes*, which they describe as "explanatory" accounts of sound changes. It is this distinction that results in the assessment of only eight processes. (Of course, we have decided in this text to ignore any possible distinction between phonological rules and phonological processes.)

Test: *Assessment of Phonological Processes— Revised (APP-R)*

Author: Barbara W. Hodson

Date of Publication: 1986

Sample and Method of Elicitation: The subject is asked to name 50 objects, pictures, and body parts. Each stimulus item is designed to assess more than one phonological process.

Scoring: A score sheet is provided which lists the target words, a phonetic transcription of each word, and columns for each of the 40 processes and patterns examined. The examiner phonetically transcribes the child's responses on the score sheet and places checks in the columns corresponding to the process exhibited in the child's production of each word. Although over 40 processes and patterns are assessed, 10 processes are identified as "Basic Error Patterns." Percentage of occurrence is determined for the 10 basic processes. The percentage of occurrence is used to determine a "Phonological Deviancy Score" and a severity rating.

Time required: The *APP-R* requires about 20 minutes to gather the sample and an additional 10 minutes to complete the scoring. A computer software program (*CAPP*) is available which reduces the time for scoring.

Processes Examined:

Basic Patterns
Syllable reduction
Cluster reduction
Singleton obstruent omission
  Prevocalic
  Postvocalic
Stridency deletion
Velar deviation
/l/ deviation
/r/ deviation
Nasal deviation
Glide deviation

Other patterns
Prevocalic voicing
Postvocalic devoicing
Glottal replacement
Backing
Stopping
Affrication
Deaffrication
Palatalization
Depalatalization
Coalescence
Epenthesis
Metathesis
Vowel deviation
Assimilation
  Nasal
  Velar
  Labial
  Alveolar
Substitutions of /fvsz/ for /θ/ and /ð/
Frontal lisp
Dentalization of /tdnl/
Lateralization

Comment: The *APP-R* allows the examiner to determine the presence of a fairly large set of rules and patterns. Many of the processes in this test such as coalescence are not seen commonly in other tests. Hodson also has defined some of the more commonly occurring patterns in a slightly stricter manner. For example, whereas many tests identify a pattern called final consonant deletion, Hodson discusses post-vocalic obstruent omission. This particular description allows for the occurrence of the rule in compound words such as "too*th*brush." A standard set of objects for this test is now available.

Test: *Khan-Lewis Phonological Analysis (KLPA)*

Authors: Linda Khan and Nancy Lewis

Date of Publication: 1986

Sample and Method of Elicitation: The speech sample for the *KLPA* consists of the 44 words from the Sounds-in-Words subtest of the *Goldman-Fristoe Test of Articulation* (Goldman & Fristoe, 1986), a spontaneous picture naming task. The examiner phonetically transcribes the child's entire response to each stimulus item.

Scoring: The transcriptions of the child's productions are examined for the presence of 15 phonological processes. The score sheet contains an illustration of how each process would affect each of the target words. The examiner marks the processes exhibited in each of the target words. The frequency of occurrence of each process is tabulated, and a four-point severity rating is then determined for each process. A percentile rank, speech simplification rating, and age equivalent are determined and summarized on the face of the test form.

Time required: Between 15 and 40 minutes.

Processes examined: The *KLPA* examines 15 processes. Twelve of these processes are typically seen as part of normal phonological development, three processes are not seen in normal development.

Processes seen in normal development
Deletion of final consonant
Initial consonant voicing
Syllable reduction
Palatal fronting
Deaffrication
Velar fronting
Consonant harmony
Stridency deletion
Stopping
Cluster simplification
Final consonant devoicing
Liquid simplification

Processes not seen in normal development
Deletion of initial consonants
Glottal replacement
Backing to velars

Comment: The *KLPA's* greatest contribution may be that it was among the first sources of a norm sample for phonological processes. The norm sample consisted of 852 children and is reported to be proportionally similar to the general population in terms of geographic, gender, and racial distribution.

Some instruments allow the examiner to perform a traditional substitution-, distortion-, omission-type analysis as well as a phonological analysis. Two of these instruments are described:

Test: *Assessment Link Between Phonology and Articulation (ALPHA)*

Author: Robert J. Lowe

Date of Publication: 1986

Sample and Method of Elicitation: A total of 50 black and white drawings are used to aid the examiner in eliciting target words in an imitative sentence format. The child's production of the target word is transcribed phonetically in the appropriate column on the test form. Sound omissions are indicated by a − and distortions by an ✕.

Scoring: Each sound error in the word-initial and word-final position is recorded in the appropriate column on the "Phoneme Errors" section of the test form. Errors are then examined to determine which of 15 phonological rules might account for the sound change. Using the "Phonological Process Analysis" portion of the test form, check marks are placed in columns corresponding to the phonological process(es) that would account for each sound change noted. The author indicates that not all children require a phonological process analysis. Guidelines are provided in the manual to aid the examiner in determining whether to perform a process analysis or to stop after phoneme errors analysis. In addition to identifying processes, *ALPHA* provides scores for percent of occurrence of processes, percentile rank, and a standard deviation profile.

Phonological Processes Examined: Fifteen processes are examined by this instrument:

Consonant deletion
Syllable deletion
Stridency deletion
Stopping
Fronting
Backing
Alveolarization
Labialization
Affrication
Deaffrication
Voicing Changes
Gliding
Vowelization
Cluster reduction
Cluster substitution

Time Required: The author states that the sample can be collected in 10 to 15 minutes. Scoring varies depending on whether the process analysis is performed, but the entire test can be scored in 30 minutes.

Comment: The *ALPHA* presents extensive statistical and normative data which allow the examiner to compare each subject's results to a norm sample. The norm sample for the test consisted of over 1,300 children; all, however were from the Midwest or Pennsylvania.

Test: *Bankson-Bernthal Test of Phonology (BBTOP)*

Authors: Nicholas W. Bankson and John E. Bernthal

Date of Publication: 1990

Sample and Method of Elicitation: Color pictures are used to elicit production of 80 stimulus words. The examiner phonetically transcribes the entire word on the test form. If spontaneous picture naming does not elicit the appropriate response, the examiner may use modeling. A space is provided to indicate whether a word was elicited by modeling.

Scoring: The test provides an opportunity for the examiner to obtain three inventories: The Word Inventory reflects the percentage of words correctly produced and is designed to be a quick determinant of whether a more detailed analysis is needed. The Consonant Inventory provides an indication of misarticulations in the initial and final positions of words. The Phonological Process Inventory allows the clinician to examine the speech sample for the occurrence of 10 phonological processes. Examples of common phonological processes observed for each word are included on the test form.

Time Required: 15 to 20 minutes.

Processes Examined: The authors claim that this test probes the 10 phonological processes that occur most frequently. Those processes are:

Assimilation
Cluster simplification
Weak syllable deletion
Stopping
Depalatalization
Gliding
Final consonant deletion
Deaffrication

Vocalization
Fronting

Comment: The *BBTOP* claims a standardization sample of more than 1,000 children. This allows raw scores to be converted to percentile ranks for the Word, Consonant, and Phonological Process Inventories. Twenty-eight items from the *BBTOP* have been incorporated by the authors into a screening test, the *Quick Screen of Phonology* (1990), which screens for the presence of the same 10 processes.

At least two published assessment instruments include a phonological process analysis but incorporate additional procedures which move them in the direction of a microanalysis. These two instruments are *Procedures for the Phonological Analysis of Children's Language (PPACL)* (Ingram, 1981), and *Phonological Assessment of Child Speech (PACS)* (Grunwell, 1985). *PPACL* provides instructions and forms to assist the examiner in performing a phonetic analysis, an analysis of homonomy, a substitution analysis, and a phonological process analysis. The phonological process analysis includes 27 common processes. The type of speech sample upon which the analysis is based is left to the examiner. PACS is based on a sample of 100 different words from a suggested sample of 200–250 words in a connected speech sample. Instructions are provided for the completion of three types of analyses; a phonetic analysis of error productions, a contrastive analysis, and a phonological process analysis which includes 12 processes.

As can be seen from the previous descriptions, some instruments assess a large number of rules while others assess a very limited number. The justification for the selection of processes and patterns is generally included in the manual that accompanies the instrument. Comparison of different instruments is made even more difficult because different authors frequently refer to the same patterns or processes by different names. For example, the sound changes in the following three words represent a pattern in which the final consonant is not produced.

/bot/ → /bo/; /kaɪt/ → /kaɪ/; /bɛd/ → /bɛ/

As can be seen, this pattern would be described differently by different test instruments, as follows:

Deletion of Final Consonants (*PPA, KLPA*)

Final Consonant Deletion (*NPA, BBTOP*)

Consonant Deletion (*ALPHA*)

Postvocalic Singleton Obstruent Omission (*APP*)

Or consider the following example: Depending on the test instrument, /tɛləfon/ → /tɛfon/ might be variously described as

Syllable Reduction (*APP, KLPA*)

Syllable Deletion (*ALPHA*)

Weak Syllable Deletion (*PPA, BBTOP*)

Unstressed Syllable Deletion (*NPA*)

It becomes clear that it is up to the clinician to become knowledgeable as to what a given test author has meant by a label or pattern name used in his or her test instrument. Only then can the results be interpreted validly.

Computer Analysis

Sharon W., a speech-language pathologist from Chicago, Illinois, has had a particularly difficult day at her job. After coming home, she decides to take a quick nap. During this nap, she dreams about this particularly troublesome little 6-year-old boy named Fang who has 23 rules and says only one word intelligibly: *no*. Although she is evaluating his speech for the first time, Sharon, quite incredibly, has a smile on her face. She sits at a table, shows Fang several pictures, talks with him for a bit, and then calmly walks toward the other side of the room, where a computer printer is noisily spewing forth paper. As Sharon reaches the printer, the noise ceases and she tears off the printout of Fang's transcript and a completed phonological analysis. After she dismisses Fang, she walks to her supervisor's office where she is immediately notified that her request for a raise in salary to $221,000 per year has been approved. . . . Back at home, Sharon dreams on, with a blissful smile on her face. . . .

Unfortunately, technology has not yet reached the point where we can elicit a conversation sample from a client and then simply walk to a computer and pick up a print-out of the finished phonological analysis. However, even today, microcomputers can provide valuable assistance to clinicians engaged in phonological analysis.

In recent years, several computer software packages have been designed which are capable of performing various phonological analyses on a speech sample. A detailed description of these computer programs is beyond the scope of this chapter. A summary of the most widely used packages may be found in Masterson and Long (1991). We feel, however, that some mention of these programs should be made here. The software packages currently available vary greatly in terms of the speech samples allowed and the type of output provided. The simplest package may be the *Computer Analysis of Phonological Processes (CAPP)* (Hodson, 1985) which accepts as input only the consonants of the 50 words in Hodson's *APP-R* (1986) and provides a single page of output which includes the percent of occurrence of 10 basic phonological processes, a phonological deviancy score, and a suggested treatment objective. More complex programs, such as *Programs to Examine Phonetic and Phonologic Evaluation Records (PEPPER)* (Shriberg, 1986) and the *Profile of Phonology (PROPH+)* portion of *Computerized Profiling* (Long & Fey, 1991) accept as input single word or connected speech samples. These latter programs provide several types of analyses, including a phonetic inventory, type-token data, syllable shapes, and measures of percent consonants correct, in addition to an analysis of selected phonological processes. What is important to remember for the purpose of this discussion is that the analysis provided by these computers is the same kind of analysis performed by humans simply done more quickly. Unfortunately, this means that the clinician is still responsible for gathering and transcribing the speech sample, and then has the added responsibility of entering the phonological data into the computer. Further, some computer analyses are actually more limited than human analysis because of constraints in terms of the input and the capabilities of the software to recognize variations and atypical patterns.

In summary, the possible value of computerized phonological analysis lies in expected time savings for the analysis, and a potential for obtaining and organizing large amounts of data in a more systematic fashion than can normally be undertaken given other forms of analysis. However, the problems inherent in computerized analysis are not unexpected. The output can be no better than the input. Since the input is usually limited to a preselected number of phonological rules, the final analysis may be limited indeed.

Informal Assessments

Many clinicians use informal methods of identifying phonological patterns in addition to, or in place of formal tests. Of course each clinician who does this probably does it a bit differently. The typical pattern often involves administering a speech sound inventory and transcribing the entire set of single word responses. A spontaneous speech sample is recorded and transcribed. Finally, a list of specific words designed to probe for the consistency of patterns noted in the other samples is administered. The clinician then examines the sample for the presence of patterns of which she may be aware.

Such informal methods are probably best used simply to confirm the presence of patterns noted in formal testing or to explore variability in identified rules. The reasons for restricting informal samples of this type are that informal samples frequently do not contain sufficient variety in phonetic context, syllabic structure, or semantic and syntactic complexity to provide an accurate picture of a child's phonological patterns. Also, many of the children for whom a phonological analysis is most needed exhibit moderate to severe intelligibility problems. It is quite difficult to identify patterns or processes when the target utterance is not known to the examiner. Shriberg and Kwiatkowski (1985) have provided the following guidelines for spontaneous speech sampling:

1. The examiner must have the flexibility to shift stimuli and questions in order to keep the child talking.
2. Intelligibility can be increased by increasing control over the content of the child's utterances.
3. The child's output should be monitored for repeated use of the same vocabulary and the stimuli should be varied to increase the number of word types.
4. The child's cognitive and affective states should be monitored during the evaluation.

Although these suggestions are quite helpful, they still do not ensure that the sample obtained will be adequate to examine factors known to affect phonological production such as variations in syntactic complexity (Panagos, Quine, & Klich, 1979), pragmatic factors (Weiner & Ostrowski, 1979; Campbell & Shriberg, 1982) and semantic complexity (Camarata & Schwartz, 1985). Finally, there is evidence that some children may avoid words that contain problem sounds or difficult syllable structures (Stoel-Gammon & Dunn, 1985). Therefore, it may require an extensive speech sample and a sizable investment in time to get a child to produce particular phonological structures.

Conclusion

There are a number of formal instruments and computer software packages available to assist the speech-language pathologist in conducting a phonological analysis of a child's phonology. There are also published suggestions for structuring an informal assessment of this type as well. Regardless of how many phonological rules are assessed, these techniques still limit the analysis to a finite set of predetermined patterns. If we believe that children are active participants in the learning of their phonology and master this skill by creative trial and error and hypothesis testing, then it seems likely that many children will develop idiosyncratic rules or patterns that have yet to be described in the literature. Most formal tests of phonology are either unable to identify such creative patterns or lead the examiner to make an incorrect pattern identification.

✦ PART III ✦

Phonological Intervention

Author's Note: The concept of phonologically based intervention is
in its infancy. In fact, so little has been talked about in this area, that
there has been some discussion about whether there really is any
difference between traditional and phonological approaches to
therapy. Rest assured that there is; or at least there should be.
However, the abysmal state-of-the-art has left us with few guidelines and fewer areas of professional consensus. Because the
attempt here will be to present as purely phonological a concept of
therapy as is possible, the reader may find the following chapters
somewhat more controversial than the first 2 parts of this book.
That's OK. After all, the procedures to be presented have been
shown to work time and time again over the last 15 years.

In short, there's little doubt that the seeds of our future concepts
of therapy lie somewhere in this garden, even if we do not yet
know which of the seeds will ultimately bear fruit.

CHAPTER 11

Relationship Between Traditional and Phonological Intervention Approaches: Motor Versus Cognitive Learning

Laurie P. was a 36-year-old speech-language pathologist in a large hospital in eastern Pennsylvania, when she received her first opportunity to learn how to play a musical instrument. Because she had never received any music lessons, she was asked to participate in an experiment. Very simply, she was going to be taught how to play the piano in one easy lesson in front of 100 other clinicians. She walked nervously to the front of the filled room, looking warily at the little hand-held electric piano. After greeting Laurie and thanking her for taking part in the experiment, the instructor played 7 notes on the piano ("Twinkle, twinkle, little star . . . "). Laurie was asked to copy what she had seen and heard. So far so good. The instructor played the same 7 notes again and then added 7 more (". . . how I wonder where you are"); Laurie again was asked to imitate the entire 14-note sequence. Following success at this level, additional notes were added little by little until finally Laurie was able to play the entire 42-note song on her own.

To thunderous applause, Laurie began to move back to her seat—until she was abruptly stopped by the instructor.

"Not so fast," he exclaimed. "That's just one song. I said I was going to teach you to *play the piano*. So come on back."

Laurie started walking back uncertainly. The instructor, as confident as ever, stated, "OK, now that you know how to play the piano, try another song—the *Star-Spangled Banner*."

Laurie looked from the instructor to the piano and back up to the instructor again. The room was hushed. "Go ahead," the instructor urged. Laurie again looked down to the keyboard, took her pointing finger and pushed down a note. A long pause followed.

"I can't," she said at last.

"What do you mean you can't? I just taught you how. Now try again," the instructor ordered.

"No, I really can't do it."

At this point, the instructor knew that the battle was lost. However, he was a good enough clinician to know that it was a good idea to leave the client with some success.

"OK, forget the *Star-Spangled Banner*," he said supportively. "Let's just try *Twinkle, Twinkle Little Star* once more."

Laurie looked back at the piano somewhat relieved. She played the first 7 notes correctly but then she forgot what came next. Stumbling around the keyboard, she made several errors on the song she had supposedly mastered a few minutes earlier. But the instructor, rather than being upset, now appeared to be positively thrilled. He now had an "explanation" for his lack of teaching success. It was obvious. The inconsistency, the searching movements.

"Ah ha!" he exclaimed. "Index finger apraxia!"

Back to Reality

Actually, this short story is only partially meant to be tongue-in-cheek. In reality, there's a very close connection between why Laurie couldn't play more than that one song and why traditional modes of articulation therapy have yielded such mixed results. We will discuss this connection soon. But first, let's return to Laurie for a few moments. "Index finger apraxia" is a ludicrous attempt at an explanation for her difficulties. But there are some other possibilities that immediately come to mind.

1. *Perhaps the instructor was a poor teacher.* Yet he wasn't. Insensitive perhaps. Maybe not very knowledgeable about learning. But Laurie learned what she had worked on—at least initially. And she learned the song very quickly. No, his teaching was adequate.
2. *Maybe Laurie was learning disabled—or retarded.* After all, she demonstrated one of the prime characteristics of learning disability or mental retardation—the ability to learn one thing but no ability to generalize. Unfortunately, in a group of certified speech-language pathologists, this explanation is as ludicrous as was the apraxia hypothesis.

No, there are no simple answers for Laurie's problem. Instead, a fuller consideration of learning in general is needed.

Types of Learning

The fairly recent discipline of cognitive-behavior modification[8] provides a good framework for our consideration of learning in general and Laurie's problem in particular. How do we learn something new? We have two methods available to us.

First, there is *rote learning*. Rote learning involves practice and the establishment of habits. Simply, it is doing something over and over again until you learn it. When might you use this type of learning? If you are learning a song on the piano perhaps. Or if you are learning to say a particular phrase in a foreign language. Basically, you use rote learning any time you want to learn one or a few particular target behaviors.

Now, there is nothing wrong with rote learning. In truth, it can be very valuable, depending on what your goal is. For example, it is probably the best way to teach *Twinkle, Twinkle Little Star*. In fact, we could formulate a rule: *rote learning allows for the quickest learning of a particular target behavior.* And rote learning would work best, even if you wanted to teach 5 or 10 or even 20 songs. The only problem is, there's little generalization of this learning. Why? Because the person has not learned the system of rules and regulations underlying this target behavior. And there's no need to do so—unless you want the person to be able to sit down at a piano and play any unheard piece of music. Then, the person with only rote learning would be in trouble.

Another example of rote learning: Some of you may still remember this or a similar dialogue from high school French or Spanish:

---

[8]This discussion is a simplification and adaptation of concepts presented within the discipline of cognitive-behavior modification. For those interested in studying some original souces more closely, see works by Meichenbaum (1977) and/or Kazdin (1978).

Bonjour, Jean. Comment vas-tu?
Tres bien, merci. Et toi?
Pas mal, merci. Qui est-ce?
C`est un ami.
Ah, comment s'appelle t'il?
Il s'appelle Paul.
Present nous, veux-tu?
Jean, je voudrais te presenter Paul Martin.
Bonjour, Paul. Ou vas-tu?
Au coeur de francais.
Ah, tu vais de francais? Nous aussi.
Et bien. Allons y.

Many of us spent countless hours memorizing dialogues such as this one. Did we learn how to speak French? Most likely not. Although this type of rote memorization was probably the best way to get us to recite the dialogue, it was probably the worst method for teaching us to speak a foreign language.

The second way we can learn to do something new is through *cognitive learning*. Cognitive learning involves teaching an understanding of the rules and regulations underlying a particular target behavior. When is this type of learning valuable? If you want to be able to play any song at the piano, without much practice. Or if you want to be able to converse in a foreign language, not just say some phrases.

Unfortunately, there is a cost to cognitive learning. Cognitive learning usually results in slower initial learning of target behaviors. But there is a payoff because much generalization of learning results. Again, both types of learning—rote and cognitive—have value, depending on your goal. If your goal is to teach one or a few particular target behaviors, rote learning is best. If, on the other hand, your goal is to teach a skill or ability involving many target behaviors, perhaps even hundreds, then cognitive learning is most appropriate.

To look at the same thing in a slightly different way, for each of the two different types of learning, the *locus of learning* is different. In rote learning, the locus of learning is mostly in the organ of production. For example, in learning a song on the piano, the locus of learning is in the fingers (helped by visual cues). In speaking a foreign phrase, the locus of learning is in the mouth. On the other hand, for cognitive learning, the locus of learning is in the child's cognitions—in the brain, if you will.

Now, what does all this have to do with articulation? Just about everything. The goal of traditional articulation therapy has been the *production of target sounds* either in isolation, words, or other units. We never tried to teach the system of rules and regulations underlying the production of the sounds. Why? Because we didn't use this system ourselves when evaluating articulation. What is this underlying system? The rules for place, manner, voicing, context, structure, semantics, and linguistics that form the basis of American English phonology (as presented in the *Model of Parameters of Articulatory Constraint*).

So, in traditional articulation therapy the locus of learning has been the child's mouth (or articulators). That helps to explain why oral-motor approaches have been so predominant in our history of speech therapy. You might wonder, "If this approach wasn't optimal, why did children learn?" Because eventually, through practice, children learned the rules for American English phonology on their own. But often it took a very long time. As in most rote learning situations, obtaining initial production in isolation was quick and not difficult. (For example, there isn't a clinician around who could not get the child to produce the *k* sound by clamping her fingers on the child's tongue tip and then providing models.) But generalization and transfer was always difficult.

If the concept of a child teaching himself the rules of phonology (despite our supposed "help") is a bit difficult to accept, consider this analogy: the self-taught musician who has never had any formal training. And just to carry this a bit further, what is the system of rules and regulations underlying music that this self-taught musician has had to learn? The western scale and the relationships between notes in that scale, including factors such as intervals, chords, and preferred keys. (The western scale is different from the eastern scale—accounting for the substantial differences between the sound of western music and that of purely eastern, or oriental, music.)

In contrast to traditional modes of articulation therapy, the goal of therapy from a phonological perspective is not production of target sounds, but instead involves a conceptualization or understanding of the system of rules and regulations underlying American English phonology. Once again, production of target sounds is considered unimportant. Instead, what is important is developing understanding (and eventual production) of the underlying rule—regardless of the sounds produced.

In this newer form of articulation therapy, the locus of learning is the brain, or the child's cognitive system. The underlying thesis of all this is that *once the child understands the rule-bound contrast between his production and the correct production, it will be easy to facilitate improvement.* Initial learning may be a bit slower, but the payoff will come in quicker generalization. In reality, this is just what proponents of phonologically based intervention have seen.

To get a little more concrete, there are several differences between traditional and phonological frameworks for therapy. Below is a brief discussion of these differences.

1. In phonologically based therapy, *the major emphasis is not the sound; instead it is teaching the child (or adult) a rule.* So the goal of therapy is not to encourage the client to produce certain idealized sounds, but to get her to change her system of phonological rules. As such, specific sound errors are sometimes accepted and rewarded if the correct rule is exhibited by the client. Also, in most circumstances, therapy involves working on many sounds at once. For example, for stopping of fricatives, the child may be working on the contrast between all fricatives (i.e., *s, sh, th, f, v,* etc.) and all stops simultaneously. For deletion of final consonants, all final sounds may be considered fair game.[9]

2. Whether or not you teach one or many sounds at once, in phonologically based therapy *the rule is always taught in the context of its contrast*. So if you're trying, for example, to teach the concept of frication to a child with stopping of fricatives, you never just teach the concept "blowing"; instead you teach "blowing" and "popping" at the same time. And you want the child to shift repeatedly between both sides of the contrast. (As you'll soon see, in the program to be described in Chapter 13, even at higher levels of production the concept of contrasting the two images remains.)

3. *No value judgments are made regarding correct or incorrect production of particular sounds.* The contrast pairs are presented as equal alternatives rather than one right and the other wrong.

4. In phonologically based therapy, *there should be a de-emphasis on motoric manipulation or placement of the articulators.* Thus, the client is given absolutely no instruction at any time relating to how to produce a given sound. Many traditional motoric approaches—for example, phonetic placement, use of mirror, or motor exercises—are not only not used, but even are viewed as counterproductive.

---

[9]It should be noted that at least one investigator in clinical phonology, Barbara Hodson, doesn't necessarily believe in working on all sounds of a given contrast simultaneously. In Hodson and Paden (1983), a "cycle approach" is described whereby sounds for a given side of the contrast are worked on one at a time in Cycle 1 before being combined in later cycles. More on "cycles" will be discussed in Chapter 13.

Even in placement errors, motoric manipulation is de-emphasized. For example, we would never say "Put your tongue . . . " to a client, although we might stress front versus back (of a car, perhaps). The thesis of all this is that the child *has* the motor capacity to produce any sound. So it makes no sense to teach him as if he doesn't (have that motor capability).

5. *Modeling and the need for direct imitation on the part of the client is avoided* if possible (although, as we will see it cannot always be avoided and delayed imitation must be used in certain cases).

6. *No more than one phonological rule is expected to be altered in a given word at one time.* This creates some interesting problems that make some of us schooled in traditional techniques quite nervous. For example, if the client has stopping of fricatives (she says /tʌm/ for *thumb*) and then suddenly starts saying /fʌm/ for *thumb*, she's correct! Why? Because she has correctly produced the feature that you want.

7. In most phonologically based intervention, *there is a de-emphasis on auditory discrimination training.* For years, auditory discrimination training has been an important part of many traditional therapy programs. Even today, many clinicians swear by the importance of this sort of training. Yet there is virtually no research to support the value of discrimination training in articulation improvement. (See Bernthal & Bankson, 1993 or Shelton, 1978, for a summary of the relevant research.)

In short, most phonological approaches to therapy avoid any auditory discrimination training. Even Barbara Hodson, whose current work in phonology has extensive auditory ingredients (she recommends "auditory bombardment," perhaps a remnant of her early work with deaf children), avoids any reference to auditory discrimination. In

our own approach (to be described fully in Chapter 13), although we do have a stage called Semantic Identification, for which listening is a prerequisite skill, no auditory discrimination instruction takes place.

Distinguishing between Traditional and Phonological Frameworks for Therapy

Unfortunately, the clear, idealized distinctions drawn here between traditional and phonological therapeutic paradigms do not often appear in the current phonological literature. In fact, Fey (1992) observed that even the strongest advocates of phonological analysis regress to some use of more traditional, or motor-oriented approaches, when discussing therapy! So Hodson and Paden (1983) in their section on therapy, recommended that the clinician use "whatever cues . . . are required for correct utterance [sic]" (p. 67), including, presumably, phonetic placement or other traditional techniques. And Young (1983), even while stressing the importance of a phonological approach, stated that if the child has initial difficulty, "traditional articulation techniques may be applied" (p. 50). Finally, Creaghead (1989) went so far as to say, "the choice of targets for therapy is the primary distinction between these (phonological) approaches and the traditional ones. To some extent, any approach may be used for teaching the target sounds" (p. 204).

This tendency to embrace traditional motor-oriented therapy techniques even while proclaiming the importance of a phonological framework for working with children with speech disorders has created a real dilemma for clinicians attempting to understand clearly the differences between the alternative models. Ironically, in the sentences immediately following this quoted passage, Creaghead (1989) presented two principles of phonologically based therapy that provide a good test for whether a phonological paradigm is indeed being followed:

1. *Principle of Rule-Governed Knowledge*—states that if children are going to learn the phonological rules of their language, they must be presented with circumstances that allow them to *discover* those rules.

2. *Principle of Communicative Function*—states that for therapy to be successful, children must be given opportunities to see the relationship between appropriate phonological output and effective communication.

To these principles, Fey (1992, 1995) has added another:

3. *Principle of Treatment by Sound Class*—states that programs that are phonologically based concentrate on remediation of classes of sounds that seem to be treated similarly by clients. Thus, all phonologically based programs target errors at the feature or rule level, not at the isolated sound level.

Traditional procedures such as phonetic placement do not meet the test of these three principles; unfortunately, neither have many of the therapy procedures described thus far in the phonological literature. If, indeed, the value of our recently developed phonological framework for speech disorders is to be fully realized, we need to be more consistent in our recommendations for therapy, and must resist the temptation to "regress to our past learning" when faced with unanswered questions within the therapy room.

It is hoped that this chapter has helped to clarify somewhat the distinctions between traditional and phonological approaches to therapy. These distinctions should become clearer yet, as the discussion of therapy continues over the next three chapters.

CHAPTER 12

Therapeutic Procedure Based on Minimal Pairs

As stated in the author's note at the beginning of Part 3, state of the art phonological approaches to therapy are currently quite unimpressive. Thus far, only two major categories of approaches stressing *conceptualization* rather than motor production have been described. The first one has been written about extensively in the literature and thus will be presented only briefly here.

Ferrier and Davis (1973) were among the first to present a treatment approach for articulation disorders that required that the child learn to distinguish between "meaningful minimal contrasts" in pairs of words. This approach has since been described in greater detail by Weiner (1981) and then Young (1983) and is now referred to colloquially as the "minimal pairs" approach. (Although we have, in our lighter moments, described this procedure as the "Increasing Frustration" or the "Heightening Ambiguity" approach. You will see why shortly.)

The minimal pairs approach is probably best understood through a description of one typical use: Trying to teach a consonant-vowel-consonant (CVC) syllable structure to a child who currently only produces CV utterances. (In other words, the child has deletion of final consonants.)

Prerequisites

- Need pairs of words that differ by only one feature—the feature that you're trying to get the child to conceptualize.

  Examples: bow—boat (see Figure 12–1)
  pie — pipe

- These words must be picturable. So word pairs such as *kuh—cup* would be a problem unless you made *kuh* picturable in some way. (See Figure 12–2 for an example of how this might be done.)
- The clinician is expected to devise many of these minimal pairs.

Step 1

- Put minimal pairs in front of the child.
- Either ask the child questions about the words that help to illustrate their meanings ("Which one sails on the water?") (Young, 1983) *or* label the words and instruct the child to point to the item being named (Weiner, 1981; Young, 1983).
- This probably won't be very difficult for the child; after all, he will most likely already be familiar with the words being used.

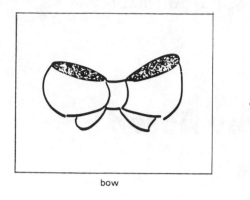

Deletion
of
final
consonants

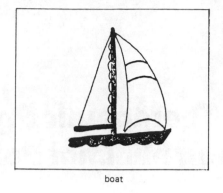

bow

boat

Figure 12–1. Sample minimal pair for deletion of final consonants.

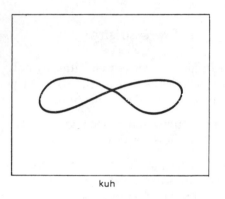

Deletion
of
final
consonants

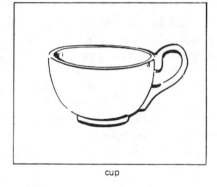

kuh

cup

Figure 12–2. Minimal pair using one nonsense drawing.

- According to proponents of this approach, this step heightens the contrast auditorily and teaches the child to hear the contrast.

Step 2

- In this step, the roles are changed in the game.
- Put 3–5 of each member of the contrast pair in front of the child (e.g., 3 *bows*, 3 *boats*).
- Tell the child *you'll* now pick up the picture *he* tells you to pick up. (For the

child to "win," he has to get you to pick up all of the pictures.)
- Tell the child to start. What will he say first? Probably *bow*. Then he will try to ask for the other picture. But what will inevitably come out? Again *bow*. In fact, he will keep saying the CV word until all the CV pictures are picked up. Usually his frustration level will begin increasing during this stage.
- Finally, all the CV pictures will be gone. When the child tries to ask for the *boat* now, and says /bo/, the clinician will of course respond, "I don't see another *bow*. Tell me what to pick up next, so that you

can win." At this point, the child will usually become highly frustrated.

Step 3

- When frustration occurs, teach the child to produce the target response by either heightening the contrast or underlining the meaning differences between the words.
- The thesis is that the desire at this time to learn the contrast will be very high on the part of the child. So you are using this frustration and/or ambiguity in therapy.[10]

NOTE: Advocates of a minimal pair approach become extremely vague as to exactly how to do the teaching at this point. Young (1983) advocated increased use of modeling and a repetition of the attempt to contrast meaning. ("You called this one *bow*. But remember, the other picture was *bow*. This one sails across the water; it's a *boat*. Say *boat*.") However, if the child still doesn't produce the target, no further instructions are provided. Weiner was more eclectic, saying about this point of frustration, "Any way that you can teach the child to produce the final sound at this point is OK" (Weiner, 1983). It is noteworthy that both Young and Weiner were prepared to "regress" to traditional procedures at this point, in order to stimulate production.

Step 4

- Repeat Steps 1–3 with other minimally contrasting word pairs until the child can easily produce both sides of the contrast.
- Once the contrast is learned, the child will start generalizing on his or her own.
- Eventually start increasing the response requirements so that final consonants are produced in phrases, sentences, and ultimately, spontaneous conversation.

Now, keep in mind that this example illustrates only one possible use of the minimal pairs approach—to eliminate final consonant deletion. In reality, the procedure can be used with any rule. Figure 12–3, for example, illustrates a possible minimal pair if the rule being worked on is fronting of velars.

Comment

The minimal pairs approach has many advocates. There is at least some research supporting its effectiveness (e.g., Monahan, 1986; Weiner, 1981a; Young, 1983) and many clinicians in the field have reported positive results for clients who have received minimal pairs therapy. Yet, we no longer use minimal pairs in our own clinic, for several reasons. First, we see no value in frustrating the child, even if the desire to learn is higher at that point. We believe there are other ways to teach

---

[10]In his workshops on phonological analysis, Weiner (1983) has offered the following example which illustrates the "value" of frustration in this approach. He tells the story about a darling, well-behaved 5-year-old girl who deleted final consonants. He put down 6 pictures (3 *bows*, 3 *boats*) and had a special surprise for her if she could get him to pick up all the pictures. Of course, she said /bo/ at first and Weiner picked up the first *bow*. Two more /bo/ productions and Weiner picked up two more *bows*. She said /bo/ once more and Weiner looked at her with puzzlement and said, "I don't see another *bow*." The girl looked down at the pictures, up at Weiner, and then he could see small tears in the corners of her eyes, now beginning their way down her cheeks. Back at the workshop, Weiner snaps his fingers and says to the audience, "At this point, I knew I had her." He then relates how he asked the girl, "Do you want me to help you make *boat*? The girl nods "yes" tentatively. Weiner says, "You see, the word *boat* has a tail on the end. Can you make it with a tail? It's like this—*boattt*"(with an exaggerated, highlighted final consonant).

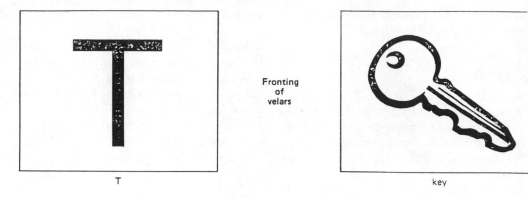

Figure 12–3. Sample minimal pair for fronting of velars.

the child meaningful contrasts, which do not require heightened ambiguity. Second, most current descriptions of minimal pairs therapy represent a skeleton of an idea, rather than a full therapeutic regimen. For example, there is no clear indication as to what the clinician should do if the child can hear the contrasts, but doesn't produce them immediately (something that occurs frequently). Suggestions to revert to traditional motor-oriented procedures at this point represent a betrayal of the theoretical framework underlying minimal pairs in the first place—and even these suggestions are vague. Likewise, the preferred sequence of steps is unclear. Once the child has produced the target correctly, is the concept of meaningful contrasts dropped (as Young, 1983, implied) or are there additional steps where the child actively contrasts the target and the incorrect production meaningfully? How many word pairs are needed to enhance and ensure generalization? Four, as Weiner (1981) implied? Three, as Young (1983)

implied? More? Less? What if the child produces the correct side of the contrast but the incorrect sound—for example, a child who previously deleted final consonants now says /bop/ for *boat*? Is it judged correct, as Weiner (1981) suggested? Or does the clinician try to correct the sound error, as Young (1983) implied?

With all of these unanswered questions, it becomes clear that, at least thus far, *there is no one standardized minimal-pair approach.* Of course, many clinicians have developed their own individualized procedures based on the minimal pairs concept and have claimed substantial success. That is why this review is included here. The concept of using meaningful minimal contrasts is sound theoretically and the purpose here is not to discount or minimize the success that some clinicians are currently having with the technique. If we don't use the technique in our clinic, it is because we have found a procedure that works better for us and our clients. A discussion of that procedure forms the basis of the next two chapters.

CHAPTER 13

Therapeutic Procedure Based on Imagery

The second major therapeutic approach that stresses conceptualization rather than motor mimicry is imagery. In this procedure, the clinician helps the client learn the contrast by presenting a variety of semantic prompts or images. By attaching a label to each side of the contrast, the goal is to give sounds an identity to which the child can relate. (This stage will be called *semantic identification*.) The type of imagery used will depend on two factors:

1. *Type of contrast you are trying to teach*— We'll talk shortly about the fact that the use of imagery is not new; in fact, it has been used periodically throughout the era of traditional therapy. But the images have not always matched the type of contrast in the past. For example, one typical image that was used for a client with a frontal lisp (*th/s* substitution) was the image of a snake sound. But the problem in a frontal lisp is one of placement, not manner. So an auditory image focusing on the acoustic output of a snake was probably inappropriate. Regardless, the goal is for the image to match the contrast in as logical a fashion as possible.
2. *What the client can understand*—It's obviously unwise to try to teach the child a label for a concept that he or she cannot

understand. (Although in all fairness, we have observed that the specific labels used seem to be less important predictors of success than how those labels have been taught.)

The wealth of images available to you is limited only by your imagination and the ability to transform abstract phonemic features into images understandable to the client. Let's consider some possible examples:

Stopping of Fricatives
- *Running* vs. *dripping*—A beautiful example of how the use of imagery is far from a new concept lies in the fact that this image contrast was first described more than 10 years ago by Weiner and Bankson (1978). They combined auditory and visual imagery by bringing the child to a sink and turning the faucet full on and then almost off to demonstrate *running* sounds (fricatives) and *dripping* sounds (stops).
- *Popping* vs. *blowing* or *flowing*— Again attributed to Weiner (1983).
- *Popping* vs. *windy*—One of the contrasts we use most often today; children seem to respond better to the term *windy* than either of the others noted.

- *Spitting* vs. *raining*—OK, so it sounds weird. But we stumbled across this contrast almost by accident and it has been very effective, especially with hard-to-motivate boys. . . . We *do* recommend a raincoat, however.

Fronting of Velars

- *Front* vs. *back*—This is not one of our favorites because for some clinicians this contrast stimulates an unconscious urge to say, "Put your tongue . . . . " As this latter instruction is a death knell for phonologically based therapy, we often stay away from *front* versus *back*. However, several clinicians have reported success with this contrast, so if you can avoid the temptation to regress to a motor-oriented approach, it might be effective.
- *Tippy* vs. *throaty*—This is our favorite and most successful contrast for fronting of velars; it works well with children as young as 2.5 years old.

Deletion of Final Consonants

- *Open* vs. *closed*—This is probably the most popular contrast currently in use for this rule. Not particularly interesting or inspired but it seems to work.
- *Tail* vs. *no tail*—Some clinicians like this contrast very much. The problem arises in using the same word (i.e., *tail*) in both sides of the contrast. This forces the child to make the distinction on the basis of the word *no*, perhaps placing a particular strain on children with accompanying language deficits. One innovative way of overcoming this problem has been to use an animal with a tail (e.g., *monkey*) and an animal without a tail (e.g., *frog*) and to call sounds with final consonants *monkey* sounds and those without *frog* sounds.
- *Driveway* vs. *garage*—Clinicians using this contrast present two pictures—one illustrating a car on a driveway with an open garage at the end of the driveway and the other illustrating a car inside the closed garage. This contrast has been of more interest to older children than either of the previous sets of images.
- *Sticky Sam* vs. *Missing Mo*—A highly imaginative contrast developed by a clinician in the Orange County School District in California. She drew two pictures, one having all limbs, the other missing his right eye, arm, and leg. Utterances without final consonants were labeled *Missing Mo*, those with final consonants *Sticky Sam*. This clinician reported great success with this contrast. It is cited here to illustrate once again that some of the best contrasts are probably still inside your head rather than in this book.

Cluster Reduction (within words)

- *Friendly* vs. *lonely*—The client is taught that friendly sounds always go together whereas lonely sounds are all by themselves. This is one of the most popular and most effective contrasts available to teach clusters.
- *Buddy* vs. *lonely*—Same concept, but for older boys.
- *Friendly* vs. *nerdie*—An extremely popular and motivational contrast for boys older than age 5. Anytime you can include some of the slang terminology used among the kids themselves, you increase motivation substantially. And as we'll see in Chapter 15, motivation is probably the most important determinant of how successful any intervention will be. For some reason, boys older than the age of 5 love the label "nerd"—so why not use that?

All of these attempts to come up with images have one thing in common: the desire to reduce sounds and/or syllable structures to something that a child can understand. The goal, then, is to give the sound or feature a *semantic referent*: this semantic referent becomes a code word that allows for communication between the clinician and the child about a certain mode of speech production. Once again, the only guidelines for image construction are:

1. Make sure you develop two images, one for each side of the contrast.
2. Make the images interesting and/or motivational for the child.

3. Try to create images that the child can relate to, or at least understand.

Because image construction is an important part of the pretherapy process, the Clinical Mastery Exercise on page 292 has been developed. Before reading any further, take some time to complete that exercise and then check your answers with the suggested answer sheet in the Appendix. And remember—there is no right or wrong; as is usual in therapy, whatever works is automatically right and whatever doesn't— well, you know the rest.

Clinical Mastery Exercise: Developing Image Contrasts

One of the most important aspects of imagery therapy is the development of appropriate image contrasts. While there is no way to know with certainty which image contrasts will work best for a particular client (and thus there are no *wrong* image contrasts), it might be helpful to obtain some practice in coming up with images for some specific rules. For your benefit, some of the images we've used more often are included on the answer sheet in the Appendix. But remember, there's nothing magical about the possibilities we've presented; some of our best image contrasts have come from people like you, learning about imagery for the first time. So give it a shot!

Rule		Example		Image Contrasts
A. Stopping of Fricatives	/tʌn/	for *sun*		popping-blowing spitting-raining
1. *h*'ing of stops	/hi/	for *key*		_____ _____
2. lateral lisp	lateral /sup/	for *soup*		_____ _____
3. cluster reduction	/bɪdɔg/	for *big dog*		_____ _____
4. gliding of *1*	/jæmp/	for *lamp*		_____ _____
5. labial assimilation	/pʌp/	for *cup*		_____ _____
6. alveolarization of fricatives	/sʌn/	for *fun*		_____
	/su/	for *shoe*		_____

Therapy Regimen Based on Imagery

It was mentioned earlier that imagery has a long history in traditional therapy. For example, Lousie Binder Scott was well-known for her creation of images for each of the speech sounds (e.g., see Scott, 1952) — and the "snake sound" has held an honored place in the field of speech pathology.

So then, you might be thinking to yourself by now, what's the big deal? As we'll soon see, the key to this different form of therapy is merging the use of imagery with several principles of phonological intervention that have been or will be discussed. This will all become clearer as we discuss the regimen, an outline of which appears in Figure 13–1.

** • STEP 1—*Semantic Identification of the Image Contrast* (Two stars).

  1. In this step, your major goal is to teach the child to identify semantically both sides of the contrast in nonsense syllables. It is important that you begin in nonsense syllables, that you do not break it down to an isolated sound level (even if the client is having some initial difficulties), and that you avoid real words at all costs during this early training. (We'll talk about why later in this chapter.)

     At first, you will generally want to use only one vowel in your nonsense syllables. Although we usually begin with the vowel *ah*, some clinicians have reported beginning with other vowels successfully, most notably *ee*. Also, at first you will want to use only one member from each contrast group. So if the rule you're working on is *stopping of fricatives* and your contrast is *popping* versus *blowing*, your initial stimuli might be /pa/ versus /ʃa/.

It is particularly important to limit yourself to just these two stimuli at first. At this stage, the client is learning a connection between a newly learned label and a nonsense utterance. This connection can best be developed if the set of possibilities is limited at first.

NOTE: When the client is first learning to identify the contrast, we usually use pictures as additional cues to help teach the new concepts. An example of simple, clinician-drawn pictures for the *friendly-lonely* contrast used for cluster reduction appears in Figure 13–2. One thing to watch out for: whereas it is permissible for the client to point to the correct picture when identifying a particular nonsense syllable, you also want the child to label the side of the contrast verbally. In other words, have the child say *friendly* or *lonely* in addition to pointing to any pictures. (Of course, if the client is unintelligible, it will not be said correctly; however, this is not important as long as you can decipher what the client is trying to say.)

STEPS FOR THERAPY USING IMAGERY

STEP 1 · IDENTIFYING THE IMAGE CONTRAST

    a) *Nonsense syllables with* <u>*ah*</u>*; one member of each contrast group*

        EXAMPLE: *RULE: Fronting of velars*
                    CONTRAST: Tippies vs. throaties
                    STIMULI: /ta/ vs. /ka/

    b)*Nonsense syllables with* <u>*ah*</u>*; many members of each contrast group*

        EXAMPLE: *STIMULI: /ta/, /da/ vs. /ka/, /ga/*

    c) *Nonsense syllables with many vowels; one member of each contrast group*

        EXAMPLE: *STIMULI: /ta/, /ti/, /tu/ etc. vs. /ka/, /ki/, /ku/ etc.*

STEP 2 · PRODUCTION OF CONTRAST IN NONSENSE SYLLABLES

        a) *Usually just necessary to tell child to be teacher*
            • *Don't instruct placement*
            • *Try to avoid imitation*

        EXAMPLE: *STIMULI: "You be the teacher & give me a tippie. Now you give me a throaty."*

            • *Production at first, usually with only one vowel - That's fine!!*
            • *Production at first, usually with only one member from each contrast group - That's also fine!!*

        b) *After child can produce consistently one member from each group with one vowel try to*
          stimulate production of other vowels.
            • *Again, try to avoid imitation; perhaps use masked imitation"*

        EXAMPLE: *"Can you make a tippie with /i/?"*
                      or
              "I'll make a sound with a throaty; you make it with a tippie"

        RULES FOR THIS STEP
            - *Never teach just one part of contrast pair; have child go back & forth.*
            - *Periodically return to identification activities (so that image of contrast is overlearned).*
            - *When child can identify perfectly, start making mistakes in your identification of him.*

STEP 3 · IDENTIFICATION OF CONTRAST IN WORDS
        a) *Don't go anywhere near this step until steps 1&2 have been mastered*
        b) *Probably best to start with CV words*
        c) *Avoid words with mixed cues*

        EXAMPLE: *Good starting words for tippy/throaty: key, toe, two, cake, toad, go*
                      Poor words for tippy/throaty: cat, talk, dog, coat

STEP 4 · PRODUCTION IN WORDS
        a) *Point out to child the ambiguity between his production and correct production*

        EXAMPLE: *"You made a tippy; I thought you said that was a throaty"*

        b) *Fairly quick learning at this point*
        c) *Use easier words first (CV); expand little by little*

Figure 13–1. Steps for Therapy Using Imagery *(continues)*

RULES FOR THIS STEP
- *Continue production of both sides of contrast; randomly intersperse words or have child produce word in both ways.*
- *Correct sound production is not goal here; production of contrast is goal.*

EXAMPLE: *RULE: Deletion of final consonants*
            CHILD SAYS: /kʌk/ for /kʌp/ - correct!

(GRADUALNESS PRINCIPLE)

STEP 5 · IDENTIFICATION IN PHRASES (OPTIONAL)
a) *Child identifies whether you used (tippy) or (throaty) in your phrase*

EXAMPLE: *STIMULE:"I see a tey (key)"*

b) *Usually at this stage child will be correcting your errors.*

STEP 6 · PRODUCTION IN PHRASES
a) *Start off with stereotyped phrase productions*
      ("I see a_____"; There's a big_____")
b) *Progress to less stereotyped phrases*
c) *Continue to make errors periodically and have child correct*
d) *Continue to use both sides of contrast; stress that he's made the word with a good (tippy) or (throaty)*
e) *You'll see extensive generalization into conversation at this point.*

STEP 7 · PRODUCTION IN CONVERSATION
a) *If steps 1-6 have gone correctly, child will usually start this step at 70% or more correct.*
b) *Goals of this stage:*
    - *Point out remaining errors and have child correct.*

EXAMPLE: *CHILD: "I see a tey"*
            CLINICIAN: "You see a tey?" (questioning prosody)
            CHILD: "I see a key"

- *Heighten reinforcement for spontaneously correct sounds.*
            ● *Bell*
            ● *Noisemaker*
            ● *Chart*

- *Make errors periodically and have child correct you.*
- *Create opportunites for child to unlearn overlearned words.*

Figure 13–1. *(continued)*

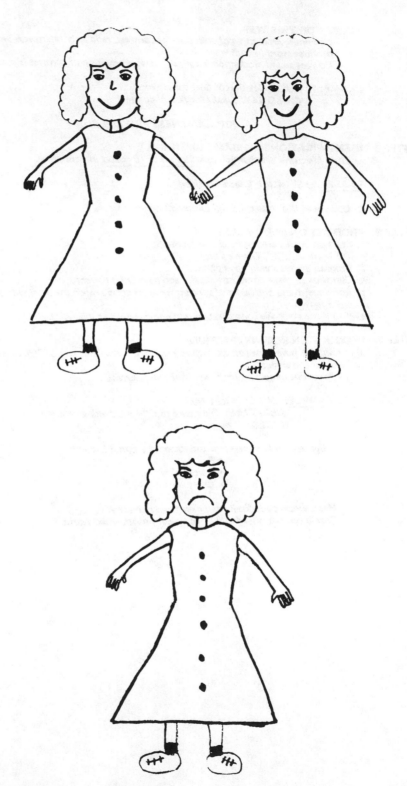

Figure 13–2. Clinician-drawn *friendly-lonely* pictures.

Finally, although we use pictures most often, we have on occasion used objects and/or body movements to accompany the syllable production, rather than pictures.

2. After the child can label the two nonsense syllables correctly with 100% accuracy, it's time to add additional members from each contrast group. So if the rule again is stopping of fricatives, you might add /ta/, /ka/, and /da/ to your *popping* stimuli and /sa/, /fa/, and /za/ to your *blowing* stimuli.

   Notice that at this stage, the stimuli are still limited to only one vowel. Also note that not all members of the *popping* or *blowing* contrast groups need to be presented at this point; instead, just a broad cross-section of syllables representing both sides of the contrast is necessary. Keep in mind—the goal here is to expand modestly the child's definition of the new labels, not to have him identify every possible member of the contrast pair.

3. After the client can correctly identify several members within each constrast group with one vowel, it is time to add additional vowels. At this point, however, you want to revert to only one member from each contrast group again—preferably the same sounds that were used in A. So given our *popping— blowing* contrast, the stimuli

at this state would be /pa/, /pi/, and /pu/ on the *popping* side and /ʃa/, /ʃi/, and /ʃu/ on the *blowing* side. Once again, it's not necessary for the clinician to include every vowel in the stimuli presented; a cross-section of different vowels (e.g., /a/, /i/ and /u/) is usually sufficient.

Additional notes—Step 1

• If the client has problems at any stage, go back to earlier stages until, if necessary, you are back to one member of each contrast group, with one vowel.

• Although we are only interested in identification at this point, you may see some production on the child's part, especially if he repeats aloud the syllable you've presented prior to telling you what side of the contrast it is. *If he produces the contrast correctly, do nothing.* Don't let him know that he has produced it correctly; just evaluate his identification. (You are, of course, allowed to cheer loudly to yourself—as long as he doesn't hear it.) *If*, on the other hand, *he produces the contrast incorrectly, stop him from trying to imitate your production* and have him concentrate only on labeling.

• This step often looks like auditory discrimination to clinicians first learning about the procedure. It is not. Though listening and discrimination skills *are* prerequisites to semantic identification, the key is matching particular phonemic output with a concept or label. You will see proof of this before the end of this chapter.

• Notice that there is no point at which the client is asked to identify nonsense syllables with both a variety of vowels and several members from each contrast pair. Although an additional step of this sort probably wouldn't hurt the client, we do not find it to be necessary.

- Do not go on to Step 2 until the child has responded with 100% accuracy at the highest level of Step 1. This will represent a change in pattern for some clinicians who regularly use an 80% criterion to move on. However, our data indicate that an 80% figure is not sufficient to create a base for future learning. Later in the chapter we'll talk about one exception to this 100% rule, but barring that exception, our advice is to require 100% mastery before moving on.

** • *STEP 2—Production of Both Sides of Contrast in Nonsense Syllables* (Two Stars)

    1. At this stage, the client will more often than not produce both sides of the contrast on his own when given the opportunity to do so. What works often for us is to tell the client that it is time for *him* to be the teacher. If working on stopping of fricatives, for example, you might say, "How about if *you* be the teacher? Give me a *popping* sound."[11] Once he has done this and you have identified his production correctly, you then say, "OK, now give me a *blowing* sound." (Notice that your initial request is for the syllable he already produces. *Then* you ask for the other side of the contrast.)

    2. If the client produces both sides of the contrast immediately, great; continue practice

at this level. If not, follow these guidelines scrupulously:

a. Do not instruct placement.

b. Try to avoid modeling and the need for imitation. Your goal is to get the child to produce both sides of the contrast on his own. Unfortunately, the use of modeling often works against this goal because by its nature it encourages motor mimicry. As we'll see, if after some period of time the child cannot get it on his own, then we may produce a brief model. But at first, try to avoid it totally.

c. Avoid spending time on unsuccessful activities. If the child is unsuccessful upon first request, have him try again. If there is still no success, go back to Step 1 (Identification) for a while before trying again. The key is to avoid having the child get to the point where he thinks he can't do it. We've seen many children who have not produced both sides of the contrast correctly until their third session of trying. It is the encouragement along the way and the lack of time spent on unsuccessful attempts that have kept these children in their problem solving modes until the third session. (In our later section on trouble-shooting, we

---

[11]Even though we are working at the syllable level, we use the word "sound" with our children, mostly because it's easier to pronounce and more easily understood by most children than the word "syllable." So when we refer to "popping sound" in our descriptions, we are referring to units (either syllables or words) that contain a sound having the popping feature.

will talk about what can be done if the client still isn't successful by the third or fourth session.)

3. When the client eventually does produce both sides of the contrast, it will usually be with only one vowel. That's fine. The early productions will also usually include only one member from each contrast group. That's also fine. So a typical set of early productions from a child working on stopping of fricatives might be /pa/ and /sa/. Until the client fully masters these early productions, don't push for production of any other syllables.

4. After the client can produce both sides of the contrast consistently with one vowel, try to stimulate production with other vowels. There are several possible ways to do this. (Once again, if possible, you want to avoid imitation learning):

   a. Sometimes a client will produce a different *popping* or *blowing* nonsense syllable if you say something as simple as, "That was a good blowing sound. Can you give me a different blowing sound?" This works especially well if you have just recently been doing some extra practice in identification of different *popping* and *blowing* nonsense syllables.

   b. *Delayed imitation*—purposely go back to a few minutes of nonsense syllable identification. When the client identifies the production correctly, say

something like, "Yes, that was a different (blowing) sound." After doing this a few times, go quickly back to, "Okay, now you make a (blowing) sound." When he is successful, say, "Remember when I made a different (blowing) sound? Now *you* make a different (blowing) sound."

   c. *Masked imitation*—this is probably the most effective of the three procedures. You say to the client something like, "OK, now I'll make a (blowing) sound—/si/—you make it (popping)." In this case, you'd expect the child to say /pi/ or /ti/; in other words, a *popping* sound with a vowel /i/. Then you might want to continue. "Good, now I'll make a popping sound—/tu/—and you make it (blowing)." After doing this with several vowels for both sides of the contrast, the client will be effectively producing several different nonsense syllables for each side of the contrast.

Your ultimate goal is for the client to produce each side of the contrast on command with two or three different vowels.

Additional notes—Step 2

• You may have noticed that there is no step where you try to get the client to produce other members of the contrast groups. In other words, if you are working on *popping* and *blowing* sounds, the client might be producing /pa/ and /ʃa/, and /pi/ and /ʃi/, and /pu/ and /ʃu/, and maybe even /pʌ/ and /ʃʌ/. But there's no formal attempt to get her to produce different *popping* sounds (perhaps /tu/ or /ki/) or different *blowing* sounds (e.g., /sa/ or /fi/). Of course if she does produce some other *popping* or *blowing* sounds on her own, great. But we have found that with most children, there's really no need to push for production of other members of the contrast group; that stage will come soon enough. If you want to try informally to stimulate other contrast group members, fine. But we have found that it's not really necessary.

- When a client who is working on a stopping of fricatives, for example, first produces a blowing sound, many clinicians have a tendency to get excited and try to push the child to produce many more *blowing* sounds in a row. This is probably a throwback to our traditional frameworks, which encourage this type of drillwork, so that the client doesn't "forget" how to produce this new sound. It is also counterproductive.

  In short, you never want to teach just one part of the contrast pair. Instead, always teach a sound and its contrast during the same step. Have the client shift back and forth on command between *popping* and *blowing* syllables rather than having her produce just one or the other in a drill-like manner.

- Even though you are now at the production level, periodically return to semantic identification practice. In fact, we start off every session with a short period of semantic identification, and just for a change of pace, we'll sometimes include an identification activity in the middle of a session. This additional practice serves two purposes: First, it allows for the image con-

trast to be overlearned. Second, it prepares the client for Step 3, which will also require identification.

NOTE: Some of the best therapy results when identification and production are combined in turn-taking games. To accomplish this, a competitive game is devised whereby forward movement on the game board occurs after correct identification and/or production of the appropriate contrast. So, for example, the client might draw a card that indicates "blowing." If she correctly produces a *blowing* sound, she moves forward in the game. If the clinician then correctly identifies the client's production she also moves forward. Then the task shifts and the clinician draws a card. At higher levels of this task, the clinician can start making mistakes in identification or production; this will be more difficult cognitively for the client and will help solidify the learning that is taking place.

- *STEP 3—Semantic Identification of the Contrast in Words*
  1. It is very important that you do not begin this step until the child has mastered Steps 1 and 2. Why? We'll go into this more fully later in the chapter, but simply, it is important that the client's semanto-phonological system be bypassed during the early learning process. In other words, we want to avoid the client's own system until we're certain that he has developed

the ability to alter his production pattern on command.

2. Our goal at this stage is to have the client identify both sides of the contrast in real words. This will not be difficult for him if Steps 1 and 2 have been mastered, but this practice in identification of the contrast in real words forms an important base for the production that will be required in Step 4.

3. In order to ensure a semantic connection, we generally present picture cards along with the verbal stimulus. So if we were working on stopping of fricatives, we might present a picture of a piece of pie, say "pie" and then ask the client to label it *popping* or *blowing*. We would then present a picture of a shoe, say the word and again ask the client to correctly identify it.

4. Stay at this level until the client can identify the contrast in real words with 100% accuracy.

Additional notes—Step 3

• Although it's not vital, at first it may be helpful to present easier words to the client. For example, words having a consonant-vowel (CV) syllable structure might be easier for the client to identify than words having a CVC construction. Of course, this suggestion only works for placement or manner rules; if you are working on a structural or contextual rule, you will have to present more difficult words right from the beginning.

• Avoid words that contain both elements of the contrast. Of course, this guideline necessitates that the clinician pay extremely close atten-tion to stimulus selection for the client. For example, *goat* would be a poor word choice if working on fronting of velars because it contains both a velar and an alveolar. Likewise, *soup* would be a poor word for stopping of fricatives because it contains both a stop and a fricative. *Sun*, on the other hand, would be fine because the initial sound is a fricative and the final sound is neither a fricative nor a stop. In order to further clarify this issue, Table 13–1 contains several suggested good and bad words for a number of the most frequently occurring rules.

• Have the child identify the contrasts in the initial position only. We have found that most children tend to generalize to other word positions on their own; only on very rare occasions have we had to teach in anything other than initial position. (Of course, this guideline does not apply to structural rules that involve the medial or final position; in these cases, the clinician should obviously target the position with which the client is having difficulty.)

• Use only simple, single-syllable words as stimuli (unless, of course, you are working on a rule that involves longer words, e.g., deletion of unstressed syllables). Once again, we've found that clients tend to generalize quite easily on their own to longer, more complex words.

* • *STEP 4—Production of Both Sides of the Contrast in Words* (One Star)

1. At this point, the client theoretically should be able to produce either side of the contrast on command. (She learned this in Step 2.) So present her with pictures representing both sides of the contrast. Now, let's say you

TABLE 13–1. Appropriate and inappropriate stimuli for some common rules.

Rule	Good Words		Poor Words	
Stopping of fricatives	• sun	• boat	• soup	
	• cup	• see	• frog	
	• shoe	• four	• fit	
	• fire	• fish	• sheep	
Fronting of velars	• cake	• keep	• cat	• kiss
	• go	• cough	• goat	• shake
	• cup	• cook	• talk	• gas
	• kick	• game	• catch	• can
Deletion of final consonants	• top	• book	• Any word with	
	• cat	• toy	final cluster	
	• cup	• soup	(e.g., nest,	
	• frog	• boy	fast)	
Gliding of liquids	• look	• why	• yellow	
	• light	• low	• wall	
	• red	• one	• year	
	• yes	• read	• roll	

are working on *popping* and *blowing* sounds, and you present her initially with a picture of a shoe. How is she going to produce this word? Incorrectly, of course; she will probably say /tu/. Why? Because you've intruded into her semanto-phonological system and she will respond in a manner that is consistent with that system.

2. When the client is wrong for the first time, point out the ambiguity to her between her production and yours. We usually instruct our clinicians to scrunch up their face quizzically and to say something like, "Hmm . . . you made a (popping) word, I thought you said it was a (blowing) word; try to make it (blowing)." Then we instruct the clinicians to do nothing; just sit and wait for

a bit. The goal is for the child to correct herself. In fact, sometimes you will even see a client actively trying to problem solve. What is most important is that you don't show the client how to make the word; let her figure it out for herself.

3. If the client does not produce the word after a few attempts, there are several options for the clinician:
   a. You can return to identification of words again for a while, followed by another attempt at production.
   b. You can go all the way back to production of nonsense syllables again; ask the client to make any (popping) sound. Then have her make a (blowing) sound. After she does so a number of times, return to the word level. Start with

one (popping) word. Then go to the (blowing) word and say, "Now be careful; this one is a (blowing) word." Again let her try to work it out herself.

c. If the client says, "I can't do it" at any point in the process, your primary responsibility is to show and convince her that she can produce the feature. Keep in mind, she has already done it (albeit at the nonsense syllable level). What is left for her is essentially a cognitive task; she has to overcome the ambiguity inherent in assaulting her current phonological system. So it's important that the cognitive task be attempted; that the client not "give up" (which is what "I can't do it" essentially signals).

4. Once the client has "figured out" how to produce that first word, you will see fairly quick learning for the other words you present. Start off with easier words (i.e., CV), then progress to more difficult words (CVC).

5. Toward the end of this word production level, you can start introducing words that have both sides of the contrast. For example, if you're working on stopping of fricatives, you would not have used the word *soup* early on, but you can do so once the client has mastered the problem-solving needed to produce the blowing feature on command. In fact, the client may notice that the word "is

both *popping* and *blowing*." There is one thing to keep in mind, however. Our experience has been that the initial sound in a word has the most perceptual importance or salience for the client. So, unless you are working on a syllable structure rule, select your stimuli on the basis of the initial sound in the words.

Additional notes—Step 4

• Don't use words more complex than a CVC syllable structure at this stage. (Again, of course, unless you are working on a structural rule that requires longer syllable structures.) We've found that it's unnecessary to present more complex words at this level; they will receive sufficient practice with different syllable structures when they get to the phrase level.

• Continue to encourage production of both sides of the contrast throughout this step. The best way to do this is to randomly intersperse the two types of words. For example, if working on stopping of fricatives, a typical order of picture presentation might be as follows: *tie, sun, gun, four, zoo, cow,* etc.

Another way of encouraging the client to shift between both elements of the contrast is to have her produce a given word in both ways. Continuing with the *popping-blowing* contrast, for example, you could present a picture of a shoe and then ask the client to produce the word first with a *blowing* sound (/ʃμ/) and then with a *popping* sound (/tu/). We have found that this mode of interspersing the sides of the contrast is not as effective in promoting generalization as is presenting two types of words, as previously discussed. It is also somewhat more difficult for the child. However, some clinicians find this variation valuable, so it's included here.

- When engaged in Step 4, it is important to remind oneself continuously that correct sound production is not the goal. Instead, it is the production of the correct side of the contrast that's important. So for a client working on stopping of fricatives, if she originally said /pɔr/ for *four*, and when trying to make a *blowing* sound comes up with /sɔr/, she is considered correct! In fact, the use of any fricative in the word initial position would make the client's response correct. As stated earlier, this idea of accepting errors is difficult for many clinicians. Yet as we'll see soon when talking about the *gradualness principle* (Ingram, 1976), it's a primary ingredient of effective phonologically based therapy.
  - STEP 5—*Semantic Identification in Phrases*
    1. This stage is now considered optional. Although we used to recommend semantic identification in phrases for all clients, numerous clinicians have recently reported dropping this step, with no decrease in therapeutic effectiveness. Because we continue to believe that some children can benefit from additional semantic identification practice, the step is still included as part of the regimen. However, it is up to you to decide whether to include it in your client's therapy.
    2. At this level, the client is presented with a picture and a short phrase is uttered about the picture. (For example, a child may be presented with a picture of a dog wearing a shoe. The clinician might then say, "The dog is wearing a /tu/.") The child is asked to identify which side of the contrast has been produced.
    3. The child will most likely have no difficulty with this task. In fact, he will often, on his own, begin correcting your errors (e.g., "No! The dog is wearing a /ʃu/"). This is great, and forms the basis of an activity that can be devised for Step 6, whereby the clinician and child take turns during a competitive game, producing the word in a phrase and monitoring the other "player" for errors.
- STEP 6—*Production of Phrases*
  1. Have the client begin by producing stereotyped phrases in which only the last word changes. Some examples:
     "I see a _____."
     "The dog is wearing a _____."
     "There's a big _____."
     At this stage, make sure all of the words in the phrase reflect correct production of the rule you're working on. For example, if working on stopping of fricatives, in the phrase, "I see a shoe," both *shoe* and *see* should be produced with *blowing* sounds.
  2. Eventually have the client progress to less stereotyped phrases, for example, those produced during picture description.
  3. Continue to provide the client practice with producing both sides of the contrast, providing liberal reinforcement for appropriate production of each side. When reinforcing verbally, continue to

use the contrast names that the client has learned. For example, say, "Yeah! That was a great (blowing) word," once again underlining the identity of the production, even at the phrase level.

4. If the client says a target word incorrectly, make certain that she corrects herself before continuing. Do not emphasize the fact that she was wrong; instead, indicate that she produced the other side of the contrast. Example: "I think you said that with a (popping) word; now say the same thing with a (blowing) word."

Additional Notes—Step 6

- It is a good idea to set up a turn-taking activity or game whereby you say the word incorrectly and the client corrects you. This is not only highly motivating for a child, but it requires a higher level of attention and cognition for her to recognize and then correct your errors. This higher-level task will enhance generalization.

- You will start seeing extensive generalization into conversation at this point on the part of the client. However, the extent of generalization depends on how will you handle correction procedures. The better you are at stopping the client when she has used the wrong side of the contrast and having her correct this output, the more generalization you will see.

  - *STEP 7—Production in Conversation*
    NOTE: If Steps 1–6 have been mastered, enough generalization will typically have taken place so that the child will at this point produce the correct side of the contrast appropriately at

least 70% of the time. Adults will often be at 90% or more. As such, your major goal for Step 7 is to extend and complete the generalization process.

1. While playing and/or talking with the client, stop him every time he produces the wrong side of the contrast. A good way to do this is to put your hand over his hands. This will usually stop his verbal output and cause him to look at you. When he does, you repeat the phrase he just incorrectly produced in the same way he produced it but with a questioning prosody (e.g., "putting on his /tuz/?"). This should be enough for the client to change his production on his own. The key is, don't let any errors get by.

2. Even while monitoring for errors and stopping the client whenever an error is made, you also want to heighten reinforcement for spontaneously correct productions. So, if working on stopping of fricatives, for example, you now heighten the reinforcement for spontaneously produced *blowing* sounds. There are a number of possible ways to do this. You can simply ring a bell every time she produces a (blowing) sound and periodically accompany the bell with "good (blowing) sound." Alternately, we have used noisemakers, stickers, slash marks in a chart, marbles dropping in a can, or just a piece of paper with "correct" and "incor-

rect" columns for adults. Essentially, anything that takes note of the client's correct productions is satisfactory. This combination of a positive consequence for correct productions along with mild punishment (i.e., stopping the forward flow of communication) for incorrect productions is effective in promoting total generalization.

3. In order to promote continued listening skills on the part of the client, make periodic errors in your conversational speech and create an incentive for the client to correct you.

4. Even after a child has come close to mastering both sides of the contrast, she will often continue to regress to her old pattern on certain overlearned words. It's important that the clinician create some activities that will help the child unlearn these overlearned words. Consider the following example:

Joey P. had just about finished his work on fronting of velars. In fact, there were only two lingering problems he had: He continued to say /ote/ for *okay* and in the phrase *time to go*, he would regress to his old production /taɪm tu do/. In order to help Joey unlearn these overlearned words, the clinic supervisor came into the therapy room one day. She sat down to play with Joey and the clinician, talking about how she'd heard that Joey was making

some great *throatie* sounds. After a minute or so of play, the supervisor made a move as if to leave and said /ote—taɪm tu do/. Joey thought this was very funny and while smiling, said to the supervisor disapprovingly, "No, it's *okay*—time to *go*," emphasizing the *throatie* sounds. The supervisor looked crestfallen and sat back for a minute looking at Joey. Then her face brightened and she again made a move to leave. "I get it," she said, "It's /ote—taɪm tu do/." For some reason, Joey thought this was funnier than the first time. He again stopped the supervisor from leaving and, believe it or not, this little scene was re-enacted over and over again for 17 minutes. Sometimes the supervisor would say, "You show me; I can't get it." At other times, she might say excitedly, "Oh, I get it now," but in all instances, she would end with /ote—taɪm tu do/, and be "forced" to stay in the room. When Joey started to lose interest after 17 minutes of the same thing, the supervisor finally said it correctly and left the room. From that time on, Joey never misarticulated those two overlearned words again. Generalization was complete.

Without implying that this particular scenario would work every time, it's important that the clinician devise at least *some* strategy to help the child unlearn any overlearned misarticulations, if they exist. The goal is 100% accuracy.

Guidelines for Phonologically Based Therapy

Certainly not every element of the therapeutic regimen just described is of equal importance. For example, although it is vitally important that the clinician avoid telling the client where to put his tongue during attempts at production, it is probably not as vital that only single syllable words be used early in the learning process. So, then, how do you determine what is most important? You can get some idea by rereading the last half of Chapter 11, which discusses the differences between traditional and phonological frameworks for therapy. However, there are also several therapeutic guidelines that help to suggest the most significant aspects of the program. Let's discuss these guidelines now:

1. Work at production at the syllable-level first. Don't, under any circumstances, encourage production of isolated sounds. Although some traditionally based investigators recommended the syllable as the place to start in therapy (e.g., see McDonald, 1964a), much traditionally based therapy began at the isolated sound level (e.g., see Van Riper, 1972). Unfortunately, our experience has indicated that encouraging production of isolated sounds is one of the most counterproductive things that can be done in therapy. Why? Because it reduces the production to solely a motor behavior, devoid of any linguistic significance. For a perfect example of how working in isolation can actually hurt the therapy process, consider the following situation which most of us have encountered at least once in our careers:

The child we're seeing has stopping of fricatives, so he says /tʌn/ for *sun*. Using a combination of phonetic placement, instructions to close his teeth, and auditory stimulation, we've finally gotten to the point where the child can produce the /s/ sound. He can even now produce some nonsense syllables appropriately. So we try to get him to produce the sound correctly in *sun*. He makes a long, strong /s/ sound and then follows it with /tʌn/, his original way of producing the word. And no matter what we try to do to get him to change it, we cannot stop him from producing /ssstʌn/.

As stated, we have all encountered this frustrating situation in our past clients. Happily, this problem doesn't occur with the therapeutic regimen just described, at least partially because working at the syllable level is more appropriate linguistically.

2. Use nonsense syllables and words early in therapy. Once again, this guideline has been suggested previously in the field of articulation. However, there have always been clinicians and writers who have felt that it is more meaningful for the child to use real words early in therapy. And curiously, this latter belief has achieved some renewed popularity recently, insofar as most minimal pairs procedures begin at the word level.

Certainly it is possible for a child to learn a new contrast while beginning at the word level. But is it advisable to start there? Probably not. To understand why, it's valuable to consider what we are asking of the client. In essence, any client with a speech problem has to do two things:

1. He must unlearn an old pattern of sound production.
2. He must learn a new pattern of sound production.

If we begin the learning process at the real word level, we are asking the client to both unlearn his old pattern and learn his new pattern at the same time. On the other hand, by beginning the process at the nonsense level, the client can first learn the new pattern free from any interference caused by his current semantic system. Then, by the time he gets to real words, he still has only one thing to master—the unlearning of his old pattern. In other words, the use of nonsense syllables allows us to bypass the child's past mislearning during the early acquisition stage of therapy. This, of course, makes more sense from a behavioral science perspective and unsurprisingly, it facilitates the therapy process.

3. Anything is permissible in the attempt to heighten the contrast for the client during early learning. Anything. You can get louder, you can use your body, anything. Remember, the goal is for the client to be able to identify semantically both sides of the contrast. If you can help facilitate achievement of this goal by adding additional cues, thus making it easier for him to remember the two sides of the contrast early on, then why not do it?

4. Always teach semantic identification before any attempt is made to stimulate production. Why? Because it's important that you provide the child with a *semantic referent* that will allow you to communicate with her (and vice versa) about what she is hearing and then producing. (Another added benefit of establishing semantic referents is that it helps the clinician avoid the trap of labeling productions "right" or "wrong," a bit of parental value judgment that rarely, if ever, helps the therapy process.)

What about the complaint that "semantic identification" is no more than auditory discrimination with a fancy name. Is it really? To find out, try this experiment on an adult friend of yours. Tell the friend that you're going to teach her some new words. Then hold up a pen, and say, "This is a *saskwatch*." Next, hold up a ball and say, "And this a *mewhippy* (/məwɪpi/)." Finally, have the friend alternately point to *saskwatch* and *mewhippy* as you name them.

Perhaps even have her label the item for you. Can you call this little experiment an auditory discrimination task? Well, certainly auditory discrimination is a prerequisite skill, but since your friend undoubtedly can already discriminate auditorily all the sounds in those words, her only remaining task is to learn the new semantic referent or label.

Likewise, in *semantic identification*, whereas auditory discrimination is a prerequisite skill, the child, if she can understand her mother saying, "Let's go get some ice cream," undoubtedly has sufficient auditory discrimination abilities, and the task becomes one of learning new semantic referents, or vocabulary.

5. Do not work on more than one rule in a given word at one time. We've already talked about this several times. But because we have found that this is the single most difficult element for clinicians to accept and internalize, it bears repeating. Remember, many words produced by a client will have more than one simplification rule working at the same time. Some words have as many as four or five rules. As a simple example, consider the child who has the following two rules in her system:

• Velar assimilation
• Stopping of fricatives

How will she say the word *sick*? Probably as /kɪk/. Now let's say that in therapy, you're teaching the child to eliminate the velar assimilation first. What production will you now have to accept as correct? Right! /tɪk/ for *sick*. In other words, you will have to accept and reinforce an incorrect production. If you tried to make the child say *sick* correctly immediately, you'd be asking her to alter two rules at once. And this she generally will not do.

Another example: Another child has deletion of final consonants and thus says /bo/ for *boat*. Often after the child first learns the concept of final consonants, her first production will be /bop/ for *boat*. Again, this should be reinforced initially as correct; later on, you can work on the remaining rules.

As stated, this concept of accepting incorrect productions from the child (as long as she correctly produces the rule) is the most difficult for clinicians to deal with. We seem to have an aversion to reinforcing errors, even if we know it's only going to be for short periods of time. Yet, this is one of the most important guidelines for phonological therapy. As Ingram (1976) stated in his *gradualness principle*, children learn things gradually, not in one "fell swoop" (p. 151).

The only way to avoid the need to reinforce errors is to choose as stimuli only "golden words" (see Chapter 7), that is, words that have only one rule working at a time. But this solution is more illusory than practical because many clients have so many rules in their system at one time that it becomes difficult to find enough golden words.

In summary, when doing phonologically based therapy, it's important that you keep the gradualness principle in mind. Only require that your client produce correctly the rule that you're working on. And be mindful of the fact that you may have to reinforce sound errors if you want the client to learn the rule you're trying to teach.

Priorities for Intervention—Where Do You Start in Therapy?

If the client that you're seeing has only one rule affecting his speech, the issue of where to begin therapy is obvious. But with clients who demonstrate several rules at once, the question of which rule(s) should be worked on initially becomes more difficult. Unfortunately, although suggestions have been presented in the lit-

erature (e.g., see Ingram, 1976, Edwards, 1983, or Hodson and Paden, 1991), many of these suggestions are difficult for the clinician to follow and in many cases even contradict one another. There is one suggestion, however, that has been mentioned by numerous authors, and forms the basis of the only guideline that we use for choosing rules to work on: *Select for initial therapy those rules resulting in the greatest unintelligibility.*

Unfortunately, by itself, the unintelligibility guideline is not very helpful. After all, which are the rules that affect intelligibility the most? Regrettably, no empirical data exist that could definitively answer this question. However, after many years of experience, we have devised a hierarchy that we believe accurately evaluates the effect on intelligibility of different types of rules.

Priority 1—Syllable Structure Rules (except for cluster reduction within words)

These rules result in the most unintelligibility and include the following:
- Deletion of final consonants
- Deletion of unstressed syllables
- Cluster reduction across words

This last rule especially accounts for those clients who are fully intelligible to the clinician when given a traditional single word articulation test, but are quite unintelligible in conversation. The only syllable structure rule not included in Priority 1 is cluster reduction within words (e.g., /tar/ for *star*). Because the bulk of the word shape is available for these words, intelligibility is not as severely affected—which is just as well because cluster reduction within words is a later disappearing rule in normal children, whereas these other syllable structure rules normally disappear very early.

Priority 2 — Assimilation Rules

Assimilation rules will also render a child's speech almost totally unintelligible. However, at least the entire word shape is available to the listener, allowing for at least some guessing on the basis of context. Rules that fall into this Priority 2 category include:

- Velar assimilation
- Labial assimilation
- Alveolar assimilation
- Nasal assimilation
- Sound preference rules (e.g., "*h*'ing of stops")

Priority 3—Placement Rules

Children having only placement rules are usually not totally unintelligible. However, it often takes very close listening and many contextual cues to decipher the client's full meaning. Some rules included in this category:

- Fronting of velars
- Backing of alveolars

Priority 4—Manner Rules

Because so many cues are already available to the listener (correct syllable structure, correct placement), manner rules only partially impede intelligibility. What is interesting, however, is that even though these rules are designated Priority 4 here, many clinicians (mistakenly) work on these rules first—probably because they are easier to teach than any of the rules from Priorities 1–3. Anyway, rules that belong to this category include:

- Stopping of fricatives
- Denasalization
- Gliding of /1/

Priority 5—Rules That Disappear Late in Normal Children

There are several rules that technically fall in the categories of Priorities 1–4, but that have only limited effect on intelligibility. Most of these rules occur both in children who are developing normally and in children who are speech disordered; in children who are developing normally, they usually disappear on their own without the need for intervention. These rules include:

- Cluster reduction within words
- Lisping (i.e., *th* for *s* substitution)
- Gliding of *r*
- Stopping of voiced *th* (e.g. /dɪs/ for *this*)

Priority 10—Voicing Rules

What happened to Priorities 6 through 9? They do not exist. But even they should be exhausted before working on voicing rules. In as early as 1966, Susan Ervin-Tripp, after reviewing the literature, concluded that voicing contrasts were among the last to develop in normal phonological development (Ervin-Tripp, 1966). Yet many clinicians report working on voicing with their clients with speech disorders. The bottom line is, we have yet to see any child or adult (except for nonnative American speakers or speakers with organic problems such as hearing loss, cerebral palsy, or adult apraxia) who has come to the end of therapy and has still had a problem with voicing. We believe that inevitably, if we just work on other rules, the client will learn the voicing contrast on his own. What this means is that if you're currently working on voicing, before you have worked on the client's other rules, you are probably wasting time. More than 10 years ago, this author began offering a $100 reward to any clinician at his workshops who could present evidence of a native American, nonorganically impaired client who had voicing rules as his final speech problem. After several thousand clinicians, that money is still untouched.

The bottom line? If the client has any other errors in his speech, work on those before you do his voicing problem.

Intermission

At this point, you've been presented with the basics of phonologically based therapy. Unfortunately, you probably have more questions now than you did before you began reading these chapters on therapy. In order to try to help flesh out this skeleton, the next chapter is devoted to addressing some of the most important issues of concern to speech-language pathologists when they first begin to use phonologically based therapy. More importantly, a large section of the next chapter will discuss the problem of, "What happens if it doesn't work immediately?" In fact, dealing with this latter issue is vital if you're determined to avoid that dreaded disease—regression to past learning. Have a good break!

CHAPTER ◆ 14

Implementation of Phonological Procedures

For most clinicians, nothing is quite as difficult as attempting a new therapeutic procedure for the first time. In fact, uncertainty, discomfort, and self-doubt mark most good clinicians' attempts to try something new in therapy. The reasons are understandable. The new procedure "feels" foreign and has not become internalized. And these unsettled feelings often remain for quite a while — mostly because there is no expert nearby to tell her whether or not she is following the procedure correctly. To add to this problem, far too often clinicians are provided with a detailed if not programmed therapeutic regimen only to find that additional "real world" questions begin to arise as soon as the procedure is attempted. The frequent lack of answers to these more practical questions and issues may then leave the clinician in a quandary as to how to continue implementation of this new approach.

The purpose of this chapter is to try to ease this sometimes uncomfortable process of clinical growth and discovery. To this end, several typical problems and issues often associated with the implementation of a phonological approach to therapy will be examined. However, as you will see, the discussion will soon expand beyond the limited scope of clinical pho-nology to consider some more general questions that frequently arise as part of the therapy. As such, of course, some of it may not be relevant either to your particular caseload, or even to your own clinical style. On balance, however, just your full consideration of these issues should enhance your initial experiences with phonologically based therapy. And this will undoubtedly translate into greater success with your own clients.

Organizational Issues

Issue 1: Age to Begin Therapy

The year is 1995. A typical, everyday mother and father have visited a typical, everyday pediatrician. They are concerned about their son—a 4-year-old who seems to understand everything that is said to him but "cannot produce any sounds correctly." The parents cannot understand anything their child says and they are worried. The pediatrician attempts to allay their fears, assuring the mother and father that their son is still young and will "outgrow" his speech problem.

Even today, the frequent first response of a medical doctor to a parent's complaint of speech problems in a 3-, 4-, or 5-year-old child is "he (or she) will outgrow it." In fact, it wasn't too many years ago when speech-language pathologists gave the same advice, especially with 2- or 3-year-olds. And with good reason. Because until recently, speech-language pathologists have lacked two important pieces of data that would help prove the need for early intervention:

1. Data on when speech simplification rules disappear or are no longer used by normal children.
2. Data on the efficacy of early intervention for children with speech disorders.

Until recently, clinicians have had to rely on data for individual sounds to determine whether a child's speech delay warranted intervention. The problem is, results from the several studies assessing individual sound development have been widely variant, most likely due to differences in experimental design. Thus, Prather, Hedrick, and Kern (1975) found that the /t/ sound is normally acquired at 2 years 8 months of age, whereas Templin (1957) established the age of acquisition at 6 years of age. Wellman, Case, Mengart and Bradbury (1931) indicated that the /f/ sound was acquired at 3 years of age whereas Poole (1934) found the acquisition age to be 5 years 6 months. Even Smit, Hand, Freilinger, Bernthal, and Bird (1990), in the most ambitious and far-reaching study of speech sound development in over 30 years, found differences when they tried to match the experimental design of Templin, the best-regarded study of the past generation. For example the /dʒ/ sound was found to be acquired between the age of 4 and 4 years 6 months by Smit, et al., whereas Templin indicated development of the /dʒ/ sound at 7 years of age.

Of course, for those interested in phonology and the development of phonological rules, there are serious questions whether data on development of individual speech sounds has any meaning or importance at all for clinical intervention. In fact, it can be argued that speech sound development is dependent on and subservient to the disappearance of phonological simplification rules. Unfortunately, data on the disappearance of these phonological rules in normal children is thus far sparse, indeed.

Nevertheless, several studies over the last 10–15 years have begun to create a picture of the elimination of these simplification rules in children (e.g., see Dyson & Paden, 1983, Grunwell 1987, Preisser, Hodson & Paden, (1988), and Stoel-Gammon, 1987). Putting the results of these studies together allows us to begin devising some guidelines that should help us decide better when to begin therapy with our children with phonological disorders.

1. Children who are developing normally by and large get rid Fronting of Velars, Deletion of Final Consonants and most Assimilation rules (except on over-learned words) by age 2 years 6 months. This suggests that if you see a 3-year-old child who still has either or all of these rules, then this child is substantially behind his or her peers in phonological development and probably should be recommended for therapy, despite the young age.
2. Children who are developing normally by and large eliminate their regular use of Cluster Reduction, Gliding of /r/, and Vocalization of /ɚ/ by the age of 4 years 6 months. This age, of course, is much younger than we have traditionally been led to believe, especially for the rules involving the /r/ sound. In fact, for many years in our clinic, we accepted unintelligible children for speech therapy at the age of 2 years 6 months to 3 years and regularly dismissed them before the age of 5 years or so, if their only lingering problem

was an /r/. What we began finding, however, distressed us. Inevitably, the parent would contact us one to one and one half years later, telling us that the /r/ problem was still there, requesting that we again begin therapy. We also found another thing, which we have not yet tested empirically, but which we are intuitively becoming more certain of all the time. When we waited until the child was age 6 years or more to begin therapy for /r/, even children who had been extremely successful in earlier therapy were now more resistant to change than were children at the age of 4 years 6 months, who worked on /r/ as their last of several rules targeted in therapy. The reason was, these now 6-year-old or older children were by now extremely aware of their "inability" to produce the /r/ sound, and like many therapists who work with children at this stage, we had a tougher time overcoming this "mindset of failure." For the younger children, on the other hand, "rambo-wimp," or whatever contrast we decided to use, was just a new contrast, and the /r/ sound was not yet viewed by the children as impossible to produce.

3. There are several rules that children who are developing normally rarely, if ever, demonstrate. These rules include Gliding of Fricatives, Deletion of Initial Consonants, Systematic Sound Preferences (e.g., *h*'ing of stops), and any overriding Assimilation problem where all sounds are reduced to one position in the mouth. Obviously, then, if a child demonstrates any of these rules, regardless of age, chances are that his or her speech will not improve without intervention and it is important to recommend therapy.

In the future, as more research is conducted, our knowledge of what is normal regarding the development and disappearance of phonological rules will undoubtedly expand. Until that time, the previous guidelines are a good beginning in helping with the decision-making process.

There are two additional factors to consider prior to recommending early therapy for children with speech disorders. The first consideration is *efficacy*. Recommending speech therapy before the age of 3 years is only valid if this will result in the child being relieved of a speech disorder either in a shorter period of time or at an earlier age than would occur if the child were referred at a later age. Fortunately, both ingredients seem to be occurring. A later section in this chapter will focus more fully on the issue of efficacy.

A second factor to consider is *normalization*. Shriberg, Kwiatkowski and Gruber (1994) defined normalization as "the process and behaviors by which speech becomes normally articulate over time" (p. 1127). Speech-language pathologists for many years have expressed concern about whether children's speech might have normalized even without intervention. In other words, has the agent of change for children with speech disorders been the speech-language intervention or has it just been the passage of time, or maturity? When intervention took many years, following the use of a traditional framework, it was natural to worry whether intervention or maturity was the agent of change. With the use of a phonological framework, however, it becomes easier to demonstrate that intervention is indeed the agent of change, at least in most children. For example, 54 children with speech delay who had not received any intervention at the time of first assessment were studied by Shriberg et al. (1994). These children averaged 4 years 3 months of age. Obviously, none of these children had normalized on their own by the age of 4 years 3 months. These same children were again studied one year later (at an average age of 5 years 3 months). Of the 54 children, the speech of only 10 had normalized in the intervening year. Thus, there was an 82% probability of nonnormalization by the age of 5 years 3 months. Yet most efficacy research for phonologically based therapy indicates normalization within one and one half years or less for most clients. As such, if results of both the normalization and efficacy studies are generalizable to other children, phonologically based therapy is indeed the agent of change for children with speech disorders, because maturity and/or other factors will result in speech normalization by 5 years 3 months of age only 18% of the time.

In summary, it is probably best to start phonologically based therapy for children with speech disorders as soon as possible after you decide that he/she is significantly behind most other children phonologically. Do not wait for maturation to "cure" most of these speech disorders because for many, if not most, of these children, it will not happen.

Issue 2: Group Versus Individual Therapy

In most of the research supporting the efficacy of phonologically based procedures, therapy has been conducted on an individual basis. Unfortunately, this standard is not possible in some settings. For example, many, if not most, public school clinicians must see their clients in groups, if their entire caseload is to be served. Fortunately, this is not a problem. Not only can the therapy procedures described in the last chapter be used with groups, but the argument might be made that it's preferable to do so.

Consider this situation. A clinician has two children on her caseload who have Final Consonant Deletion, but they also

have some fricatives in their speech repertoires. Two other children have Stopping of Fricatives, but put final consonants into their speech. Why not create a group for these four children? You can work on two rules at once; at any given time two of the children can serve as indirect models for the other two. All of the children will have periodic easy success interspersed with periods of challenge. Of course, one might expect that progress would be somewhat slower given this situation, because only half of each child's total time in therapy is focused on his or her own individual speech problem. However, the benefits of having peers as models and "being the advanced speakers" for at least half of the therapy process may compensate for this expected deceleration of progress.

In short, there is no reason to avoid the use of groups when you implement phonologically based therapy. If you group your children carefully and follow the procedures and guidelines closely, you should have mostly equivalent results, whether working with one or four clients.

Issue 3: Use of Parents

Using parents to implement or, more commonly, to supplement therapy is very much in vogue at present. There are several reasons for this. First, parents frequently want to be involved in the therapy process—especially if the child is of preschool age. Second, the underlying thesis of much preschool speech and language intervention is that communication is best developed in the naturalistic context (e.g., see McCormick & Schiefelbusch, 1984). What could be more natural than including the most significant persons in the preschooler's communicative environment—his or her parents? Finally, in this time of budget cutbacks and limitations of insurance coverage, third party payers are often reluctant to bear the full cost of speech-language intervention. As such, the use of parents becomes attractive, indeed, from the perspective of cost effectiveness.

All of that being said, we sadly have not had much success in using parents as surrogate therapists. Perhaps the largest reason for this has to do with why you are reading this book at this time. Think of all the new learning you have had to absorb in order to begin to master clinical phonology and you can begin to appreciate the difficulties in teaching that information to parents. If you as a professional or near-professional experience trepidation at the thought of accepting and reinforcing incorrect sound productions, as you will periodically have to do when using a phonological approach, imagine how a parent will feel. In fact, some parents have particular difficulty understanding the concept of working on rules, not sounds, and just can't understand why we are not just telling the child where to put his or her tongue.

For these reasons, we typically do not use parents in our therapy programs. Initially, we will usually explain to the parents that we are not worried about the child's ability to produce sounds. He produces lots of sounds, we explain, just not the exact sounds we want him to produce, when we want him to produce them. We comment on the fact that the child has developed his own system of speech rules; the only problem is that these rules differ from the speech rules we would like for him to have. Our goal as speech therapists, we say, is to get the child to understand the differences between his rule system and the rule system of those around him. Once we achieve this understanding, we conclude, it will be easy to stimulate the child to alter his production of individual sounds.

After this explanation, we usually tell the parents to sit back, relax, and come to us if they have any questions. Often, the parents we have seen seem noticeably relieved when we tell them that they will not have to be part of the therapy process.

At other times, a given parent may insist upon working with the child at home. In these instances, we will explain the contrast we are working with, give a list of syllables for each side of the contrast, and then have the parent and child work on *identification only*, in syllables.

Finally, the form illustrated in Figure 14-1 was developed by a public school preschool clinician (McLain, 1989), in order to explain the basics of phonologically based therapy to parents as well as to provide them with a description of the contrasts used and the steps to be undertaken during the therapy process. We find the form to be clinician-friendly yet helpful in addressing typical questions of parents during the course of intervention.

Issue 4: Meeting State/School District Guidelines for Service Provision

Most states, and by extension, school districts, have well-defined criteria that must be met before service is provided to children with speech impairments. Unfortunately, in most states, these criteria are still stated in terms of speech sound development. This creates a predicament for public school clinicians who believe in a phonological approach but need to qualify their children with speech disorders according to state guidelines.

Fortunately, the solution to this problem is fairly simple. Chances are you will have administered one of the well-known single-word articulation tests in order to help compile your speech sample (e.g., the *Arizona Articulation Proficiency Scale [AAPS]*, Fudala, 1970). You can use the speech sound data generated from that administration along with results from one of the well-known studies of speech sound development to support whatever clinical decision you feel is appropriate. For example, if you want to support a decision in favor of intervention for a 5-year-

---

CONCEPTUAL CONTRAST THERAPY

NAME: _____ DATE OF BIRTH: _____ CA: _____ _____

DATE: _____

CONTRAST NAME: _____

In order to help your child learn correct production of:

We will be using a contrast approach. I will introduce the concept of:

vs.   sounds.

(i.e.

At first, I will ask your child to identify my productions of the contrast at the nonsense syllable level
(e.g. _____ =

_____ =

Once he/she is able to do so accurately 95% of the time, I will ask your child to produce either a
_____ or a _____ sound. When your child is able to produce the contrast accurately 95% of the
time in nonsense syllables, we will move to words (e.g. _____ =

_____ =

Eventually we will progress to the sentence and finally conversational level. At these higher levels, I will
encourage your child to use more and more sounds (i.,e. their speech goal), and less and less of the
undesired sound. This approach helps your child to better internalize/understand the concept of how to
produce the sound correctly (e.g. changing his way of thinking about the sound). It is important that
your child does not think of one side of the contrast as being worse or better than the other; rather, your
child will learn that there are *2 different* types of sounds.

Please feel free to contact me if you have any questions regarding the contrast therapy approach.

Thank you,

Figure 14–1. Clinician generated form for parents.

old child with Gliding of /r/, use the well-known normative data of Templin (1957), which indicated normal acquisition of the /r/ sound by the age of 4. If you would like to support a decision in favor of therapy for a child aged 4 years 6 months with Stopping of Fricatives, use normative data from the recent study by Smit et al. (1990), who found the normal age of acquisition for most fricatives to be 4 years of age or younger.

In summary, even though most state guidelines for service provision do not consider phonology, there are ways for the astute clinician to work around this deficiency.

Issue 5: Use of Phonologically Based Therapy When the Client has Only One or a Few Sound Errors

Most discussion and research concerning the use of a phonological paradigm has centered around children with multiple speech errors. This has led many clinicians to assume that if a child has only one or two speech errors, a phonological approach is unneeded. In fact, we have frequently heard clinicians report that if a child has many errors, they use a phonological approach, if the child has one or two errors, they use a traditional approach. Even Hodson and Paden (1983), perhaps the primary early influence for many clinicians in their use of clinical phonology, stated that their phonological approach was "neither appropriate nor realistic in cases of mild articulation disorders" (p. xvii).

The question is, why should the *quantity of errors* exhibited by the client prescribe the clinical framework? We have explained our

and large passed over clinicians working with adults. There are at least two reasons for this. First, the caseloads of most clinicians working with adults are composed of fewer clients who have primary articulation problems than the caseloads of clinicians working with children. Second, in those adults who do have primary articulation problems, the dysfunction has frequently been precipitated by a known neurological insult. Thus, the adult who demonstrates apraxia or dysarthria secondary to acknowledged neurological dysfunction has a verifiable motor problem. As such, any articulation problem demonstrated by this adult would be best treated using a traditional framework, right? Maybe . . . and then again, maybe not. Consider the adult with dysarthria who has slowed, imprecise movements of the articulators, resulting in several speech errors consisting of imprecise tongue tip contact and frequent omission of alveolar sounds, especially at the ends of words and in clusters. Are all of these client's errors directly caused by the dysarthria? We find that the answer to this is usually no. Although the dysarthria has indeed created motor difficulties for the client, there is not always a 1:1 relationship between the motor difficulties and the resultant phonological system of the client. In fact, many, if not most, of the adults with verified motor problems that we have seen for therapy have had phonological overlays to their primary motor-caused articulation deficits and have benefited greatly from therapy combining elements of traditional motor-oriented intervention with features from phonologically based approaches.

There is one other group of adults with which we have used phonological procedures with great success—adults with dialectical variations. Over the last 30 years, educators and speech-language pathologists have come to agree that most American English dialects are neither substandard nor the result of structural deficiency but instead reflect a logical, rule-governed system of phonological features usually related to the speaker's first language. For example, Black English dialect is thought to represent a fusion of features from African and European languages (Iglesias & Anderson, 1993). Likewise, dialects from various immigrant groups are usually related to the phonologies of these nonnative speakers' first language. For example, consonant clusters are not a part of Japanese phonology. It is unsurprising, then, that when Japanese persons start speaking English, they tend to reduce these clusters, not only within words, but also across words (so *big boy* would become /bɪbɔɪ/, with the /gb/ cluster reduced to /b/).

Overall, we have had much success using phonologically based procedures with a wide variety of adults with dialectical variations, including individuals from Japan, China, Taiwan, Vietnam, Cambodia, Russia, Mexico, and Italy. The important thing to remember is that the speech of an individual with a foreign dialect, like that of a child with phonological disorders, is not randomly generated but is instead the result of a series of rule-based simplifications of the accepted American English phonological system. Approach it in this way and you will undoubtedly have greater success with your clients.

Issue 7: To Cycle or Not to Cycle

Hodson and Paden (1983) are without a doubt the investigators most responsible for the wide dissemination of concepts of clinical phonology to clinicians in the field. As part of their program, they introduced an organizational strategy that they called "Cycles." In describing this newly developed organizational strategy, Hodson and Paden stated that they "do not continuously target the phonological pattern until it has reached a predetermined criterion. Rather, [they] restrict focusing on a pattern

to only a few weeks (usually two to four), using a different phoneme or sequence each week" (p. 56). Using this strategy, then, the clinician would work on several patterns sequentially until a cycle was completed (usually within the space of 15 weeks or so). The clinician would then return to and work on those same patterns in subsequent cycles until target patterns were incorporated into the child's speech.

As can be seen, the cycles approach seems at variance with the therapy program discussed in the last chapter. Indeed, in our own therapy, although we may work on two rules during the same session, we will continue work on these same two rules in subsequent sessions until 100% mastery is achieved by the child, prior to moving on to additional rules. Thus, we have never attempted Hodson and Paden's (1983) cycle approach in our own work. Nevertheless, many clinicians to whom we have spoken speak highly of their own experiences with the cycle approach.

The bottom line is probably this: Because the cycle approach is an organizational strategy, it can likely be used with any intervention design. Thus, we believe that if the use of cycles is an important part of your current therapeutic repertoire, there is no reason not to continue using cycles, even if you use the imagery approach described in the previous chapter. There is one provision, however. Although it seems acceptable to begin working on new rules before the child has mastered the first rules he or she is working on, it is important that you continue requiring 100% mastery of each step within a given rule in the therapy program, prior to going on to a more difficult step.

Therapeutic Issues

Issue 8: Using Phonologically Based Therapy for the First Time

As discussed at the beginning of this chapter, it is a disconcerting and uncomfortable experience for anyone to use a new intervention technique for the first time. And so it will likely be for you, the first time you try to use the therapy program presented in Chapter 13. There are some things you can do, however, to minimize the discomfort.

First, realize that performing successful phonologically based therapy relies on mastery of three prerequisite skills on the part of the clinician:

1. Phonetic transcription
2. Ability to categorize sounds into dimensions of place, manner and voicing
3. Ability to perform a phonological analysis.

As stated in Chapter 3, these skills are the tools of our trade, as much as the scalpel is a surgeon's tool or knowledge of precedent is a lawyer's tool. So make certain you feel secure in these areas prior to undertaking phonologically based procedures.

Second, recognize that you will undergo periods of fear and discouragement—especially if your client has had a particularly awful session. These emotions are normal, but try to resist the "tendency to revert" which often accompanies these emotions. Whenever we are placed in a challenging and uncomfortable situation, we tend to easily revert to what we know best, what will lessen this feeling of discomfort. So it is with therapy. Most clinicians who try phonologically based therapy for the first time have periods where they want nothing more than to use a tongue depressor, put peanut butter on the child's alveolar ridge, or perhaps suture the child's tongue tip to the roof of his mouth. During these periods, it is important to remember the reason that you're trying these phonological procedures; that traditional procedures have not been very successful anyway. So again, resist the very normal temptation to revert to your old procedures. You will be glad you did.

Finally, and perhaps most importantly, pick your initial client(s) carefully. Keep in mind, you are giving this alternate form and framework for therapy a test. Make certain it is a fair test. For example, don't pick a 16-year-old boy with an /r/ problem who has had 13 years of speech therapy for your first test. Likewise, picking a 9-year-old child who has had 7 years of intervention and is still unintelligible is not a particularly fair test. In the long run, you may want to attempt phonologically based therapy for both of these individuals. But do yourself a favor and avoid using this new procedure with your hard-core cases until you are more comfortable with it: Instead, the ideal client for a first test is a 2- to 4-year-old child with multiple phonological errors who has not had previous therapy. If you do not have access to children that young, at least choose a child of any age who either has had very little previous intervention or has not been negatively affected by the intervention he or she has had. (As we will soon see, a child's belief that he *cannot* make certain sounds, is one of the greatest impediments to learning to produce those sounds.)

Issue 9: Getting Around Previous Therapy

All other things being equal, we would rather see a child, regardless of his or her age, who has not had previous therapy, than one who has. To understand why, consider the following two children. Each child has incorrectly produced the word *shoe*, pronouncing it /tμ/. You say to Child #1, "Not quite. Say *shoe*," to which Child #1 responds, perhaps a bit impatiently, "That's what I just said." Child #2, on the other hand, when asked to repeat the word, says "I can't say that." We find that children like Child #1 are our dream clients. Their entire phonological systems can be changed, seemingly without their having any idea that any changes have taken place. Children like Child #2, however, have developed mindsets of failure for certain sounds; they absolutely *know* that they are incapable of producing certain sounds and there is very little you can do as a clinician to convince them otherwise. As such, any attempt they make to produce the misarticulated sound becomes a half-hearted and usually unsuccessful effort on their part to mimic motorically what they think you are doing in your mouth. These latter individuals are not particularly good candidates for any type of therapy, whether traditional or phonological, but at least because a phonological approach does not focus on individual sounds, but instead considers group of sounds, and because a phonological approach is more concerned with contrasts, rules, and images rather than sounds, there is a chance that you can fool or "trick" the child into bypassing his needs to try to blindly imitate a motor movement. A real-life example will illustrate this.

Shanda was a 10-year-old girl who had an /r/ problem. She had had 4 years of therapy in the public schools for this /r/ problem, as well as several summers of speech therapy at a university clinic nearby. It seems that every procedure ever developed in the field of speech pathology for amelioration of /r/ problems had been tried at least once with Shanda without success. Ms. Sanders, her new clinician, had just attended a workshop on clinical phonology and wanted to try some phonologically based therapy with her clients, but knew that Shanda was not a good candidate for a phonological approach, so she continued her use of traditional procedures with Shanda and Karyn, the other girl in her group (who actually had already produced several correct /r/ syllables). After one more month of little success, Ms. Sanders consulted another clinician in her district who was well-versed in phonologically based procedures, and asked her if she had any ideas for therapy.

After much consideration, the other clinician suggested this: Ms. Sanders was to create a story about two princesses in a foreign land. Princess #1 was a strong princess who ruled her city in a very powerful fashion. Princess #2 was a very weak ruler who was loved by her people but was too weak to fight off foreign invaders. Princess #1 was named *Oshroo* /aʃrμ/ (spoken in a sharp, harsh manner) and Princess #2 was named *Oshwoo* /aʃwμ/ (spoken in a frail, delicate manner). Ms. Sanders was to create a story about how the two princesses joined forces and learned the importance of both qualities (hardness and softness). For the Identification stage of the therapy program, *Oshroo* was designated hard and *Oshwoo* soft. Each of the princesses also had two sisters: *Oshwee*, *Oshwah*, *Oshree*, and *Oshrah*. By the end of the first stage of therapy, Shanda and Karyn had to identify with 100% accuracy whether Ms. Sanders was talking about one of the hard sisters or one of the soft sisters.

On the first day of production, when Shanda was asked to produce the name of the hard princess, she said *Oshroo* correctly on her first attempt. The clinician knew enough not to get overly excited, but a resource specialist who shared the room with Ms. Sanders and knew the two girls blurted out "Wow, Shanda, that was a great /r/ sound." Happily, this inadvertent comment created no problem because both girls had been in therapy long enough to be very aware of what sound they were working on. What is most interesting, however, was Karyn's (the other client's) response to the resource specialist. She said, in a huffy manner, "Well, Ms. Sanders tricked her into it." And indeed she had. She brought Shanda to the point where, for a brief period, she forgot she was working on trying to produce the /r/ sound. Once she stopped trying so hard, the sound was produced correctly (albeit in a nonsense syllable, preceded and followed by similarly produced sounds).

Epilogue: Shanda was dismissed from speech therapy 4 months later, almost 5 years after she had first been diagnosed with an /r/ problem. The key element in the success here? Creating a way to bypass not only past therapy, but Shanda's predisposition to work hard at trying to mimic a motor movement. Over the years, we have tried many things to try to "trick" children with hard-core problems and long histories of unsuccessful therapy into producing sounds without working so hard, from embedding the target sounds into complex nonsense syllables, to getting the child to lie on the floor with her eyes closed, to encouraging alternative motor movements of the hands and/or legs during production of, say, "ripping" and "whipping" sounds, etc. Some have worked better than others but the purpose has remained the same throughout: Try to create the conditions to bypass the child's learned phonological helplessness which is usually manifested by rigid patterns of motor mimicry.

Issue 10: Getting Stuck (Part I)

It has long been our experience that every time we become just a little too comfortable or self-assured with our clinical skills, a new child enters our life and single-handedly proves to us just how much we still have to learn. So it seems to be with clinical phonology. Even though we have been using phonologically based procedures for almost 15 years now, we periodically see a child who doesn't respond like he or she is "supposed" to. After trying many different things, we finally reach the point where we realize we are stuck—it isn't working and we don't know where to go. This and the next section are dedicated to sharing with you some of what we have learned over the years about being stuck, why we sometimes get stuck, and some possible ways to become unstuck. It is possible for you as a clinician to sometimes unwittingly exacerbate a stuck condition. Often this occurs because you want so

much for the client to be successful that you push too hard. When this pushing doesn't work, it is easy to lose confidence in this fairly new procedure that you are using. Finally, if the lack of success goes on too long, you will be tempted to revert to your past learning—to techniques you have used in the past. There are two ways to avoid this trap and perhaps undo an early stuck situation before it gets too serious:

1. *Avoid spending too much time on unsuccessful activities*—One of the greatest truisms ever uttered has important implications for clinicians in the field: "The greatest predictor of future behavior is past behavior." What this means is that if a child has incorrectly responded twice in a row, his or her chance of responding incorrectly a third time is quite high, *unless you change something in the therapeutic procedure*. If a child has been wrong five times in a row, she has virtually no chance of being correct on her next attempt, again unless you change something that you are doing.

   Relating this theme to the therapy regimen presented in Chapter 13, if you reach a new step and the child is incorrect once or twice, go back to earlier successful activities for a while until you are ready to attempt the new step a second time. When this second attempt is made, again only go forward if the child is successful fairly quickly. If he or she is not, return once again to earlier successful activities. We have seen children who have spent entire sessions incorrectly responding to a new step every time it is introduced, only to respond correctly at the beginning of a subsequent session. The key is, by not spending too much time on unsuccessful or incorrect responses, the child does not build up negative emotion towards the activity itself, and will continue working actively towards the desired response.

2. *Internalize the mindset of "Isn't" rather than "Can't"*—It is very common for a clinician to express that a given child *cannot* perform a particular behavior correctly. When working in the area of phonological disorders, unfortunately, this expression might result in a mindset that will affect how you try to fix up a problem. For example, it is clear that there is a substantial difference between saying "Johnny cannot ride a bicycle" and "Johnny is not riding a bicycle." In the former case, you will probably look for causes of Johnny's bicycle disability, and try to ameliorate those underlying causes. In the latter example, your "therapy technique" will be different—you will introduce Johnny to a bicycle, explain to him it's workings (system of rules and regulations underlying bicycle riding behavior) and hopefully get him to try to the bicycle, trying to present it in small enough steps so that he is successful.

In phonology also, there is a substantial difference between saying "Carol cannot produce velar sounds" and "Carol is not producing velar sounds." The former statement implies that something is wrong in Carol's mouth whereas the latter phrase is only a statement of fact implying nothing. It becomes clear that a clinician who has a mindset of "cannot" will more likely revert to some traditional motor-oriented techniques when the client is stuck, to try to overcome the implied disability. Alternately, a clinician who has the mindset of "is not" will feel more comfortable when using a phonological approach, which essentially relies on the clinician creating conditions for the client to learn the behaviors *on her own.*

In summary, then, it is important that you internalize the "is not" mindset for your phonological clients. This will help assure that when your client gets stuck, you will not also become stuck—using an ineffective traditional paradigm.

Issue 11: Getting Stuck (Part II)— Troubleshooting

You will recall that several steps in the therapy regimen presented in the last chapter were starred. In fact, Steps 1 (Identifying the Image Contrast) and 2 (Production of the Contrast in Nonsense Syllables) received two stars each; Step 4 (Production in Word) received one star. These stars are meant to indicate areas of possible breakdown in the therapy process. Steps 1 and 2 are double starred because most breakdowns occur at these stages, and Step 1 and 2 breakdowns tend to be more difficult to deal with than Step 4 breakdowns. Let us consider each source of possible breakdown separately.

** *Step 1 (Identifying the Image Contrast)*—Although this step has been assigned two stars, it should, by rights, be an easy step. After all, all you are doing as a clinician is getting the child to associate a manner of sound production with a label, or name. It should not really be that difficult. The problem is, learning a semantic association such as this requires attending ability. Thus, for some children you will be put in a situation of having to teach attention skills, at the same time you're trying to develop phonology. Although it is not that difficult to do, it is important that you be fully aware of where the obstruction is occurring in therapy.

There are four types of children with problems that you are likely to encounter at a Step 1 breakdown: *Single Sally, Random Rick, Lazy Larry,* and *Inconsistent Ichabod* (or *Icky,* for short). As you will see, each of these children demonstrates different behaviors, requiring that you, the clinician, create different strategies to overcome the problem behaviors.

Single Sally gives the same answer over and over again regardless of the side of the contrast you have produced. For example, if working on *tippies* versus *throaties* for Fronting of Velars, you might say /ta/ and Sally will say *tippie*; you then say /ka/ and Sally says *tippie*. In fact, all she says is *tippie*.

Random Rick has a related but somewhat different problem. Rick gives different answers from presentation to presentation, but they are randomly generated. So you might present /ta/ and he will say *tippie*; you then present the same syllable a second time and this time he says *throatie.*

The key for both Sally and Rick is the same. Get them to the point where they can name one side of the contrast consistently. Then introduce the other side of the contrast with an extra cue (either make your voice louder or change duration or introduce another outside cue). An example of a typical clinical interchange follows:

Clinician: /ta/ is *popping* /ʃa/ is *blowing*. /ta/ is *popping* What is /ta/?
R or S: *Popping.*
Clinician: Good. What is /ta/— *blowing* (said softly) or *popping*?
R or S: *Popping.*
Clinician: Great. What is /ta/— *blowing* or *popping*?
R or S: *Popping.*
Clinician: Very good. Now what is /ʃa/? (said loudly and with long duration. Clinician also puckers lips into blowing posture).
R or S: *Blowing.*

After the client learns to label *popping* and *blowing* sounds with the addi-

tional cues, those cues are then faded.

Lazy Larry is a third type of child who's a little more difficult to work with, because part of the time you think he knows it. Larry always gives the answer he gave previously if he was reinforced. If the clinician tells him he is wrong, he changes to the other side of the contrast. In other words, he takes all of his cues as to rightness or wrongness from the clinician's judgments of his response.

For a child like Larry, the solution is to get him to listen more closely to the clinician stimulus rather than the clinician reinforcement. The best way to do this is to add additional cues to both sides of the contrast so that Larry cannot miss the differentiation. For example, for Stopping of Fricatives, if working on *popping* versus *blowing* sounds, present the /ta/ syllable softly with short duration. Make the /ʃa/ syllable loud in volume with a long duration on the fricative. If necessary, add one or two more cues to facilitate differentiation. Once Larry starts responding correctly, fade the cues systematically.

Inconsistent Ichabod presents a different type of problem. He can only seem to get to 70–80% correct overall. He will get 5–8 responses in a row correct, but then might miss one or a few items in a row. In short, Icky seems to "have it" and then just as easily seems to "lose it." He might do particularly well at the beginning of the session and poorly later. Or he might do well after a break, but then "lose it" suddenly after a couple of minutes' work.

The tendency of some clinicians when faced with this problem it to go on to Step 2, without ever getting to a 100% criterion on Step 1. You want to avoid this tendency if possible, because if the child has not truly mastered identification of both sides of the contrasts, she will have trouble later in therapy. Instead you may want to do something called *chunking*.

Chunking involves breaking down the client's output into chunks of response interspersed with some reinforcing activity. For example, in Icky's case, tell him all he has to do is answer 5 in a row correct and then he will be able to take a break and play with a favored toy for a few minutes.

After his break, have him respond for another chunk of 5 items. Have another break, then return for 5 more items and then repeat this scenario for a final 5 items. Icky has had to respond correctly only 5 times in a row for each stage. But overall he has responded correctly 20 times in a row. The law of probability tells us that his chance of doing this accidentally, without knowing the concept, are less than 1 in 1,000,000. Finally, there is nothing magical about a chunk of 5 responses. For children with particular attention difficulties, you can have chunks as short as 2 responses. The only problem with this is that you need 9 therapy breaks to get up to 20 correct responses, as opposed to the 3 breaks needed with a 5-response chunk. Of course, your other option is cutting down the total number of correct responses in a row that you want from 20 to 10. This lowers the odds of the child answering the items correctly just due to chance from 1 in 1,000,000 to 1 in 1000, pretty paltry odds in and of itself.

Finally, all of the problems we have addressed for Step 1 thus far have been attention problems of one type or another. There is another factor that might create difficulty at Step 1—*the appropriateness of the contrast that you have selected.*

Ideally, you want to make certain that your contrast is appropriate both for the level of your client and for what you are trying to teach. Avoid using a contrast where you are forced to teach the child a cognitive concept, prior to his or her being able to use the contrast. For example, we once saw a clinician who wanted to use *front* and *back* as the contrast for Fronting of Velars, but her client had difficulty with the concepts of *front* and *back*. So she took time away from phonological intervention to try to teach *front* and *back* with a car, running into problems with deixis, which had nothing to do with the phonological concept of *front* and *back*. The child was getting nowhere until she decided to change the concept to *tippie/throaty*. The child "took off" with this newly introduced concept and mastered Step 1 in a few sessions.

In short, if you have exhausted other possible problems at Step 1, you may want to consider changing your contrast. For some reason that we cannot put our finger on at the moment, some contrasts are particularly problematic for certain children, whereas those same children respond well with a different contrast.

** *Step 2 (Production of Contrast in Nonsense Syllables)*—This is the only other step that has two stars. It is unsurprising that this step would create some challenges for the clinician. After all, the client is being asked to produce a feature she has not produced before, often in a sound that she has never before produced. Interestingly, however, if we eliminate "motor problems" as a possible cause for a client's difficulties (as we usually do), one other factor seems to keep arising as the prime culprit for breakdowns at this stage—*motivation* on the part of the client (or reinforcement on the part of the clinician—the other side of the same coin). Most of the children with phonological disorders that we have seen for intervention have by and large been happy, self-satisfied individuals. In fact, we cannot remember the last time a 3-year-old child came to us requesting therapy. Instead, it has usually been the child's parent, or teacher, or physician, or perhaps another speech clinician, who has recommended that the child be evaluated. In short, it is basically the adult culture around the child that wants the child to alter the way he or she is speaking. The child, in most cases, has no real intrinsic desire to do so.

The goal of Step 2 is to motivate the child to try to produce some (what are for her) new nonsense sounds. Because you are not telling the child *how* to produce the sounds, she has to be sufficiently motivated to want to try and figure out on her own how to produce them. The major function of the clinician at this stage is to try to kindle this motivation.

A fairly recent true story has helped to underscore for us the vital importance of motivation at this stage of therapy: Terri E. was a speech clinician for a local school district who would be described by many as a local expert in clinical phonology. She had taken several courses in clinical phonology, had attended most public presentations on the topic, and had been extremely successful in using the procedures with the clients on her caseload. She was known for the rapid improvement of her clients and quickly became the district resource for other clinicians with problems in implementing phonological procedures.

One day, Terri gave us a call for advice. She had a particular child on her caseload, Jason, age 4 years 6 months, who was working on Fronting of Velars and was stuck at Step 2. No matter how many times she tried to get him to produce a *throaty* sound (e.g., /ka/), Jason could not do so. Terri was a good enough clinician that she did not push Jason too hard when he missed. If he missed two, or at most three, times in a row, she went back to Identification for most of the rest of the session, with perhaps one more attempt to stimulate production. We asked Terri some questions:

- Was he at 100% in Identification before you went on to Production? *Yes.*
- Was he showing any signs of frustration, or working too hard? *No.*
- Did he seem motivated during the sessions? *Yes.*

We were worried. We had never before been faced with an unsuccessful client when the therapy program had been accurately used. And to make matters worse, here was one of the most skilled clinicians we knew reporting on this failure.

After thinking for a while, we proposed a course of action for Terri that, frankly, we weren't sure was going to work. Terri was encouraged to create what we called a "Surprise Reward." She was told to purchase a toy that Jason would enjoy and then wrap the toy in nice wrapping paper and a bow. She was further instructed to bring the wrapped toy into the following session and tell Jason that the first time he made a good *throaty* sound, he would get the surprise. Terri was then told to go back to Identification and try Production no more than once a session.

On the day the surprise was first brought in, Jason was unsuccessful in producing a *throaty* sound. On the first day of therapy post-surprise, Jason came into the session, and according to Terri, took his seat, glanced at the surprise, and then said /ka/ to the clinician (in a very non-pragmatic way), all within 60 seconds of entering the room. Terri was somewhat stunned because she had not asked for any response from Jason, but she recovered fairly quickly, said "Wow" and gave Jason his surprise. Jason was now on his way.

Since that time, we have recommended the use of the "Surprise Reward" on six other occasions. Not all clients have responded as quickly as Jason (for one client, with an /r/ problem, the surprise sat there for three sessions before the fourth session when the client, a young girl, came in and announced "I can make a *growly* sound now"). Nevertheless, every client previously stuck at Step 2 has indeed responded correctly following introduction of the surprise.

One warning: It is important that you resist the temptation to use this surprise gift idea unless you truly believe there is no other alternative. If used regularly it will not only bankrupt you as a clinician, but it will deprive you of a "secret weapon" to use when you are faced with a last resort situation. We have never had to use it more than once with a given client and we hope we will never have to. (We are not certain it would work twice.) But we have had proven to us once again how important the issue of motivation/reinforcement is.

Luckily, there are things that can be done to optimize your everyday reinforcement paradigm. For example, it is important to become aware of some of the warning signs that signal the need for increased reinforcement. Most of these warning signs take the form of comments on the part of your clients which foreshadow imminent problems. Most clinicians have heard these warning signs at one time or another:

- "I don't want to"
- "Not *that* again"
- "Is it time to go yet?"
- "How much more do we have to do?"
- "I can't do that" (when you know the child can)
- Telling stories on irrelevant topics

These are all signs of a need for increased reinforcement. The key is to pick up on these warning signs quickly enough so that you can alter the motivational structure.

Finally, there are a few other guidelines that if followed carefully, will enhance not only the phonologically based therapy you undertake, but the rest of your clinical work as well:

1. As much as possible *make your reinforcement short term* (the end of each session is ideal; perhaps even shorter for clients who have particular attention problems).
2. *Change reinforcers frequently.* Ideally you want to create an array of effective reinforcers and change them frequently enough so that the client doesn't get bored with them.
3. *Avoid relying on problem reinforcers*, such as saying "good" (without any backup reinforcer), using tokens without any payoff, or competition if the client has no hope of winning.
4. It is particularly effective to *make the reinforcement part of the activity*. That is why stimulus materials such as board games are so popular.
5. Don't be afraid to *create and use unusual surprises* on a periodic basis to help increase the client's

motivation. For example, fast-food gift certificates work wonders for teenagers.

There is one final comment to be made. Most of what has been written here about reinforcement applies to children. What we often tend to forget is that adults are not immune from the need for reinforcement. Certainly there is often self-reward working on the part of adults. Yet we have rarely met any adult who cannot have his or her motivation increased further through the use of various clinician strategies like charting or contracting.

In summary, reinforcement and motivation are extremely important factors that help to determine how successful your intervention will be, phonological or otherwise. If you are stuck in therapy and after trouble-shooting have dismissed all other factors, chances are the problem lies in this area.

* *Step 4 (Production in Words)*—This is the final step that sometimes can be a source of breakdown. However, the problems encountered here are not usually as difficult to remedy as those already described for Steps 1 or 2.

Theoretically, this step should not pose any problems at all for the new learner. After all, the client has already shown that she can produce both sides of the contrast (albeit in nonsense syllables). The problems then arise for one of two reasons. Either:

1. The client *thinks* that she is unable to produce the target.
2. The client hasn't yet attempted to incorporate her new learning about the contrast into her phono-linguistic system.

Either way, the problem is usually fairly easy to handle. First, it is your role as clini-cian to convince the child that she can produce both sides of the contrast. (She has done it already, albeit in nonsense syllables.) Second, if necessary, go back to either Identi-fication in Words (Step 3) or Production in Nonsense Syllables (Step 2), and practice those earlier steps if desired for a while before trying Step 4 again. It is at this Step 4 stage that the child will have to overcome the ambiguity that exists between how she produces a particular word, and how the world around her produces that same word. Once this ambiguity is conquered once or twice, you will begin to see rapid generaliza-tion of correct production.

Issue 12: Working with Vowel Problems

Until now, we have not dealt with vowel problems to any great extent, for three rea-sons. First, only children with the most severe phonological disorders demon-strate significant vowel problems, and many of these children with severe speech problems exhibit no significant vowel problems at all. Second, vowel deviations are often very closely related to the conso-nant misarticulations a client is exhibiting. For example, you will often find that the most severe vowel distortions occur in the context of liquid and glide targets (whether or not the client is producing the liquids or glides correctly). Finally, vowels are much tougher for the clinician to tran-scribe reliably than are consonants. As such, many clinicians pay particular atten-tion to vowel problems only when they are so prominent that they cannot be ignored. Nevertheless, vowel difficulties requiring attention and intervention do occur and it is important that we consider them.

Overall, vowel problems should be approached similarly to consonant prob-lems; that is, you want to describe the mis-articulation in terms of how it differs from the target vowel when considering the parameters of articulatory constraint. Pay close attention to the placement and manner parameters, analyzing factors such as tongue height, tongue position in the mouth roundedness, vowel duration, and perhaps lingual tension. Also pay attention to the context parameter to determine whether you are truly seeing a primary vowel difficulty or if surrounding sounds may be culprits, that is, causing the vowel problem. If context is indeed contributing to the vowel misarticulation, you may want to work initially on the surrounding consonants, to see if the context-caused vowel problems will clear up on their own.

The most common manifestation of vowel problems is some form of neutralization whereby high and low vowels might move towards the middle of the mouth and front or back vowels might become more centered. Additionally, lip rounded vowels might lose their roundedness, tense vowels might become more lax and longer vowels might become shorter in duration.

An image approach can be used profitably with vowel problems in much the same way it is used with consonants. Create images for the contrast pair you are working on and them proceed through the therapy regimen. There may be one or many vowels included for each side of the contrast, depending on the specific contrast. For example, if the client's problem is lack of lip rounding, one side of the contrast might include all lip rounded sounds ($/\mu/$, $/o/$, $/ɔ/$, $/ʊ/$) and the other side, all the remaining vowel sounds.

Finally, foreign dialect cases often present individuals with vowel problems. Usually these vowel problems do not greatly affect intelligibility so the decision of whether or not to target vowels in speech therapy is often made by the clients who have to decide for themselves how important they feel it is to alter their accents.

Issue 13: The Problem with /r/

Our experience has indicated that /r/ continues to be the bane of many clinicians in the field. In fact, the growth of clinical phonology over the last 20 years has seemed to have little or no success in slowing the development of gray hairs in clinicians who must work frequently with /r/ problems.

Before continuing, it is important to state that we *have* had substantial success in using a phonological approach with /r/. We will discuss this shortly. However, it is just as important to communicate that this success has not been unqualified. In fact, we now believe that when it comes to phonemic learning, the /r/ sound may work somewhat differently than the other speech sounds, at least for older children. This being said, we are also convinced that a phonological approach remains the best option, short of the development of a foolproof alternate methodology.

When we first started seeing children for phonologically based intervention, we would typically see them for the first time sometimes between the age of 2 years 6 months and 3 years 6 months. Usually by the time these children were nearing 5 years of age, they would be fully intelligible with only gliding of /r/ (e.g., /wed/ for *red*) or vocalization (e.g., /mʌðo/ for *mother*) as a lingering problem.

After a few years, however, we started noticing a disturbing pattern. The parents of these children dismissed at 4 years 6 months or 5 years were inevitably showing up at our clinic once again when the children were now 6 to 8 years of age, with the same lingering problems: gliding of /r/ and vocalization. Virtually no progress had occurred in the intervening years. Of course, bringing these children in again for therapy at the age of 7 or 8 created some new problems: the children were now inevitably aware of their speech problem, changing much of the dynamic of therapy that had existed previously. Also, these children had now experienced their speech disorder for 2 additional years, strengthening the deviant pattern and making change more difficult.

Realizing that /r/ seemed not to normalize on its own and seeing the greater problems emanating from leaving the /r/ sound untouched for 2 years, we decided that we would no longer dismiss children who were otherwise phonologically normalized with lingering /r/ problems from therapy. Instead, we would continue to see them for phonologically based therapy until their /r/ problems were eliminated.

We found that children even as young as 4 years 6 months responded very favorably to the phonologically based therapy for /r/, if it was presented as a continuation of the earlier therapy. Most of these children were dismissed with normalized /r/'s after a few months. This, of course, contrasted greatly with the children who had been dismissed with nonnormalized /r/'s and then returned for additional intervention after a couple of years. These latter children responded erratically to renewed therapy. Some responded very quickly to the renewal of phonologically based therapy. Others struggled, with many of them exhibiting the obstructive rigidity of other older children we had seen for remediation of /r/. For some of these latter individuals, we even reverted to trying more traditional methods in the attempt to establish an /r/ sound. (You see, even we were not immune to "regression to past learning" when we were in a bind.) These traditional techniques were also unsuccessful and for all of these "hardcore /r/" children we eventually established the /r/ sound using a phonological procedure, usually by tricking them in some way into bypassing the tendency to "try too hard" (see again the discussion on this topic earlier in this chapter).

Is there indeed a difference in the way /r/ is learned from the way other phonemes are learned? At this point, our best answer is that we don't know, but we tend to think not—at least at early stages. Our therapy results over the last 10 years lead us to believe that at early ages, /r/ works very much like other sounds. However there is at least one substantive difference for /r/; it is the only consonant that is produced without a well- defined valve point within the oral cavity; in fact, this may account for the great variability that exists from person to person in their motor postures for /r/. We believe that after a certain age or set of environmental experiences, a child realizes that he or she is unable to produce the /r/ sound. What sets in, we believe, is a "learned helplessness" that manifests itself in an inflexible lack of rear-tongue muscle movement during attempts at /r/. After several years of this, the learned behavior has become rigid and unvarying and it takes something extraordinary to break the cycle. Although we believe that there are some traditional methods that sometimes work at this stage with some children, our experience has convinced us that it is more effective to use phonological procedures and try to trick the child into bypassing the learned helplessness. However, we remain open to the possibility that at some point a sure-fire, can't miss traditional technique will be developed. Until that time, we remain committed to trying to eliminate /r/ problems phonologically before the learned helplessness has set in, at the end of the normal course of therapy, even if the child is only 4 years 6 months of age. Further, we will use a phonological approach even if we see a child with an /r/ problem for the first time at age 10— because it seems to be more effective.

For more information on the subject of learned helplessness, which has been studied extensively in the discipline of special education, see Seligman (1975), or Pearl, Bryan, and Donahue (1980).

The Efficacy of Phonologically Based Intervention Procedures

Walking up and down the aisles of the Exhibit Hall at any American Speech-Language-Hearing Association (ASHA) annual convention can be an overwhelming experience. The speech-language clinician is faced with table after table of books, materials, equipment, and people promoting new games, activities, and techniques, all geared towards helping you with your caseload. New therapy techniques and/or materials are published by one company or another almost daily. Do they work? Are they all effective? Absolutely not. Are some of them effective? Certainly. But which ones? Without efficacy data presented by the author or publisher, it is impossible to tell; the clinician thus is forced to rely on her judgment rather than empirical data.

It is easy to develop a therapeutic technique; it is much more difficult to demonstrate its effectiveness. For this reason, we believe that this may, indeed, be the most important section in this book.

Is phonologically based therapy effective? As important, is it more effective than traditional procedures for assessment and intervention with individuals with speech disorders? These are vitally important questions. Unless the use of a phonological paradigm is superior to the use of a traditional framework, there is little reason to learn the material presented in this text.

For several years, proponents of a phonological framework have claimed remarkable results for their clients with speech disorders. For example, Hodson and Paden (1983), Monahan (1986), and Weiner (1981), among others, have presented data indicating that many children who previously might have attended therapy for several years, given the severity of their disorder, were now being dismissed in 12–18 months after being exposed to phonologically based therapy. Hodson

(1992) reported on her successful treatment of over 200 such children during a 17-year period.

The problem is, the bulk of these data have come from case studies, case presentations, and informal reports; there have been no group data to support the claims of remarkably quick speech improvement by proponents of phonological analysis and intervention—until recently.

In 1988, we were awarded a grant from the California State Department of Education in order to investigate the efficacy of a phonological approach in treating children with speech disorders. When initially deciding on the methodology for the study, we had a problem. Because we believed that the use of a phonological approach accelerated the therapy process, we could not ethically withhold this treatment from a control group, in order to evaluate its effectiveness. We were left with only one option—to use a retrospective research design. What we ended up doing was comparing a group of 19 children who had received a traditional treatment paradigm from 1975–1981 with 17 children who received therapy based on the phonological procedures described in this text from 1982–1988.

It should be noted that the use of a retrospective design introduced some possible threats to validity. For example, all clinicians were masters degree students in Communication Disorders. Because of the different dates for the treatments, children in the traditional group were served by different clinicians, who were supervised by different supervisors, than were children in the phonological group. Although all supervisors were ASHA certified and several years post-master's degree, and although both sets of supervisors maintained the program-imposed 33% minimum rate of supervision, there is the possibility that one group of supervisors was better trained or perhaps just more competent than the other group. Likewise, the argument could be made that clinicians seeing the phonological group children from 1982–1988 were more skillful than their peers from 1975–1981. Finally, because the data were retrospective, it was not possible to control factors such as the language abilities of the two groups, their hearing abilities, the stimulability of the children involved, or their motivation for speech change.

To balance these possible threats to validity, both groups of children were assigned to their treatment groups only on the basis of when they were seen for therapy. These children represented all children seen in the clinic during the years in question who were administered either a traditional or a phonological program of intervention. Because of the nature of the group selection procedure, then, threats to validity should have been reduced.

For example, there is no reason to believe that one group had different language or hearing abilities than the other solely as a result of when they were seen for therapy.

Prior to presenting the results of the research, one more important factor must be discussed. Originally, we were going to compare the traditional phonological groups on two factors:

1. Number of therapy sessions prior to dismissal with essentially normal speech.
2. Number of months in therapy prior to dismissal with essentially normal speech.

Measuring these factors would have been sufficient to compare the effectiveness and efficiency of the two therapy procedures, but for one problem that we observed during initial study of the client's files. It seems that very few of the children being administered traditional treatment were ever formally "dismissed" from therapy, after adequate speech improvement.

Instead, most of these children discontinued therapy prior to being formally dismissed, usually to undergo several additional years of speech services in the public schools. For this reason, we compared the two groups on one additional factor:

3. Speech disorder severity rating at the end of therapy provision.

Finally, we compared the two groups on whether there was a difference in the number of children who finished treatment with essentially normal speech.

Results

The data calculated for each group are shown in Table 14–1. As can be seen, the traditional and phonological groups were essentially equivalent prior to treatment. The age at which therapy was first provided averaged between 4 years 4 months and 4 year 5 months for both groups. Likewise, there was essentially no difference in the severity of the speech disorder for the two groups prior to therapy.

However, substantial differences between the two groups can be seen following therapy provision. For example, the severity score of the traditional group only decreased from an average of 25.95 to an average of 12.84, whereas the phonological group's severity score decreased from an average of 23.76 to an average of 1.53. By the end of therapy provision, the phonological group's severity score was significantly lower than the severity score for the traditional group.

Just as striking, this greater degree of improvement for the phonological group was seen in significantly less months of therapy (an average of 13.47 months for the phonological group, an average of 22.32 months for the traditional group).

Finally, Table 14–2 compares the number of children in both groups who did

TABLE 14–1. Means and standard deviations for each factor, by group

| | Traditional | | Phonological | | t | SIG |
	M	SD	M	SD		
Severity score-beginning	25.95	5.20	23.76	3.94	1.44	NS
Severity score-end	12.84	5.40	1.53	1.90	8.57	p<.001
Number of sessions	100.95	44.40	81.88	28.20	1.56	NS
Number of months	22.32	10.28	13.47	5.15	3.32	p<.005
Age at first therapy	52.74	10.14	52.29	11.81	.13	NS

TABLE 14–2. Number of subjects in both groups who did and did not need further therapy at the end of intervention

Status	Traditional (N = 19)	Phonological (N = 17)
Further therapy needed	17	0
No further therapy need	2	17

$X^2(1, N = 36) = 28.84, p < .001$

and did not require additional therapy after they left our clinic. As can be seen, only 2 of the 19 traditional group children were dismissed with essentially normal speech at the end of an average 22.32 months of therapy. On the other hand, all 17 of the phonological group children were dismissed with essentially normal speech after an average of only 13.47 months.

Summary

The response of children who were provided a traditional therapeutic framework was found to be vastly inferior to that of children who were administered phonologically based therapy. Children in the phonological group not only showed significantly more improvement, but they demonstrated this improvement in a significantly shorter period of time, after being provided with fewer sessions of therapy (though this latter comparison was found to be nonsignificant). For full details of the results of this study, see Klein (in press).

When the results of the study are combined with the many case reports cited at the beginning of this section, it becomes clear that phonologically based therapy is more effective and efficient than the traditionally based procedures that are still the norm for most settings. In fact, a compelling argument can be made that all speech-language clinicians should be using a phonological paradigm, at least for all of their children with multiple speech disorders. Unfortunately, as of 1995, this is, by and large, still not occurring.

✦ PART IV ✦

Related Issues

CHAPTER 15

The Question of Childhood Apraxia

Message from the Author

"Why a chapter on childhood apraxia in a book on clinical phonology?" If this question has crossed your mind, you are probably not alone. After all, as we will see shortly, the "childhood apraxia model" of articulation disorders stands in total contradiction to the phonological model that we have discussed for 14 chapters. But I have a confession to make. Prior to being introduced to clinical phonology, I was, for several years, a confirmed "childhood apraxophile." I studied whatever literature was available (actually there was very little). The behaviors seemed to be well explained. The therapy was structured and straightforward. (At the time, I was using a variation of McDonald's [1964a] sensory motor approach.) I even presented workshops to professionals in the field, teaching them how to do "childhood apraxia therapy." And if the children that underwent this therapy seemed unusually resistant to improvement, that was okay also. After all, I had an excuse—children with childhood apraxia were supposed to be resistant to improvement; that was one of their primary characteristics.

In fact, Muriel Morley, who with her colleagues is credited with origination of the concept of childhood apraxia, in 1957 listed four distinguishing characteristics of the disorder:

1. Lack of speech intelligibility.
2. Frequent family histories of speech/language disorders.
3. Awkward, uncoordinated articulatory movements.
4. Slow response to therapy.

And it wasn't as if my own clients with childhood apraxia were making *no* progress. Certainly the progess in therapy was slow, but it was supposed to be. And with my highly systematic procedure, I felt that I was at least showing better progress than many other therapists.

I probably would have remained a champion of childhood apraxia and its therapy except for one thing: I was introduced to clinical phonology, something that actually worked and seemingly sped up the therapy process, even with children who had been diagnosed as apraxic. But "old ideas die hard," a truism that has been demonstrated throughout history—from the time the world was flat, to the time when you could tell about a person's brain by feeling the configurations of the skull, to the time (less than 40 years ago) when autism was supposedly caused by a cold, nonloving mother. (As late as the early 1970s, Bruno Bettelheim, in several very popular books, was still promoting the concept of parentally caused autism.)

Unfortunately, just as old ideas die hard with others, so it was with your author.

And as late as May, 1982, I was still presenting lectures on how to do childhood apraxia therapy. But even though old ideas die hard, they usually do die eventually in people who prize intellectual growth. So by 1984, I was starting to question the existence of childhood apraxia. After all, I was seeing case after case of children diagnosed as apraxic, some of whom had previously undergone long periods of unsuccessful therapy, now suddenly showing progress after being given therapy based on a phonological model.

The problem is, even today, many clinicians remain wedded to the concept of childhood apraxia. As such, we continue to have two models or frameworks for studying severe articulation disorders in children which are totally contradictory to one another. Consider for example, the following comparison:

Childhood Apraxia Model	Phonological Model
• Organic underlying cause of articulation disorder.	• No organic underlying cause
• Child's speech behaviors occur as a result of a disordered physiological mechanism.	• Child is in full control of a system he has created, which differs from adult American English phonology.
• Child must overcome this disordered mechanism before speech will improve.	• Alternative system can be taught to child by contrasting his model with the adult model.

The purpose of this chapter is to present support for the thesis that the childhood apraxia model is an old idea that deserves to die (except, perhaps, in cases of documented brain damage, such as stroke or head trauma). As you will see, the entire notion of childhood apraxia has developed as a result of faulty reasoning. Further, there is little or no agreement as to the definition of the disorder; it is rare to find two different professionals who will agree on a set of characteristics that typify childhood apraxia. Finally, there is currently no therapeutic procedure or set of procedures designed to improve the speech of supposedly apraxic children that has been shown to be effective. In fact, one of the few areas of agreement concerning the disorder has been the fact that children labeled apraxic respond very poorly to therapy.

How then has the concept of childhood or developmental apraxia achieved such prominence among many of our profession? To answer this question, we have to turn for a bit to the disciplines of philosophy and psychiatry.

The Formulation of Syllogisms

Imagine for a moment that you are sitting in a large auditorium, in the midst of over 500 men, women, and children. All of you are waiting for the appearance on stage of Ronzonee, The Magnificent. The lights go on and suddenly a wall of fire 5-feet tall erupts in the center of the stage. Out of the smoke comes Ronzonee. As he flings his arms outward towards different parts of the audience, sheets of flame 10-feet long mysteriously explode from the ends of his fingers.

Suddenly, you begin to feel the stirrings of the one need that separates you as a human being from animals; a need that is uniquely human; a need that is particularly well developed in speech pathologists—the *need to explain what you see*. We all have this need to explain our observations. Whether we say "Ah-hah—it's a trick." Or whether we think it out more fully and reason to ourselves, "I get it—he has some sort of lighter or torch in his hand." Or whether we just conclude, "Oh —it's some sort of optical illusion." Either way, we have devised an explanation of sorts for what we have seen.

The problem is, our explanations in these circumstances are not always accurate, especially if we are seeing something for the first time. As most of us have seen magic before, we can begin to formulate a valid hypothesis as to how Ronzonee might have performed the magic trick. But 500 years ago, Ronzonee might have been declared a god—or the devil. And 500 years ago, Ronzonee's accusers would have sworn that their conclusions were logical and irrefutable.

How could something so patently absurd given a 20th century consciousness seem so logical to a 15th century mind? The answer to this lies with one of the primary methods we use to explain what we see: the formation of *syllogisms*.

The word *syllogism* is usually heard only in philosophy courses. Certainly many speech-language pathologists have never heard the term. Yet, knowledge of this term helps us to comprehend one of the mechanisms by which we explain the world around us. It also helps to explain one of the major elements of the scientific method, which underlies not only speech pathology, but all of the scientific disciplines. Finally, it helps us to understand how and why our explanations sometime go astray.

Simply defined, a syllogism is an argument or form of reasoning in which two statements or premises are made and a logical conclusion is drawn from them. Consider the following example:

Major Premise—All mammals are warm-blooded.

Minor Premise—Whales are mammals.

Conclusion—Whales are warm-blooded.

In this example, both of the premises are factually correct, and the conclusion is a logically drawn and, as we know, factual derivative of these premises.

Although the formulation of syllogisms is certainly one of our primary modes of explanation for the world around us, there are two problems that can occur in this type of deductive reasoning:

1. Inaccurate premise. If either of the premises is incorrect, the "logical conclusion" will almost certainly also be inaccurate. For example, let's look at a syllogism that might have been developed by audience members if Ronzonee had done his fire trick 500 years ago:

Major Premise—A fire can be created from what looks like nothing only by God or the devil.

Minor Premise—Ronzonee created a fire from nothing.

Conclusion—Ronzonee is either God or the devil.

Obviously, with our 20th century minds, we recognize the major premise as hopelessly flawed. Unsurprisingly, this flawed premise leads to a similarly flawed conclusion. Yet 500 years ago, when this same major premise was generally accepted by many, the flawed conclusion might have assumed the veil of fact.

2. Paleological thinking. This is a term from the field of psychiatry (e.g., see Arieti, 1966) which refers to the attempt to create a syllogism by assuming that different phenomena or objects having the same or similar characteristics, are in fact the same. Paleological thinking is best understood by studying the following example:

Major Premise—Jesus had a beard.

Minor Premise—Next door neighbor George has a beard.

Conclusion—George is Jesus.

Or to return to our earliest example:

Major Premise—All mammals are warm-blooded.

Minor Premise—Birds are warm-blooded.

Conclusion—Birds are mammals (which, of course, they are not).

In both of these cases, different individuals or animal classes having the same characteristics are considered to be identical to one another.

The Connection with Childhood Apraxia

In order to understand how all of this relates to childhood apraxia, it is valuable first to study one widely disseminated and accepted definition of *adult* apraxia:

> Certain adult patients with lesions of the left cerebral hemisphere have difficulty with the motor programming of phonemes and sequences of them, demonstrating the variable difficulty in finding the correct oral postures. This difficulty is identified as apraxia of speech. (Darley & Spriestersbach, 1978, p. 178).

This is certainly a definition with which most clinicians could agree. Darley and Spriestersbach then go on to describe a group of children with articulation problems, who seem to demonstrate the same difficulties. These children, they conclude, also present an apraxia of speech (Darley & Spriestersbach, 1978).

But let us study the syllogism arising from the authors' statements.

Major Premise—Adults with apraxia demonstrate a given syndrome of behaviors.

Minor Premise—Certain subgroups of children demonstrate the same or a similar syndrome of behaviors.

Conclusion—These children are apraxic.

What we see is a clear example of paleological thinking; in this case assuming that different groups of people having the same/similar characteristics are in fact the same. If this level of paleological thinking were used in other areas of the field of speech-language pathology, we'd quickly see the faulty reasoning. Consider this ludicrous but instructive example:

Major Premise—Adults with global aphasia demonstrate no intelligible speech/language output.

Minor Premise—Three-month-old children demonstrate no intelligible speech/language output.

Conclusion—Three-month-old children have global aphasia.

Obviously, any competent clinician would recognize the flawed reasoning arising from the conclusion that 3-month-old children have global aphasia. It thus becomes curious that many, if not most, clinicians have readily accepted the conventional explanation for childhood apraxia noted previously, despite the similar flaws in logic.

Unfortunately, the problems with conventional explanations of childhood apraxia do not end with paleological thinking. Indeed, there are two serious problems in even accepting the minor premise, that "certain subgroups of children demonstrate the same or similar syndrome of behaviors" (as adults with apraxia):

1. There has been little or no agreement as to which specific characteristics are, or should be, included in this syndrome.
2. Even if one overlooks this lack of agreement and just studies those characteristics that *are* most readily agreed upon across investigators, research has failed to substantiate any definitive subgroup of children that demonstrates these characteristics.

In support of these points, Guyette and Diedrich (1981), in what many consider to be a superb, landmark review of the childhood apraxia literature, concluded: "that there was poor agreement on the characteristics of developmental apraxia of speech; and even where there *was* agreement, data were not generally available to support the conclusions" (p. 32). And Deputy (1984), to further muddy the waters, noted that there has even been "disagreement on whether there is disagreement" (p. 6), comparing Guyette and Diedrich's (1981) sentiments with Blakeley, who claimed his *Screening Test for Developmental Apraxia of Speech* was based on a "set of symptoms that are in high agreement among authorities" (Blakeley, 1980).

In fact, a review of the childhood apraxia literature yields at least 38 characteristics that have been cited in at least one source as being differentially diagnostic for childhood apraxia. These characteristics are listed in Table 15–1. As can be seen, not only is the list extensive, but some of these supposedly differentially diagnostic characteristics actually contradict each other.

If, then, informal description based on observation doesn't result in a set of agreed upon characteristics that would help to define childhood apraxia, how about empirical research? Yoss and Darley (1974) reported on just such a research study which many have agreed comes perhaps the closest to providing an experimental design that might yield an acceptable operational definition of childhood apraxia. Briefly, they studied 30 children with moderate-to-severe articulation disorders between the ages of 5 and 10. They found a subgroup of those 30 children who demonstrated the following set of eight characteristics that reportedly distinguished them from the other children with articulation disorders:

1. Soft neurological signs.
2. Slowed oral diadochokinesis.
3. Greater difficulty with polysyllabic words.

4. Altered prosodic features, including rate and stress.
5. During imitative tasks, occurrence of a substantial number of two and three-feature errors, prolongations, repetitions of sounds and syllables, additions and distortions.
6. During spontaneous speech, occurrence of a different pattern, consisting of one place feature errors and omissions.
7. Poor auditory perception and sequencing skills.
8. More difficulty with nonspeech, volitional oral movements (Yoss & Darley, 1974).

These characteristics, Yoss and Darley (1974) claimed, constituted an empirically demonstrable syndrome of childhood apraxia. And for many years after this 1974 study, the Yoss and Darley characteristics were viewed by many as definitive. The problem is, in 1981, Williams, Ingham, and Rosenthal attempted to replicate the Yoss and Darley study. Their results? Their own words probably summarize it best: "These findings [of the replication study] are at variance with almost every conclusion Yoss and Darley reach[ed] in their study" (Williams et al., 1981, p. 503).

In short, Williams et al. (1981) found no evidence of a subgroup of children with articulation disorders who demonstrated unique behaviors indicative of childhood apraxia. In other words, none of their data could be interpreted as verifying or supporting the existence of a syndrome called childhood apraxia.

Since the Williams et al. (1981) study, several investigators (e.g., Crary, 1984; Crary, 1993; Hall, Jordan, & Robin, 1993) have attempted to better delineate the nature of childhood apraxia. But the problems remain. In fact, even two investigators who agree that childhood apraxia not only exists, but that the nature of the disorder is motorically based, cannot agree on the nature of that motor problem (see Hall, 1992; Robin, 1992).

TABLE 15–1. Characteristics Variously Designated as Diagnostic of Childhood Apraxia

1. Difficulty sequencing articulatory movements
2. Difference between voluntary and involuntary use of speech articulators
3. Normal language comprehension
4. Disordered lexical and syntactical formulation
5. Normal lexical and syntactic formulation
6. Normal imitation of sounds in isolation
7. Deficient speech sound imitation
8. Occasional disorders in reading, spelling, and writing
9. Slow improvement with traditional articulation therapy
10. Soft neurologic signs, fine and gross motor incoordination
11. No soft neurologic signs
12. Mixed hand laterality
13. No unusual handedness characteristics
14. Predominance in males
15. Family history of speech/language problems
16. Prosodic disturbances, especially of rate and stress
17. Highly inconsistent errors
18. Severity increases as length of utterance increases
19. Sound and syllable reversals
20. Particular problems with vowels/diphthongs
21. No particular problems with vowels/diphthongs
22. Presence of an oral apraxia (difficulty with volitional nonspeech oral tasks)
23. Slowed diadochokinetic rates
24. Incorrect syllable sequencing
25. Poor auditory perception skills
26. Normal auditory skills
27. Groping movements when attempting successful articulation
28. Absence of groping, searching movements
29. Reduced rate of speech
30. Asynergy in coordination of vocal tract structures
31. Multiple articulation errors
32. Normal intelligence
33. Articulation better automatically than on command
34. Child's speech development shows a deviant rather than an immature pattern
35. Greater proportion of two and three feature artic errors
36. Sound omissions a primary characteristic
37. Poor fine motor skills
38. Decreased oral awareness, oral astereognosis

The Importance of Accurate Differential Diagnosis

Why does this all matter? Does it really make that much of a difference if you say a child has developmental apraxia rather than a severe phonological disorder? In order to answer this question, it is impor-

tant that we return for a moment to our discussions in Chapter 11 on motor versus cognitive learning.

When most clinicians talk about any type of apraxia, they are referring to what is essentially an oral-motor deficiency. In any apraxia therapy then, including therapy for childhood apraxia, not only is the locus of learning thought to be the mouth, but the entire focus has become the client's mouth and how it moves. Unsurprisingly, then, therapeutic regimens developed for childhood apraxia have tended to revolve around highly systematized attempts to build oral-motor control in the child, using mostly the same procedures that have been part of the traditional repertoire for many years, only in a more systematic way. Now, all of this would be fine, if this type of therapy was successful. Unfortunately, however, one of the things that virtually all investigators and clinicians agree upon is that progress in therapy for these supposedly apraxic children is excruciatingly slow. And yet, reports indicate that phonologically based intervention is effective *even with children who have in the past been labeled apraxic*. A brief return to the group efficacy study presented in Chapter 14 (Klein, in press) highlights these findings. You will remember that a retrospective design was used to compare 19 children who received evaluation and therapy based on a traditional paradigm with 17 children who received phonologically based evaluation and treatment. Not only did children in the phonological group show significantly greater improvement in a significantly shorter period of time, but fully 6 of the 17 children in the phonological group had been diagnosed as having childhood apraxia at some point prior to beginning their phonologically based intervention. Of course, it is probable that adherents of the concept of childhood apraxia would claim that these children were misdiagnosed. Perhaps they were, but then we are getting dangerously close to basing a diagnosis on only one distinctive feature—resistance to improvement in therapy. And we believe we have

another better explanation for that characteristic or feature.

Summary

In the final analysis, we're faced with a dilemma. We have a construct—childhood apraxia—which rests on a questionable premise and has been reified through paleological thinking, or faulty reasoning. We have no agreement as to which characteristics would constitute this syndrome, even if it did exist. The one characteristic which *is* cited fairly frequently—inconsistency in speech sound production—is, in most cases, no more than a reflection of the examiner's problems in deciphering the child's rule system. Finally, we have a disorder that, by all accounts, doesn't respond auspiciously to therapy organized to tackle the supposed underlying cause. Yet, when an alternative framework is utilized—that of phonological analysis and intervention—therapeutic success is forthcoming.

The purpose of this chapter has *not* been to try to convince those of you who are having consistent therapeutic success with children you diagnose as apraxic to change what you are doing. Congratulations on your success and we would make only one request of you: Please start communicating the details scientifically to the rest of us in the community. We need to know about it!

If, on the other hand, you are like most clinicians in the field who are baffled, perplexed, and frustrated by the slow progress shown by children diagnosed as apraxic, this book has provided you with an alternative. Phonological analysis and intervention is stimulating, exciting, and important to your clients—because it works, we believe, even with children labeled as apraxic.

CHAPTER 16

The Future of Clinical Phonology

Where do we go from here? We believe that procedures for phonological analysis and intervention represent one of the most important developments seen in the field of speech-language pathology in its close to 75-year history. Although some may call this statement hyperbole, even the most jaded nonbelievers should be beginning to admit that "there seems to be something to this new approach." Since the first publication of that remarkable little volume on clinical phonology by David Ingram (1976) almost 20 years ago, there have been hundreds of reports demonstrating the greater effectiveness of phonologically based procedures. There is now one group study indicating the same thing. During that same 20-year period, we are unaware of even one case study disputing the greater effectiveness of clinical phonology. Yet we continue to hear comments like this one, from a well-respected editorial reviewer: "I would suggest, too, that clinicians who are not using a phonological approach feel they are getting (positive) results comparable to those (reports of success for phonologically based therapy). For example . . . Bernthal and Bankson (1993) say that 'traditional' approaches have 'worked for many clinicians with many clients'." Our question is, if clinicians are indeed getting equivalent results using a traditional approach, why is there no communication of this in the literature? More importantly, why are we still regularly hearing complaints from public schools clinicians concerning children on their caseloads who continue to have speech problems, yet have been in therapy for years and years? In other words, despite the claims to the contrary of this editorial reviewer, the status quo is not working very well. And there is an alternative. Isn't it about time that we as a profession begin embracing this alternative?

Several years ago at an ASHA convention, a mini-seminar was presented on the topic of a fairly new approach to laryngectomy rehabilitation—then called the Singer-Blom technique. After the presentation, several well-respected investigators in the field of laryngectomy rehabilitation and research attacked the presenter fiercely on many grounds, from lack of efficacy research, to lack of quality of what efficacy research was available, to the charge that the presenter was just trying to eliminate the need for speech pathologists, and on and on. Each of these well-respected investigators claimed the superiority of then-current techniques for rehabilitation following laryngectomy, even though most speech pathologists were aware of the shortcomings of the electrolarynx or traditional esophageal speech. Following these many negative comments, it remained for one well-respected clinician, teacher, and researcher, Dr. James C. Shanks, to provide the only balancing response. What he said, essentially, was this: It is difficult for any clinician, especially one that has been in the field for many years and has had much success with clients over the years, to accept the fact that something may be better than what he or she has been doing for so many years. It is easy for us to be skeptical; to claim that the old "tried and true" is best. I have some uneasiness about this new approach also. But it is important that we not ignore what is in front of our eyes; that we not be so protective of what we've done for so many years that we are unwilling to move ahead if it will help the clients we serve. Of course, the Singer-Blom approach is now called the tracheo-esophageal puncture (TEP) and is now accepted as a superior alternative for perhaps half of the new laryngectomies that are performed yearly.

It is important that we not let this same fear of change stop us from moving forward in the areas of articulation and phonology. The research base supporting a phonological approach is not yet complete; several questions remain unanswered. But the years of informal reports and case studies coupled with the retrospective research described in Chapter 14 make a compelling case for the efficacy of this newer paradigm. It is time that we all agree on at least the following fundamental propositions:

- That a traditional framework for assessment and intervention of children with multiple speech disorders is different from a phonological framework.
- That with the use of traditional procedures, many if not most children with multiple speech disorders have been forced to undergo several years of therapy, with no clear link demonstrated between that therapy and speech improvement, if any.

- That the use of phonological procedures seems to result in shortened time in therapy for these children with severe speech disorders.

Once we can agree on these propositions, perhaps we can then move forward to solving some of the very important questions that still exist in the area of clinical phonology. There is still much that we do not know. What has been presented in this text is only a very small step in the journey that remains ahead. More therapy techniques that rely on cognitive rather than motor learning will undoubtedly be developed. Other formal tests will be created that will allow the examiner to determine both idiosyncratic and limited rules. Better norms will be developed that will help us to make better decisions concerning which rules to work on in which order. Finally, continued research will help us to understand more fully the mechanism by which phonological disorders develop, as well as clarify the importance of other issues now being studied, such as phonological knowledge. All of these things are possible, but will become likely only when more clinicians are using a phonological methodology in their work.

For many years, what might be called a "benevolent parent" model has formed the foundation of many therapy approaches for children with speech disorders. In essence, we have tried in therapy what a good, perceptive parent would try with a child with speech disorders. If that child could not produce the /t/ sound, the good perceptive parent would try to get the child to put the tongue on the roof of his or her mouth. Even a good, perceptive parent might come up with the idea of using a mirror, or peanut butter, or a finger, or a tongue depressor, to try to stimulate the tongue movement. For many years, so did we. Now we have an alternative, and the alternative works.

Thirty years from now, if the promise of clinical phonology is realized, the provision of speech therapy services will probably look very different from the way it looks today. If phonologically based preschool or early intervention programs become available, the primary locus of service provision for these children will shift away from the elementary school, where children should be learning academic and social skills, to the preschool, where the learning of basic communication skills is entirely appropriate. No longer will fifth or sixth grade children be undergoing their fifth or sixth year of speech therapy, with some errors perhaps continuing to linger into junior high school. But for this promise to be realized, we need more clinicians who are traveling on the same path, who understand the value of clinical phonology and are willing to learn about it and give it a try. In other words, it is you,

the clinicians and students who are studying clinical phonology seriously, perhaps for the first time, who will be writing the next chapter of this saga.

Perhaps the late Charles Van Riper, one of the fathers of speech-language pathology, and possibly the best pure writer our discipline has seen, has summarized our feelings best in this quote from one of his many highly respected textbooks: "So we end this book with some of the feelings that Moses . . . must have experienced when at the end of his days he was taken up on the mountain for a brief glimpse of the promised land, a land he knew he would never enter, but one which the children of his companions assuredly would make their own." (Van Riper, 1982). This text is only a small beginning; we need your help to finish the story.

References

Albright, R. W., & Albright, J. B. (1958). Application of descriptive linguistics to child language. *Journal of Speech and Hearing Research, 1,* 257–261.

Arieti, S. (1966). *American handbook of psychiatry.* New York: Basic Books.

Bankson, N. W., & Bernthal, J. E. (1982). A comparison of phonological processes identified through word and sentence imitation tasks of the *PPA. Language, Speech and Hearing Services in Schools, 13,* 96–99.

Bankson, N. W., & Bernthal, J. E. (1990a). *Bankson-Bernthal test of phonology.* Chicago: Riverside Press.

Bankson, N. W., & Bernthal, J. E. (1990b). *Quick screen of phonology.* Chicago: Riverside Press.

Bernthal, J., & Bankson, N. (1993). *Articulation and phonological disorders* (3rd ed.). Englewood Cliffs, NJ: Prentice-Hall.

Blakeley, R. W. (1980). *Screening test for developmental apraxia of speech.* Tigard, OR: C. C. Publications.

Bowman, S. N., Parsons, C. L., & Morris, D. A. (1984). Inconsistency of phonological errors in developmental verbal dyspraxic children as a factor of linguistic task and performance load. *Australian Journal of Human Communication Disorders, 12,* 109–120.

Camarata, S., & Gandour, J. (1984). On describing idiosyncratic phonologic systems. *Journal of Speech and Hearing Disorders, 49,* 262–266.

Camarata, S., & Schwartz, R. (1985). Production of object words and action words: Evidence for a relationship between phonology and semantics. *Journal of Speech and Hearing Research, 28,* 328–330.

Campbell, T., & Shriberg, L. (1982). Associations among pragmatic functions: Linguistic stress and natural phonological processes in speech delayed children. *Journal of Speech and Hearing Research, 25,* 547–553.

Chomsky, N., & Halle, M. (1968). *The sound pattern of English.* New York: Harper & Row.

Compton, A., & Hutton, S. (1978). *Compton-Hutton phonological assessment.* San Francisco: Carousel House.

Crary, M. A. (1984). Phonological characteristics of developmental verbal apraxia. *Seminars in Speech and Language, 5,* 71–83.

Crary, M. A. (1993). *Developmental motor speech disorders.* San Diego: Singular.

Creaghead, N. (1989). Linguistic approaches to treatment. In N. Creaghead, P. W. Newman, & W. A. Secord (Eds.), *Assessment and remediation of articulatory and phonological disorders* (2nd ed., pp. 193–216). Columbus, OH: Merrill Publishing.

Darley, F. L., & Spriestersbach, D. C. (1978). *Diagnostic methods in speech pathology* (2nd ed.). New York: Harper & Row.

Deputy, P. N. (1984). The need for description in the study of developmental verbal dyspraxia. *Australian Journal of Human Communication Disorders, 12,* 3–12.

Dubois, E., & Bernthal, J. (1978). A comparison of 3 methods for obtaining articulation responses. *Journal of Speech and Hearing Disorders, 43,* 295–305.

Dyson, A. T., & Paden, E. P. (1983). Some phonological acquisition strategies used by two-year-olds. *Journal of Childhood Communication Disorders, 7,* 6–18.

Edwards, M. L. (1984). Issues in phonological assessment. *Seminars in Speech and Language, 4,* 351–374.

Edwards, M. L., & Shriberg, L. D. (1983). *Phonology: Applications in communicative disorders.* San Diego: College-Hill.

Elbert, M., and Gierut, J. (1986). *Handbook of clinical phonology: Approaches to assessment and treatment*. San Diego: College-Hill.

Ervin-Tripp, S. (1966). Language development. In M. Hoffman & L. Hoffman (Eds.), *Review of child development research* (Vol. 2). Ann Arbor: University of Michigan Press.

Faircloth, M., & Faircloth, S. (1970). An analysis of the articulatory behavior of a speech defective child in connected speech and in isolated word responses. *Journal of Speech and Hearing Disorders, 35,* 51–61.

Ferrier, E., & Davis, M. (1973). A lexical approach to the remediation of final sound omissions. *Journal of Speech and Hearing Disorders, 38,* 126–131.

Fey, M. E. (1985). Articulation and phonology: Inextricable constructs in speech pathology. *Human Communication Canada, 9,* 7–16. (Reprinted in *Language, Speech, and Hearing Services in Schools,* 1992, 23, 225–232.)

Fey, M. E. (1992). Articulation and phonology: An addendum. *Language, Speech and Hearing Services in Schools, 23,* 277–282.

Fisher, H. B., & Logemann, J. A. (1971). *The Fisher-Logemann test of articulation competence.* Boston: Houghton Mifflin.

Fudala, J. (1970). *Arizona articulation proficiency scale: Revised.* Los Angeles: Western Psychological.

Gierut, J. A. (1986). On the assessment of productive phonological knowledge. *NSSLHA Journal, 14,* 83–100.

Goldman, R., & Fristoe, M. (1986). *Goldman-Fristoe test of articulation.* Circle Pines, MN: American Guidance.

Grunwell, P. (1985). *Phonological assessment of child speech.* San Diego, CA: College Hill Press.

Grunwell, P. (1987). *Clinical phonology* (2nd ed.). Baltimore, MD: Williams & Wilkins.

Guyette, T. W., & Diedrich, W. M. (1981). A critical review of developmental apraxia of speech. In N. J. Lass (Ed.), *Speech and language advances in basic research and practice, 5,* 1–49. New York: Academic Press.

Hall, P. K. (1992). At the center of controversy: Developmental apraxia. *American Journal of Speech-Language Pathology, 1,* 23–25.

Hall, P., Jordan, L., & Robin, D. (1993). *Developmental apraxia of speech: Theory and clinical practice.* Austin, TX: Pro-Ed.

Hodson, B. (1985). *Computer analysis of phonological processes.* Stonington, IL: PhonoComp.

Hodson, B. (1986). *The assessment of phonological processes.* Danville, IL: Interstate Printers & Publishers.

Hodson, B. (1992). Applied phonology: Constructs, contributions and issues. *Language, Speech and Hearing Services in Schools, 23,* 247–253.

Hodson, B., & Paden, E. (1983). *Targeting intelligible speech: A phonological approach to remediation.* San Diego, CA: College-Hill Press.

Hodson, B., & Paden, E. (1991). *Targeting intelligible speech: A phonological approach to remediation* (2nd ed.). Austin, TX: Pro-ed.

Iglesias, A., & Anderson, N. (1993). Dialectical variations. In J. Bernthal & N. Bankson (Eds.), *Articulation and phonological disorders* (3rd ed.). Englewood Cliffs, NJ: Prentice-Hall.

Ingram, D. (1976). *Phonological disability in children.* New York: American Elsevier.

Ingram, D. (1981). *Procedures for the phonological analysis of children's language.* Baltimore, MD: University Park Press.

Jakobson, R., Fant, G. M., & Halle, M. (1952). *Preliminaries to speech analysis.* (Technical Report No. 13) Cambridge, MA: Acoustics Laboratory, Massachusetts Institute of Technology.

Kazdin, A. (1978). *History of behavior modification: Experimental foundations of contemporary research.* Baltimore, MD: University Park Press.

Kent, R. (1993). Normal aspects of articulation. In J. Bernthal & N. Bankson (Eds.), *Articulation and phonological disorders* (3rd ed., pp. 5–62). Englewood Cliffs, NJ: Prentice-Hall.

Khan, M. L., & Lewis, N. P. (1986). *Khan-Lewis phonological analysis.* Circle Pines, MN: American Guidance Service, Inc.

Klein, E. (1985, November). *Intervention strategies for remediation of phonological disorders.* Paper presented at the meeting of the American Speech-Language-Hearing Association, Washington, DC.

Klein, E. (1987, November). *Another look at childhood apraxia: It ain't necessarily so.* Paper presented at the meeting of the American Speech-Language-Hearing Association, New Orleans, LA.

Klein, E. (in press). Phonological/traditional approaches to articulation therapy: A retrospective group comparison. *Language, Speech and Hearing Services in Schools.*

Ladefoged, P. (1980). Articulatory parameters. *Language and Speech, 23,* 25–30.

Leonard, L. B. (1985). Unusual and subtle phonological behavior in the speech of phonologically disordered children. *Journal of Speech and Hearing Disorders, 50,* 4–13.

Leonard, L. B., & Brown, B. (1984). The nature and boundaries of phonological categories: A case study of an unusual phonological pattern in a language-impaired child. *Journal of Speech and Hearing Disorders, 49,* 419–428.

Leonard, L. B., & Leonard, J. S. (1985). The contribution of phonetic context to an unusual phonological pattern: A case study. *Language, Speech and Hearing Services in Schools, 16,* 110–118.

Long, S. H., & Fey, M. (1988). *Computerized profiling.* Ithaca, NY: Dept. of Speech Pathology & Audiology, Ithaca College.

Lowe, R. J. (1986). *Assessment Link between Phonology and Articulation.* Moline, IL: LinguiSystems, Inc.

MacKay, I. (1987). *Phonetics: The science of speech production.* Boston: Little, Brown.

Masterson, J. J., & Long, S. H. (1991). Computerized phonological analysis. In J. W. Bernthal & N. W. Bankson (Eds.), *Articulation and phonological disorders* (3rd ed.). Englewood Cliffs, NJ: Prentice Hall.

McCormick, L., & Schiefelbusch, R. L. (1984). *Early language intervention.* Columbus, OH: Charles E. Merrill.

McDonald, E. (1964a). *Articulation testing and treatment: A sensory motor approach.* Pittsburgh: Stanwix.

McDonald, E. (1964b). *A deep test of articulation.* Pittsburgh: Stanwix.

McLain, L. (1989). Personal communication.

McReynolds, L., & Elbert, M. (1981). Criteria for phonological process analysis. *Journal of Speech and Hearing Disorders, 46,* 197–203.

McReynolds, L., & Engmann, D. (1975). *Distinctive feature analysis of misarticulations.* Baltimore: University Park Press.

Meichenbaum, D. (1977). *Cognitive behavior modification: An integrative approach.* New York: Plenum.

Monahan, D. (1986). Remediation of common phonological processes: Four case studies. *Language, Speech, and Hearing Services in Schools, 17,* 199–206.

Morley, , M. E. (1957). *The development of disorders of speech in childhood.* Edinburgh: E. S. Livingstone.

Mowrer, D. E. (1982). *Methods of modifying speech behaviors* (2nd ed.). Columbus: Charles E. Merrill.

Panagos, J., Quine, H., & Klich, R. (1979). Syntactic and phonological influences in children's articulations. *Journal of Speech and Hearing Research, 22,* 841–848.

Pearl, R., Bryan, T., & Donahue, M. (1980). Learning disabled children's attributions for success and failure. *Learning Disability Quarterly, 3,* 3–9.

Poole, E. (1934). Genetic development of articulation of consonant sounds in speech. *Elementary English Review, 11,* 159–161.

Prather, E., Hedrick, D., & Kern, C. (1975). Articulation development in children aged two to four years. *Journal of Speech and Hearing Disorders, 40,* 179–191.

Preisser, D. A., Hodson, B., & Paden, E. (1988). Developmental phonology: 18–29 months. *Journal of Speech and Hearing Disorders, 53,* 125–130.

Robin, D. A. (1992). Developmental apraxia of speech; Just another motor problem. *American Journal of Speech-Language Pathology, 1,* 19–22.

Schwartz, R. G. (1992). Clinical applications of recent advances in phonological theory. *Language, Speech and Hearing Services in Schools, 23,* 269–276.

Schwartz, R. G., Messick, C. K., & Pollock, K. E. (1983). Some nonphonological considerations in phonological assessment. *Seminars in Speech and Language, 4,* 335–350.

Scott, L. B. (1952). *Talking time.* Chicago: Webster Publishing Co.

Seligman, M. E. (1975). *Helplessness: On depression, development and death.* San Francisco: W. H. Freeman.

Shelton, R. L. (1978). Speech sound discrimination in the correction of disordered articulation. *Allied Health and Behavioral Sciences, 1,* 176–194.

Shriberg, L. (1986). *Programs to examine phonetic and phonologic evaluations records.* Hillsdale, NJ: Lawrence Erlbaum.

Shriberg, L., & Kwiatkowski, J. (1980). *Natural process analysis.* New York: John Wiley.

Shriberg, L., & Kwiatkowski, J. (1985). Contiuous speech sampling for phonological analyses of speech delayed children. *Journal of Speech and Hearing Disorders, 50,* 323–334.

Shriberg, L., Kwiatkowski, J., & Gruber, F. A. (1994). Developmental phonological disorders II: Short-term speech-sound normalization. *Journal of Speech and Hearing Research, 37,* 1127–1150.

Smit, A. B., Hand, L., Freilinger, J. J., Bernthal, J. E., & Bird, A. (1990). The Iowa articulation norms project and its Nebraska replication. *Journal of Speech and Hearing Disorders, 55,* 779–798.

Stoel-Gammon, C., & Dunn, C. (1985). *Normal and disordered phonology in children.* Austin, TX: PRO-ED, Inc.

Templin, M. C. (1957). *Certain language skills in children.* Minneapolis: University of Minnesota Press.

Templin, M. C., & Darley, F. (1969). *The Templin-Darley tests of articulation.* Iowa City: Bureau of Educational Research and Service, University of Iowa.

Van Riper, C. (1972). *Speech correction: Principles and methods* (5th ed.). Englewood Cliffs, NJ: Prentice-Hall.

Van Riper, C. (1982). *The nature of stuttering* (2nd ed.). Englewood Cliffs: Prentice-Hall.

Van Riper, C., & Irwin, J. V. (1958). *Voice and articulation.* Englewood Cliffs, NJ: Prentice-Hall.

Webster's new collegiate dictionary (19th ed.). (1976). Springfield, MA: Merriam.

Weiner, F. (1979). *Phonological process analysis.* Baltimore, MD: University Park Press.

Weiner, F. (1981a). Treatment of phonological disability using the method of meaningful minimum contrasts: Two case studies. *Journal of Speech and Hearing Disorders, 46,* 97–103.

Weiner, F. (1981b). Systematic sound preferences as a characteristic of phonological disability. *Journal of Speech and Hearing Disorders, 46,* 281–286.

Weiner, F. (1983). *Phonological analysis and intervention.* Workshop presentation, Whittier, CA.

Weiner, F., & Bankson, N. (1978). Teaching features. *Language, Speech and Hearing Services in Schools, 9,* 29–34.

Weiner, F., & Ostrowski, A. (1979). Effects of listener uncertainty on articulatory inconsistency. *Journal of Speech and Hearing Disorders, 44,* 487–493.

Wellman, B. L., Case, I. M., Mengart, E. G., & Bradbury, D. E. (1931). *Speech sounds of young children.* University of Iowa Studies in Child Welfare, 5. Iowa City: University of Iowa Press.

Williams, D. Ingham, R. J., & Rosenthal, J. (1981). A further analysis for developmental apraxia of speech in children with defective articulation. *Journal of Speech and Hearing Research, 24,* 496–505.

Winitz, H. (1969). *Articulatory acquisition and behavior.* New York: Merideth.

Yoss, K. A., & Darley, F. L. (1974). Developmental apraxia of speech in children with defective articulation. *Journal of Speech and Hearing Research, 17,* 386–398.

Young, E. (1983). A language approach to treatment of phonological process problems. *Language, Speech and Hearing Services in Schools, 14,* 47–53.

Zemlin, W. (1988). *Speech and hearing science: Anatomy and physiology* (3rd ed.). Englewood Cliffs, NJ: Prentice-Hall.

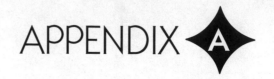

APPENDIX A

Answers for Selected Exercises

Chapter 5 Answers

FLORA DUH

CONSISTENCY CHECKLIST

Initial Rule Description: *FRONTING OF VELARS*

Rule Operating (Yes)	Rule Not Operating (No)
key cup gum pick cake cake go tow big	

Check for Consistency	Yes Words	No Words	Sig. Diff.
1. **Phonetic Context** — List vowel preceding — List vowel following — List consonant preceding — List consonant following — List other sig. non-adjacent sounds			
2. **Position** — List I, M, F for initial medial, final			
3. **Intra-class Variability** — List correct/incorrect sounds, search for intra-class patterns			
4. **Syllable Structure/ Word Length** — List syllable structures			
5. **Part of Speech/Morphological Endings** — List grammatical categories			
6. **Syllable Stress** — List U, S for unstressed, stressed			
7. **Syllable Boundary** — List words/Draw line between syllable boundaries; Note differences			

Note other factors: Elicitation mode, situational context, overlearned words, etc.

Final Rule Description: *FRONTING OF VELARS*

Raoul Schwartz

CONSISTENCY CHECKLIST

Initial Rule Description: ___*STOPPING OF FRICATIVES*___

Rule Operating (Yes)	Rule Not Operating (No)
sun zoo nose thin suit miss sheep fight very (five) five	

Check for Consistency	Yes Words	No Words	Sig. Diff.
1. **Phonetic Context**			
— List vowel preceding			
— List vowel following			
— List consonant preceding			
— List consonant following			
— List other sig. non-adjacent sounds			
2. **Position**			
— List I, M, F for initial medial, final			
3. **Intra-class Variability**			
— List correct/incorrect sounds, search for intra-class patterns			
4. **Syllable Structure/ Word Length**			
— List syllable structures			
5. **Part of Speech/Morphological Endings**			
— List grammatical categories			
6. **Syllable Stress**			
— List U, S for unstressed, stressed			
7. **Syllable Boundary** — List words/Draw line between syllable boundaries; Note differences			

Note other factors: Elicitation mode, situational context, overlearned words, etc.

Final Rule Description: ___*STOPPING OF FRICATIVES*___

Child #003

PROCEDURE FOR PHONOLOGICAL ANALYSIS — GENERIC WORKSHEET

I. <u>Take one error and choose possible parameters</u>

ERROR: *bed* ⟶ /dɛd/

ANALYSIS:
Manner? ⟶ *No*
Voicing? ⟶ *No*
Placement? ⟶ ~~Maybe~~ *No*
Context? ⟶ ~~Maybe~~ *Yes*
Structure? ⟶ *No*
Linguistic? ⟶ *Unlikely*
Semantic? ⟶ *Unlikely*

> If unclear as to whether placement or context, perform Parameter Confusion Test (See Form). Otherwise go to Step II.

II. <u>Make initial conclusion re: rule by describing the difference between target and client production.</u>

<u>*Context*</u> **PARAMETER**

Description: *When there's alveolar culprit in word, other sounds ⟶ alveolar*

Rule: *Alveolar Assimilation*

Child #004

PROCEDURE FOR PHONOLOGICAL ANALYSIS — GENERIC WORKSHEET

I. Take one error and choose possible parameters

ERROR: _cat_ → /tæt/

ANALYSIS:
Manner? ————→ No
Voicing? ————→ No
Placement? ————→ Maybe Yes
Context? ————→ Maybe No
Structure? ————→ No
Linguistic? ————→ Unlikely
Semantic? ————→ Unlikely

> If unclear as to whether placement or context, perform Parameter Confusion Test (See Form). Otherwise go to Step II.

II. Make initial conclusion re: rule by describing the difference between target and client production.

Placement PARAMETER

Description: _Velar becomes alveolar_

Rule: _Fronting of Velars_

Child #004

PLACEMENT CONTEXT PARAMETER CONFUSION CHECK

Target Word: _____ *cat*

Client Production: _____ */tæt/*

Choose Test Word: _____ *key → /til/*
    (Word in which there's no culprit; i.e no
    chance for assimilation to occur).

Error Still Occur? __X__ Yes

_____ No

Yes = Placement error; even though chance for assimilation has been
    removed, error still occurs.

No = Assimilation error; error disappears when culprit is removed.

Return to Step 1 - Generic Worksheet

Bob Alou

PLACEMENT CONTEXT PARAMETER CONFUSION CHECK

Target Word:

Client Production:

Choose Test Word:
(Word in which there's no culprit; i.e no
chance for assimilation to occur).

pot

/pap/

talk → /t>k/

Error Still Occur? _____ Yes

_____✓___ No

     Yes = Placement error; even though chance for assimilation has been
             removed, error still occurs.

    (No) = Assimilation error; error disappears when culprit is removed.

Return to Step 1 - Generic Worksheet

Bob Alou

CONSISTENCY CHECKLIST

Initial Rule Description: _Labial Assimilation_

Rule Operating (Yes)	Rule Not Operating (No)
pot big cup soup pig	

Check for Consistency	Yes Words	No Words	Sig. Diff.
1. Phonetic Context			
— List vowel preceding			
— List vowel following			
— List consonant preceding			
— List consonant following			
— List other sig. non-adjacent sounds			
2. Position			
— List I, M, F for initial medial, final			
3. Intra-class Variability			
— List correct/incorrect sounds, search for intra-class patterns			
4. Syllable Structure/ Word Length			
— List syllable structures			
5. Part of Speech/Morphological Endings			
— List grammatical categories			
6. Syllable Stress			
— List U, S for unstressed, stressed			
7. Syllable Boundary — List words/Draw line between syllable boundaries; Note differences			

Note other factors: Elicitation mode, situational context, overlearned words, etc.

Final Rule Description: _Labial Assimilation_

Chapter 6 Answers

Sissy Sassafrasser   **CONSISTENCY CHECKLIST**

Initial Rule Description: STOPPING OF FRICATIVES

Rule Operating (Yes)	Rule Not Operating (No)
soup sick feet sock shoe gas	

Check for Consistency	Yes Words	No Words	Sig. Diff.
1. **Phonetic Context**			
— List vowel preceding			
— List vowel following			
— List consonant preceding			
— List consonant following			
— List other sig. non-adjacent sounds			
2. **Position**			
— List I, M, F for initial medial, final			
3. **Intra-class Variability**			
— List correct/incorrect sounds, search for intra-class patterns			
4. **Syllable Structure/ Word Length**			
— List syllable structures			
5. **Part of Speech/Morphological Endings**			
— List grammatical categories			
6. **Syllable Stress**			
— List U, S for unstressed, stressed			
7. **Syllable Boundary** — List words/Draw line between syllable boundaries: Note differences			

Note other factors: Elicitation mode, situational context, overlearned words, etc.

Final Rule Description: STOPPING OF FRICATIVES

Sissy Sassafrasser

PLACEMENT CONTEXT PARAMETER CONFUSION CHECK

Target Word: _____ s*i*ck

Client Production: _____ /tɪt/

Choose Test Word: _____ walk ⟶ /wat/
    (Word in which there's no culprit; i.e no
    chance for assimilation to occur).

Error Still Occur? ___X___ Yes

               _____ No

Yes = Placement error; even though chance for assimilation has been
       removed, error still occurs.

No = Assimilation error; error disappears when culprit is removed.

Return to Step 1 - Generic Worksheet

Sissy Sassafrasser - Rule #2

CONSISTENCY CHECKLIST

Initial Rule Description: _FRONTING OF VELARS_

Rule Operating (Yes)	Rule Not Operating (No)
sick sock walk dog gas big	

Check for Consistency	Yes Words	No Words	Sig. Diff.
1. **Phonetic Context**			
— List vowel preceding			
— List vowel following			
— List consonant preceding			
— List consonant following			
— List other sig. non-adjacent sounds			
2. **Position**			
— List I, M, F for initial medial, final			
3. **Intra-class Variability**			
— List correct/incorrect sounds, search for intra-class patterns			
4. **Syllable Structure/ Word Length**			
— List syllable structures			
5. **Part of Speech/Morphological Endings**			
— List grammatical categories			
6. **Syllable Stress**			
— List U, S for unstressed, stressed			
7. **Syllable Boundary** — List words/Draw line between syllable boundaries; Note differences			

Note other factors: Elicitation mode, situational context, overlearned words, etc.

Final Rule Description: _FRONTING OF VELARS_

Interim Steps for Sissy Sassafrasser - 2 Rules

	Fronting of		Stopping of
<u>Target</u>	<u>Velars</u>		<u>Fricatives</u>
sick →	/sɪt/	→	/tɪt/

	Fronting of		Stopping of
<u>Target</u>	<u>Velars</u>		<u>Fricatives</u>
sock →	/sat/	→	/tat/

	Fronting of		Stopping of
<u>Target</u>	<u>Velars</u>		<u>Fricatives</u>
gas →	/dæs/	→	/dæt/

Predictions Using Sissy's Rule System

1. take $\longrightarrow$ /tet/
2. cash $\longrightarrow$ /tæt/
3. fig $\longrightarrow$ /pɪd/
4. thick $\longrightarrow$ /tɪt/
5. calf $\longrightarrow$ /tæp/
6. fog $\longrightarrow$ /pad/
7. scissor $\longrightarrow$ /tɪdɚ/

FARRELL #1

CONSISTENCY CHECKLIST

Initial Rule Description: _DEVOICING OF CONSONANTS_

Rule Operating (Yes)	Rule Not Operating (No)
d)g save d (g pig boat do zoo bad bad	

Check for Consistency	Yes Words	No Words	Sig. Diff.
1. **Phonetic Context** — List vowel preceding — List vowel following — List consonant preceding — List consonant following — List other sig. non-adjacent sounds			
2. **Position** — List I, M, F for initial medial, final			
3. **Intra-class Variability** — List correct/incorrect sounds, search for intra-class patterns			
4. **Syllable Structure/ Word Length** — List syllable structures			
5. **Part of Speech/Morphological Endings** — List grammatical categories			
6. **Syllable Stress** — List U, S for unstressed, stressed			
7. **Syllable Boundary** — List words/Draw line between syllable boundaries; Note differences			

Note other factors: Elicitation mode, situational context, overlearned words, etc.

Final Rule Description: _DEVOICING OF CONSONANTS_

Farrell #1 - 2ND rule

PLACEMENT CONTEXT. PARAMETER CONFUSION CHECK

Target Word: *sick*

Client Production: */sɪt/*

Choose Test Word: *pig → /pɪg/*
 (Word in which there's no culprit; i.e no
 chance for assimilation to occur).

Error Still Occur? _____ Yes

 _✗_ No

 <u>Yes</u> = Placement error; even though chance for assimilation has been
 removed, error still occurs.

 (No) = Assimilation error; error disappears when culprit is removed.

Return to Step 1 - Generic Worksheet

Farrell #1 – Rule 2

CONSISTENCY CHECKLIST

Initial Rule Description: _Alveolar Assimilation_

Rule Operating (Yes)	Rule Not Operating (No)
sick save dig boat bad	

Check for Consistency	Yes Words	No Words	Sig. Diff.
1. **Phonetic Context** — List vowel preceding			
— List vowel following			
— List consonant preceding			
— List consonant following			
— List other sig. non-adjacent sounds			
2. **Position** — List I, M, F for initial medial, final			
3. **Intra-class Variability** — List correct/incorrect sounds, search for intra-class patterns			
4. **Syllable Structure/ Word Length** — List syllable structures			
5. **Part of Speech/Morphological Endings** — List grammatical categories			
6. **Syllable Stress** — List U, S for unstressed, stressed			
7. **Syllable Boundary** — List words/Draw line between syllable boundaries; Note differences			

Note other factors: Elicitation mode, situational context, overlearned words, etc.

Final Rule Description: _Alveolar Assimilation_

Farrell #2- Rule 1

CONSISTENCY CHECKLIST

Initial Rule Description: _DEVOICING OF CONSONANTS_

Rule Operating (Yes)	Rule Not Operating (No)
sa(ve) d(g) boat	d(g) boat
d(g) bad	(do)
ba(d) zoo	
p(g) bad	

Check for Consistency	Yes Words	No Words	Sig. Diff.
1. Phonetic Context			
— List vowel preceding			
— List vowel following			
— List consonant preceding			
— List consonant following			
— List other sig. non-adjacent sounds			
2. Position			
— List I, M, F for initial medial, final			
3. Intra-class Variability			
— List correct/incorrect sounds, search for intra-class patterns			
4. Syllable Structure/ Word Length			
— List syllable structures			
5. Part of Speech/Morphological Endings			
— List grammatical categories			
6. Syllable Stress			
— List U, S for unstressed, stressed			
7. Syllable Boundary			
— List words/Draw line between syllable boundaries: Note differences			

Note other factors: Elicitation mode, situational context, overlearned words, etc.

Final Rule Description: _DEVOICING OF FINAL CONSONANTS_

PARSIPPANY U66

PLACEMENT CONTEXT PARAMETER CONFUSION CHECK

Target Word: *CUP*

Client Production: /pʌp/

Choose Test Word: talk → /tɔk/
   (Word in which there's no culprit; i.e no
   chance for assimilation to occur).

Error Still Occur? _____ Yes
                     X No

   Yes = Placement error; even though chance for assimilation has been
             removed, error still occurs.

   (No) = Assimilation error; error disappears when culprit is removed.

Return to Step 1 — Generic Worksheet

PARSIPPANY UGG-RULE 1

CONSISTENCY CHECKLIST

Initial Rule Description: _LABIAL ASSIMILATION_

Rule Operating (Yes)	Rule Not Operating (No)
cup soup fake sheep	

Check for Consistency	Yes Words	No Words	Sig. Diff.
1. **Phonetic Context**			
— List vowel preceding			
— List vowel following			
— List consonant preceding			
— List consonant following			
— List other sig. non-adjacent sounds			
2. **Position**			
— List I, M, F for initial medial, final			
3. **Intra-class Variability**			
— List correct/incorrect sounds, search for intra-class patterns			
4. **Syllable Structure/ Word Length**			
— List syllable structures			
5. **Part of Speech/Morphological Endings**			
— List grammatical categories			
6. **Syllable Stress**			
— List U, S for unstressed, stressed			
7. **Syllable Boundary** — List words/Draw line between syllable boundaries: Note differences			

Note other factors: Elicitation mode, situational context, overlearned words, etc.

Final Rule Description: _LABIAL ASSIMILATION_

PARSIPPANY U66-Rule 2

CONSISTENCY CHECKLIST

Initial Rule Description: _STOPPING OF FRICATIVES_

Rule Operating (Yes)	Rule Not Operating (No)
Fake Soup Sick sheep shake	

Check for Consistency	Yes Words	No Words	Sig. Diff.
1. Phonetic Context			
— List vowel preceding			
— List vowel following			
— List consonant preceding			
— List consonant following			
— List other sig. non-adjacent sounds			
2. Position			
— List I, M, F for initial medial, final			
3. Intra-class Variability			
— List correct/incorrect sounds, search for Intra-class patterns			
4. Syllable Structure/ Word Length			
— List syllable structures			
5. Part of Speech/Morphological Endings			
— List grammatical categories			
6. Syllable Stress			
— List U, S for unstressed, stressed			
7. Syllable Boundary			
— List words/Draw line between syllable boundaries; Note differences			

Note other factors: Elicitation mode, situational context, overlearned words, etc.

Final Rule Description: _STOPPING OF FRICATIVES_

Predictions Using Parsippany's Rule System

1. shop   ⟶   /pap/
2. five   ⟶   /paɪb/
3. fog   ⟶   /pab/
4. sash   ⟶   /tæt/
5. push   ⟶   /pʊp/
6. vase   ⟶   /bep/
7. calf   ⟶   /pæp/
8. bath   ⟶   /bæp/
9. fish   ⟶   /pɪp/
10. sofa   ⟶   Unknown, because of two syllables. Maybe /pop/ or /popə/

Chapter 9 Answers

CORA APPEL

PLACEMENT CONTEXT. PARAMETER CONFUSION CHECK

Target Word: *pot*

Client Production: /pɑp/

Choose Test Word: *cat* → /kæt/
    (Word in which there's no culprit; i.e no
    chance for assimilation to occur).

Error Still .Occur? _____ Yes

         ✗ No

    Yes = Placement error; even though chance for assimilation has been
            removed, error still occurs.

    (No) = Assimilation error; error disappears when culprit is removed.

Return to Step 1 - Generic Worksheet

Cora Appel - Rule 1

CONSISTENCY CHECKLIST

Initial Rule Description: *Labial Assimilation*

Rule Operating (Yes)	Rule Not Operating (No)
pot soup ship bed meat feet might come tame	

Check for Consistency	Yes Words	No Words	Sig. Diff.
1. **Phonetic Context**			
— List vowel preceding			
— List vowel following			
— List consonant preceding			
— List consonant following			
— List other sig. non-adjacent sounds			
2. **Position**			
— List I, M, F for initial medial, final			
3. **Intra-class Variability**			
— List correct/incorrect sounds, search for intra-class patterns			
4. **Syllable Structure/ Word Length**			
— List syllable structures			
5. **Part of Speech/Morphological Endings**			
— List grammatical categories			
6. **Syllable Stress**			
— List U, S for unstressed, stressed			
7. **Syllable Boundary**			
— List words/Draw line between syllable boundaries; Note differences			

Note other factors: Elicitation mode, situational context, overlearned words, etc.

Final Rule Description: *Labial Assimilation*

CORA APPEL - Rule 2

CONSISTENCY CHECKLIST

Initial Rule Description: *Stopping of fricatives*

Rule Operating (Yes)	Rule Not Operating (No)
shoot soup sock kiss shake ship nose feet	

Check for Consistency	Yes Words	No Words	Sig. Diff.
1. **Phonetic Context**			
— List vowel preceding			
— List vowel following			
— List consonant preceding			
— List consonant following			
— List other sig. non-adjacent sounds			
2. **Position**			
— List I, M, F for initial medial, final			
3. **Intra-class Variability**			
— List correct/incorrect sounds, search for intra-class patterns			
4. **Syllable Structure/ Word Length**			
— List syllable structures			
5. **Part of Speech/Morphological Endings**			
— List grammatical categories			
6. **Syllable Stress**			
— List U, S for unstressed, stressed			
7. **Syllable Boundary**			
— List words/Draw line between syllable boundaries; Note differences			

Note other factors: Elicitation mode, situational context, overlearned words, etc.

Final Rule Description: *Stopping of Fricatives*

CORA APPEL - Rule 3

CONSISTENCY CHECKLIST

Initial Rule Description: <u>Deletion of Final Consonants</u>

Rule Operating (Yes)	Rule Not Operating (No)
dog pot	feet
pig cat	might
sock shoot	come
shake soup	tame
duck kiss	
neck ship	
nose	
bed	
meat	
neat	

Check for Consistency	Yes Words	No Words	Sig. Diff.
1. Phonetic Context			
— List vowel preceding	ɔ, I, a, e, ʌ, ɛ	a, æ, u, I, o, ɛ, i, ʌ, e	No
— List vowel following	N.A. - studying final consonant only		—
— List consonant preceding	d, p, s, ʃ, d, n	p, k, ʃ	No
— List consonant following	NA		—
— List other sig. non-adjacent sounds	Visual Inspection	⟶	No
2. Position			
— List I, M, F for initial medial, final	N.A.	—	—
3. Intra-class Variability			
— List correct/incorrect sounds, search for intra-class patterns	g, g, k, k, k, k	t, t, t, t, m, d, t, t, t, p, s, m, p, z, d	Yes!
4. Syllable Structure/ Word Length			
— List syllable structures			
5. Part of Speech/Morphological Endings			
— List grammatical categories			
6. Syllable Stress			
— List U, S for unstressed, stressed			
7. Syllable Boundary			
— List words/Draw line between syllable boundaries; Note differences			

Note other factors: Elicitation mode, situational context, overlearned words, etc.

Final Rule Description: <u>Deletion of Final Velars</u>

CORA APPEL - RULE 4   **CONSISTENCY CHECKLIST**

Initial Rule Description: _NASALIZATION_

Rule Operating (Yes)	Rule Not Operating (No)

nose   pot
meat   cat
neat   shoot
might   dog
come   pig
tame   soup
    sock
    kiss
    shake
    ship
    bed
	duck
	~~feet~~

Check for Consistency	Yes Words	No Words	Sig. Diff.
1. Phonetic Context — List vowel preceding	o, i, i, aɪ, —, —	a, æ, u, ɔ, ɪ, i, ɛ, ʌ	No
— List vowel following	— — — —, ʌ, e	ɑ, æ, u, ɔ, ɪ, i, ɛ, ʌ	No
— List consonant preceding	n, m, n, m —, —	p, k, ʃ d, p, s, k, ʃ, ʃ b d.	
— List consonant following	— — — — m, m	t, t, t, g, g, p, k, s, k, p	Yes!
— List other sig. non-adjacent sounds			

2. Position
  — List I, M, F for initial
    medial, final			

3. Intra-class Variability
  — List correct/incorrect sounds,
    search for intra-class patterns			

4. Syllable Structure/ Word Length — List syllable structures			
5. Part of Speech/Morphological Endings — List grammatical categories			

6. Syllable Stress
  — List U, S for unstressed,
    stressed			

7. Syllable Boundary
  — List words/Draw line between
    syllable boundaries; Note
    differences			

Note other factors: Elicitation mode, situational context, overlearned words, etc.

Final Rule Description: _____

Predictions Using Leonardo's Rule System

1. rug   ⟶   /bʌp/
2. sand   ⟶   /tæt/
3. pig   ⟶   /pɪp/
4. feed   ⟶   /pip/
5. know   ⟶   /do/
6. zoo   ⟶   /dμ/
7. spin   ⟶   /pɪp/
8. frog   ⟶   /pap/
9. thin   ⟶   /tɪt/
10. tomato   ⟶   Unknown. Possibly /pəbepo/

List of Rules for Carmine Crayola

1. Gliding of liquids in nonfinal positions.
2. *H*ing of initial voiceless stops.
3. Deletion of final voiced velars and final voiceless consonants after following a front vowel.
4. Fronting of /g/ to /d/, /ʃ/ to /s/.
5. Cluster reduction (?) (Not really enough information).

Chapter 13 Answers

Answers for Clinical Mastery Exercise: Developing Image Contrasts

1. H'ing of stops—*happy* vs. *meany*
    huffing vs. *puffing*
2. Lateral lisp—*slushy vs. crispy*
    neat vs. messy
3. Cluster reduction across words—*long train* /aʃba/ *vs.*
    short train /aba/
4. Gliding of /l/—*rambo* vs. *wimp*
    hard vs. *short*
5. Labial assimilation—*ball* vs. *boomerang*
    twins vs. *friends*
6. Alveolarization of fricatives—*loud* vs. *quiet*
    cat vs. *snake*

Blank Work Sheets

PHONOLOGICAL RULE SUMMARY

Client: _____

Check	Target Word	Client Production	Rule(s) Operating

PROCEDURE FOR PHONOLOGICAL ANALYSIS — GENERIC WORKSHEET

I. Take one error and choose possible parameters

ERROR:
ANALYSIS: Manner? ⟶
Voicing? ⟶
Placement? ⟶
Context? ⟶
Structure? ⟶
Linguistic? ⟶
Semantic? ⟶

> If unclear as to whether placement or context, perform Parameter Confusion Test (See Form). Otherwise go to Step II.

II. Make initial conclusion re: rule by describing the difference between target and client production.

_____ PARAMETER

Description:_____

Rule:_____

III. Perform Consistency Check (See Consistency Check Form)

IV. Describe rule in Final Form

Rule:_____

V. Go to phonological rule summary, find all words for which rule is operating, and note.

VI. Perform final check

— Make sure all changes in target word can be explained by rule. If so, check the word off. If not, leave until next analysis.

CONSISTENCY CHECKLIST

Initial Rule Description: _____

Rule Operating **(Yes)**	Rule Not Operating **(No)**

Check for Consistency	**Yes** Words	**No** Words	Sig. Diff.
1. **Phonetic Context**			
— List vowel preceding			
— List vowel following			
— List consonant preceding			
— List consonant following			
— List other sig. non-adjacent sounds			
2. **Position**			
— List I, M, F for initial medial, final			
3. **Intra-class Variability**			
— List correct/incorrect sounds, search for intra-class patterns			
4. **Syllable Structure/ Word Length**			
— List syllable structures			
5. **Part of Speech/Morphological Endings**			
— List grammatical categories			
6. **Syllable Stress**			
— List U, S for unstressed, stressed			
7. **Syllable Boundary** — List words/Draw line between syllable boundaries; Note differences			

Note other factors: Elicitation mode, situational context, overlearned words, etc.

Final Rule Description: _____

PLACEMENT CONTEXT PARAMETER CONFUSION CHECK

Target Word: _____

Client Production: _____

Choose Test Word: _____
    (Word in which there's no culprit; i.e., no
      chance for assimilation to occur).

Error Still Occur? _____ Yes

                   _____ No

      Yes = Placement error; even though chance for assimilation has been removed,
           error still occurs.

      No = Assimilation error; error disappears when culprit is removed.

Return to Step 1 - Generic Worksheet

Index

A

Adult therapy, 317–318

Analysis. *See also* Generative analysis; Phonological analysis
  distinctive features (transitional model), 14–18
    "Articulatory Parameters" (Ladefoged), 18, 19
    Chomsky and Halle universal distinctive features, 15, 28
    compared with traditional, 15, 17–18
    compared with traditional and phonological analysis, 28–30
    Distinctive Feature Analysis of Misarticulation, 15
    Fisher-Logemann Test of Articulation Competence, 14, 15–16, 24
    placement-manner-voicing, 18
  error
    across sounds, 15–16
    equivalency, 12
  limits, test instruments, 25–26
  phonological. *See* Phonological analysis
    Parameters of Articulatory Constraint Model, 18–26
  place-manner-voicing, 12–13, 14–15, 18, 28, 196
  traditional, 9–14
    Arizona Articulation Proficiency Scale, 14
    compared with distinctive features (transitional model), 15, 17–18
    compared with distinctive features (transitional model) and phonological analysis, 28–30
    error description, 14
    error equivalency, 12
    Goldman-Fristoe Test of Articulation (GFTA), 9–10, 14

place-manner-voicing, 12–13, 14–15
Voice and Articulation (Van Riper & Irwin), 9, 11, 12, 13

Apraxia, childhood
  and adult apraxia, 338
  diagnostic characteristics, 340
  differential diagnosis, 340–341

Arizona Articulation Proficiency Scale, 14, 24

Arizona Articulation Proficiency Scale (AAPS), 315

Articulation
  analysis model. *See also* Analysis
    distinctive features (transitional model), 14–18
    Parameters of Articulatory Constraint, 18–26
    phonological analysis. *See* Phonological analysis
      Parameters of Articulatory Constraint, 18–26
    traditional, 9–14. *See also* Analysis, traditional
  idiosyncratic rules, 24–25
  limited rules, 25
  model for analysis, 8
  Parameters of Articulatory Constraint Model, 18–26
  phonemic difference from phonetic production parameters, 18
  phonetic difference from phonemic production parameters, 18
  place-manner-voicing, 12–13, 14–15, 18
  sound (entire) as basic analysis unit, 9, 11, 12
  "Articulatory Parameters" (Ladefoged), 18, 19

Assessment. *See also* Analysis; Exercises, Clinical Mastery; Macroanalysis of phonology; Phonetics usage; Tests; Tools
  articulation analysis, 7
  computer analysis, 272–273